Challenging Cases in Immunotherapy Related Organ Toxicities

Yinghong Wang
Editor

Challenging Cases in Immunotherapy Related Organ Toxicities

Springer

Editor
Yinghong Wang, MD, PhD
Department of Gastroenterology,
Hepatology & Nutrition
The University of Texas
MD Anderson Cancer Center
Houston, TX, USA

ISBN 978-3-031-83532-2 ISBN 978-3-031-83533-9 (eBook)
https://doi.org/10.1007/978-3-031-83533-9

This Springer imprint is published by the registered company Springer Nature Switzerland AG
The registered company address is: Gewerbestrasse 11, 6330 Cham, Switzerland

Preface

Immune checkpoint inhibitors (ICIs) have evolved as a paradigm-shifting treatment for a variety of advanced malignancies with high efficacy. ICI-induced toxicities (IOTOX), however, pose significant morbidity on already vulnerable patients with cancer and thus become a top barrier to this innovative cancer treatment.

Even in clinical practice at MD Anderson for more than 8 years, I still feel overwhelmed by complex cases every day, but simultaneously inspired by recovering patients. I'd like to quote one who benefited from fecal transplant treatment for her immunotherapy-related colitis, "I cannot state strongly enough how co-equal relief from colitis was with conquering my cancer. Both felt life threatening, and in truth, it was the colitis that nearly killed me, not cancer." Stories like this are happening almost every day in our clinic and hospital services at our institution and the same everywhere in the world.

Serving as the chair of the IOTOX Working Group at MD Anderson Cancer Center over the past 6 years, I have witnessed tremendous changes in clinical practice driven by the group, which has already made a high impact on the quality of cancer care at our world-leading tertiary cancer center. Given the preliminary successes in managing IOTOX, we feel compelled and privileged to share our practice with the peer group in the field. Our first-of-its-kind IOTOX practice handbook published in September 2022 quickly gained high recognition for its comprehensive review of 15 different IOTOX topics. Even some patients found the book informative and encouraging, thus building stronger confidence in combating cancer.

With persistent motivation and passion, we strive to continue the momentum and unite as many oncology and internal medicine providers to take on these challenges collectively. To tackle these challenging entities from a different angle, a new book focusing on unique and challenging IOTOX cases will serve as a supplement to our first book on the topic review and provide a more detailed description of the diagnosis and management. It would further enhance the understanding of the diversity of the practice and the spectrum of the disease. We also encompassed a broad territory of global academic centers to enrich the variety of toxicity cases to the maximum. We truly hope that this handbook with 65 unique IOTOX cases will add tremendous value to this emerging field and support our noble mission: "making cancer history."

I would like to extend my heartfelt appreciation to each contributor to this book; their dedication and commitment are evident that greatly helped take this project to its timely completion.

Houston, TX, USA Yinghong Wang, MD, PhD

Introduction

Since the publication of the first book in this series on the management of immune checkpoint inhibitor (ICI) therapy, edited by Yinghong Wang, MD, PhD, cancer immunotherapy has continued to expand and solidify its position as a central pillar of cancer treatment, joining surgery, radiation therapy, chemotherapy, and targeted therapy. It is no surprise that with this expansion, the number and complexity of patients with immune-related adverse events (irAE) complicating ICI therapy have grown. This second book in the series is in response to the continuing need for expert guidance in the management of ICI-related irAE. It details the management of 65 patients with particularly challenging irAE presentations, directed by clinical experts in the field of immune oncology toxicity (IOTOX) from 14 academic medical centers.

It is important to underscore that our understanding of the molecular and cellular pathogenesis of irAE remains in its infancy, even as steady progress is being made by investigators at the MD Anderson Cancer Center and other institutions around the world. In the past 2 years at MD Anderson, we have witnessed the maturation of several empirically driven guidelines into established management algorithms as evidence has accrued for their safety and benefits. These efforts will continue. In the meantime, I am confident that providers who manage ICI-related irAE will find the cases in this book very useful in helping guide their management decisions.

Division of Internal Medicine, Department of Infectious Diseases, Infection Control & Employee Health and Division of Discovery Science, Department of Molecular and Cellular Oncology
The University of Texas MD Anderson Cancer Center, Houston, TX, USA

David J. Tweardy, MD

Contents

Part I
Cardiology

Chapter 1
Complete Heart Block and Myocarditis Related to Immune Checkpoint Inhibitor Therapy

Noah Beinart and Nicolas L. Palaskas

Abbreviations

CHB	complete heart block
CK	creatinine kinase
CK-MB	creatine kinase myocardial band
CTLA-4	cytotoxic T-lymphocyte associated 4
HsTnI	high sensitivity troponin I
ICI	Immune checkpoint inhibitor
LVEF	left ventricular ejection fraction
PD-1	programmed death −1
PR interval	P wave (atrial depolarization) to the beginning of the QRS complex
ULN	Upper limit of normal

Clinical Presentation

This is a male in his 70s with metastatic melanoma who was started on combination immune checkpoint inhibitor (ICI) treatment of ipilimumab and nivolumab (combination cytotoxic T-lymphocyte associated 4 (CTLA-4) inhibitor and programmed death -1 (PD-1) inhibitor). He had a history of hypertension and hyperlipidemia but no other significant cardiovascular comorbidities. After the second dose of combination immunotherapy the patient presented to a regularly scheduled oncology visit

N. Beinart (✉) · N. L. Palaskas
Department of Cardiology, The University of Texas MD Anderson Cancer Center, Houston, TX, USA
e-mail: NIBeinart@mdanderson.org; NLPalaskas@mdanderson.org

Y. Wang (ed.), *Challenging Cases in Immunotherapy Related Organ Toxicities*,
https://doi.org/10.1007/978-3-031-83533-9_1

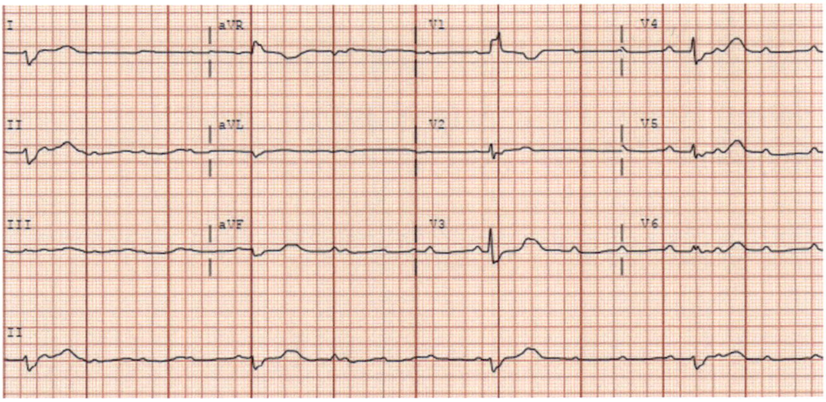

Fig. 1.1 Complete heart block with ventricular escape rhythm

and described mild dyspnea on exertion and fatigue. Vital signs in the clinic showed heart rate 90 bpm, blood pressure 126/77 mmHg, respiratory rate 18 rpm, and oxygen saturation 98% on room air. Physical exam was largely unremarkable.

Electrocardiogram (EKG) in the clinic showed normal sinus rhythm but with a new prolonged PR interval to 260 ms from baseline 200 ms. Three days later the patient presented to the emergency room with severe dyspnea and lightheadedness, bradycardia at 22 bpm, and hypotension with blood pressure 90's/60's. EKG revealed complete heart block with a ventricular escape rhythm (Fig. 1.1). Patient immediately underwent temporary pacemaker insertion.

Initial blood tests upon presentation to the emergency room revealed elevated high sensitivity troponin T (hsTnT) at 2533 ng/L (Upper limit of normal (ULN) 19 ng/L), high sensitivity troponin I (hsTnI) 3399 pg/mL (ULN 53 pg/mL, creatinine kinase (CK) 1325 U/L (ULN 308 U/L), and creatine kinase myocardial band (CK-MB) 106.9 ng/mL (ULN 10.4 ng/mL) (Table 1.1). Echocardiogram showed normal left ventricular ejection fraction (LVEF) of 55%, normal wall motion, no pericardial effusion, and normal right ventricular systolic pressure. Patient underwent a left and right heart catheterization with endomyocardial biopsy. He had normal coronary arteries, normal ventricular filling pressures, and the endomyocardial biopsy showed a dense inflammatory infiltrate with myocyte loss consistent with myocarditis (Fig. 1.2). Cardiac magnetic resonance imaging was not performed due to the presence of the temporary pacemaker.

On the first day of admission patient was started on methylprednisolone 1000 mg intravenously and the ICI therapy was stopped. On day 2 of admission due to continued complete heart block he was given upfront abatacept at 10 mg/kg which was repeated on day 3 of admission in addition to daily doses of intravenous methylprednisolone 1000 mg. On day 3 he began to have intermittent atrioventricular conduction. By day 4 he had complete resolution of complete heart block and heart rate was 70 bpm. The electrocardiogram showed a prolonged PR interval of 230 ms with a new right bundle branch block compared to baseline. The temporary pacemaker

Table 1.1 Cardiac biomarker blood values

Test	Presentation to emergency room	4 days post presentation	5 weeks post presentation
High sensitivity troponin T ULN 19 ng/L	2533 ng/L	1271 ng/L	181 ng/L
High sensitivity troponin I ULN 53 pg/mL	3399 pg/mL	721 pg/mL	76 pg/mL
Creatine kinase ULN 308 U/L	1325 U/L	456 U/L	127 U/L
Creatine kinase myocardial band ULN 10.4 ng/mL	106.9 ng/mL	15.7 ng/mL	5.3 ng/mL

ng nanogram, *L* liter, *pg* picogram, *mL* milliliter, *U* units, *ULN* upper limit of normal

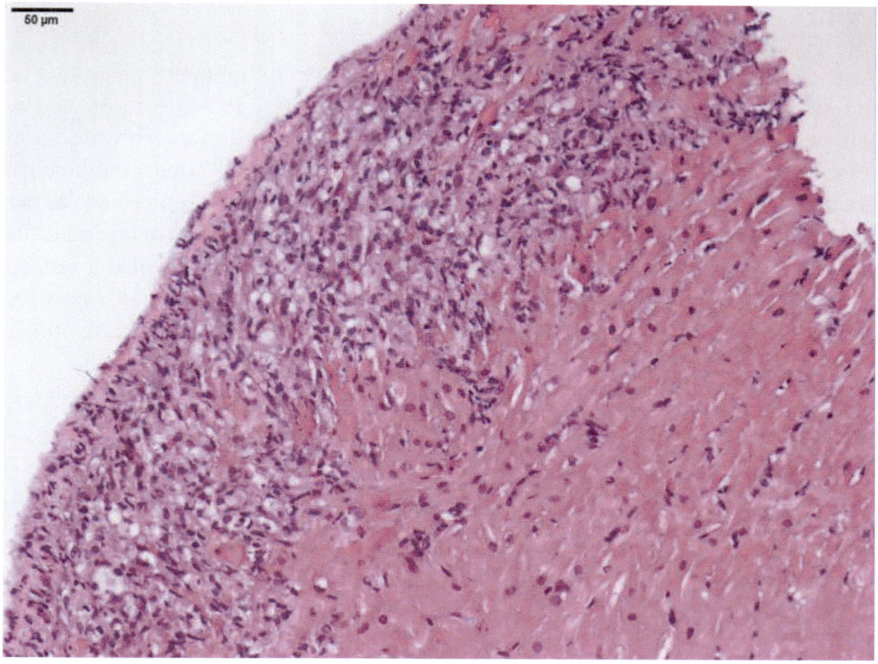

Fig. 1.2 Endomyocardial biopsy showing dense inflammatory infiltrate and myocyte loss

was removed and patient remained on telemetry to monitor for additional arrhythmias. Additionally, the cardiac biomarker blood values continued to decline (hsTnT at 1271 ng/L and hsTnI at 721 pg/mL) on day 4 (Table 1.1). Patient also transitioned to prednisone at 1 mg/kg which was tapered off over 5 weeks. He was discharged on hospital day 6 with an event monitor, a 30-day wearable ambulatory ECG device, to evaluate for arrhythmias post discharge. Given the severity of ICI-associated myocarditis presentation, patient was deemed to not be a candidate for future ICI therapy.

Clinical Outcome

At 5 weeks post discharge the patient was evaluated in clinic. Patient was asymptomatic and exercising with walking and light body weight resistance training. His vital signs were normal and physical exam was unremarkable. Labs showed hsTnT 181 ng/L, hsTnI 76 pg/mL (Table 1.1). Repeat EKG was unchanged from after the pacemaker was removed and showed persistent PR prolongation and right bundle branch block. Repeat echocardiogram was unchanged with LVEF 56%, no pericardial effusion, and normal right ventricular systolic pressure.

Summary of the Case

This is a case with metastatic melanoma on combination ipilimumab and nivolumab complicated by developing severe fulminant myocarditis. Patient presented with complete heart block requiring temporary pacemaker insertion that reversed with combination treatment of high dose steroids and abatacept. Patient remained in stable condition with normal LVEF after steroid taper without requirement of permanent pacemaker. Following the steroid taper, patient was started on the next line of therapy for melanoma which included BRAF inhibitors. He has had a durable cancer response but it is unclear whether it is due to early initiation of his next line of melanoma therapy or a lasting response from initiation 2 doses of immunotherapy. Summary of the disease course is shown in Fig. 1.3.

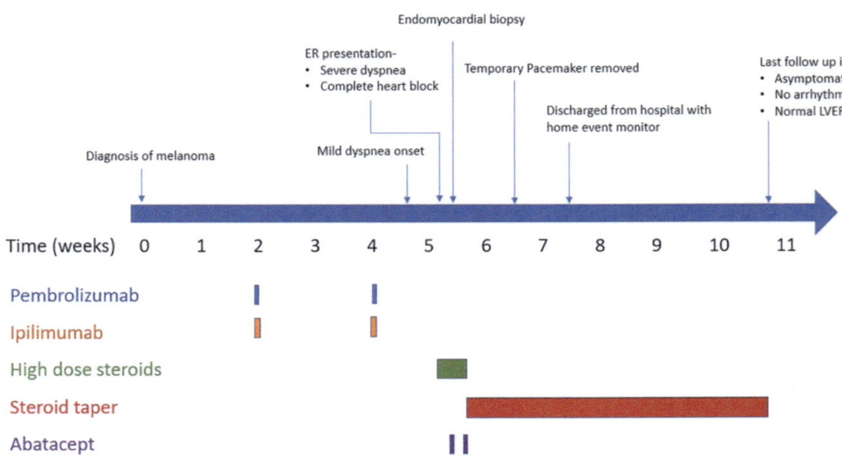

Fig. 1.3 Summary of the disease course (timepoint of 0 is melanoma diagnosis)

Discussion

ICI-associated myocarditis is an uncommon immune related adverse event (irAE) from immunotherapy with an incidence around 1% [1]. However, there is a higher mortality between 25% and 50%, compared to other irAEs [2]. Several major adverse cardiovascular events have been described to be associated with ICI myocarditis including advanced atrioventricular block even with normal LVEF [1]. This patient is unique in that the complete heart block reversed with use of immunomodulatory therapy combining high dose steroids and abatacept. The use of high dose steroids, 501–1000 mg/day for 3–5 days, is included in expert consensus guidelines for treatment of irAEs given a retrospective observational study showing that high dose steroids were associated with decreased major adverse cardiovascular events [3]. The use of abatacept, which works as a CTLA-4 agonist in opposition to the CTLA-4 inhibition from ipilimumab, has been described as a potential therapy for ICI myocarditis [4, 5]. The dosing of abatacept and long-term effect on cancer progression is not known. Currently there is an ongoing multicenter randomized controlled trial comparing abatacept versus placebo for the treatment of ICI myocarditis (NCT05335928).

Conclusion

While ICI myocarditis is an uncommon irAE, it can be life-threatening with fulminant presentations including complete heart block. Despite having a normal LVEF patients are not at reduced risk of major adverse cardiovascular events. Early identification and initiation of immunomodulatory treatment are crucial to improving outcomes of patients. Further research is needed to identify non-steroid therapy dosing and timing in order to limit adverse events and long-term steroid use in patients.

Disclosures Dr. Palaskas is supported by the Cancer Prevention Research Institute of Texas (CPRIT) RP200670, NIH/NCI 1P01CA261669-01, and the Andrew Sabin Family Foundation.

References

1. Mahmood SS, Fradley MG, Cohen JV, Nohria A, Reynolds KL, Heinzerling LM, Sullivan RJ, Damrongwatanasuk R, Chen CL, Gupta D, Kirchberger MC, Awadalla M, Hassan MZO, Moslehi JJ, Shah SP, Ganatra S, Thavendiranathan P, Lawrence DP, Groarke JD, Neilan TG. Myocarditis in patients treated with immune checkpoint inhibitors. J Am Coll Cardiol. 2018;71(16):1755–64. https://doi.org/10.1016/j.jacc.2018.02.037. Epub 2018 Mar 19. PMID: 29567210; PMCID: PMC6196725
2. Wang DY, Salem JE, Cohen JV, Chandra S, Menzer C, Ye F, Zhao S, Das S, Beckermann KE, Ha L, Rathmell WK, Ancell KK, Balko JM, Bowman C, Davis EJ, Chism DD, Horn L,

Long GV, Carlino MS, Lebrun-Vignes B, Eroglu Z, Hassel JC, Menzies AM, Sosman JA, Sullivan RJ, Moslehi JJ, Johnson DB. Fatal toxic effects associated with immune checkpoint inhibitors: a systematic review and meta-analysis. JAMA Oncol. 2018;4(12):1721–8. https://doi.org/10.1001/jamaoncol.2018.3923. Erratum in: JAMA Oncol 2018;4(12):1792. PMID: 30242316; PMCID: PMC6440712

3. Zhang L, Zlotoff DA, Awadalla M, Mahmood SS, Nohria A, Hassan MZO, Thuny F, Zubiri L, Chen CL, Sullivan RJ, Alvi RM, Rokicki A, Murphy SP, Jones-O'Connor M, Heinzerling LM, Barac A, Forrestal BJ, Yang EH, Gupta D, Kirchberger MC, Shah SP, Rizvi MA, Sahni G, Mandawat A, Mahmoudi M, Ganatra S, Ederhy S, Zatarain-Nicolas E, Groarke JD, Tocchetti CG, Lyon AR, Thavendiranathan P, Cohen JV, Reynolds KL, Fradley MG, Neilan TG. Major adverse cardiovascular events and the timing and dose of corticosteroids in immune checkpoint inhibitor-associated myocarditis. Circulation. 2020;141(24):2031–4. https://doi.org/10.1161/CIRCULATIONAHA.119.044703. Epub 2020 Jun 15. PMID: 32539614; PMCID: PMC7301778
4. Salem JE, Bretagne M, Abbar B, Leonard-Louis S, Ederhy S, Redheuil A, Boussouar S, Nguyen LS, Procureur A, Stein F, Fenioux C, Devos P, Gougis P, Dres M, Demoule A, Psimaras D, Lenglet T, Maisonobe T, De Chambrun MP, Hekimian G, Straus C, Gonzalez-Bermejo J, Klatzmann D, Rigolet A, Guillaume-Jugnot P, Champtiaux N, Benveniste O, Weiss N, Saheb S, Rouvier P, Plu I, Gandjbakhch E, Kerneis M, Hammoudi N, Zahr N, Llontop C, Morelot-Panzini C, Lehmann L, Qin J, Moslehi JJ, Rosenzwajg M, Similowski T, Allenbach Y. Abatacept/Ruxolitinib and screening for concomitant respiratory muscle failure to mitigate fatality of immune-checkpoint inhibitor myocarditis. Cancer Discov. 2023;13(5):1100–15. https://doi.org/10.1158/2159-8290.CD-22-1180.
5. Salem JE, Allenbach Y, Vozy A, Brechot N, Johnson DB, Moslehi JJ, Kerneis M. Abatacept for severe immune checkpoint inhibitor-associated myocarditis. N Engl J Med. 2019;380(24):2377–9. https://doi.org/10.1056/NEJMc1901677.

Part II
Dermatology

Chapter 2
Bullous Pemphigoid Post Immune Checkpoint Inhibitor Therapy

Hannah Y. Wang, Phyu Aung, and Anisha B. Patel

Abbreviations

BP	Bullous pemphigoid
CTCAE	Common Terminology Criteria for Adverse Events
ELISA	Enzyme-linked immunosorbent assay
HSV	Herpes simplex virus
VZV	Varicella zoster virus

Clinical Presentation

A Caucasian male in his 50s with a history of metastatic melanoma presented to the dermatology clinic for a pruritic, blistering rash of 3 months' duration. He was diagnosed with stage IV melanoma with a primary lesion of the right ear and metastases to the liver and lung 18 months prior to presentation, for which he received two cycles of ipilimumab and nivolumab combination therapy followed by 12 cycles of nivolumab monotherapy. Three months after receiving his last dose of nivolumab, the patient developed a rash on his face and bilateral forearms. Prior to his referral

H. Y. Wang
Baylor College of Medicine, Houston, TX, USA
e-mail: hannah.wang@bcm.edu

P. Aung
Department of Pathology, University of Texas MD Anderson Cancer Center, Houston, TX, USA
e-mail: paung@mdanderson.org

A. B. Patel (✉)
Department of Dermatology, University of Texas MD Anderson Cancer Center, Houston, TX, USA
e-mail: apatel11@mdanderson.org

Y. Wang (ed.), *Challenging Cases in Immunotherapy Related Organ Toxicities*, https://doi.org/10.1007/978-3-031-83533-9_2

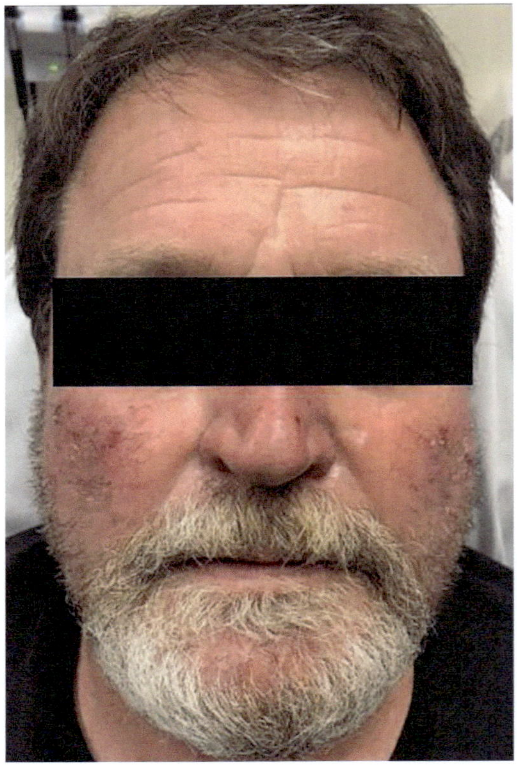

Fig. 2.1 Patient on presentation with superficial punched-out erosions and background erythema on the bilateral cheeks

to dermatology, the rash was initially diagnosed as impetigo, and he had undergone treatment with topical mometasone and oral minocycline without significant improvement. On exam, the patient had a diffusely erythematous face with superficial, punched-out erosions and vesicles on the right temple and cheek (Fig. 2.1). The bilateral forearms also had vesicles on an erythematous base.

Labs

The patient's complete blood count and complete metabolic panel were unremarkable. Results from serum enzyme-linked immunosorbent assay (ELISA) for BP180 and 230 antibodies are seen in Table 2.1.

Table 2.1 Results of serological ELISA testing

Lab	Level
BP180 antibody level	58 RU/mL
BP230 antibody level	<2 RU/mL

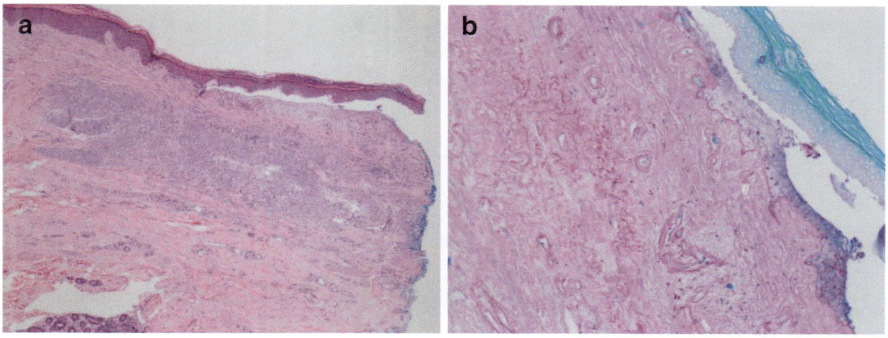

Fig. 2.2 (**a**) H&E, 40×, Lichenoid infiltrate with subepidermal split and many eosinophils. (**b**) PAS, 40×, Stain highlights the split at the basement membrane

Pathology

A punch biopsy was performed on the left forearm. Histology revealed skin with separation of the dermal-epidermal junction and underlying superficial perivascular and interstitial lymphocytic infiltrate with eosinophils (Figs. 2.2a and 2.3). A periodic acid-Schiff stain failed to reveal definite fungal organisms and highlighted the basal membrane at the bottom of the separation at the dermal-epidermal junction (Fig. 2.2b). An immunohistochemical study with VZV and HSV was negative.

Diagnosis

The rash was initially diagnosed as impetigo, which can present with a bullous morphology. However, there was a lack of honey crusting or purulent discharge when the patient presented to the dermatology clinic, and the rash failed to respond to antibiotics, making a Staphylococcus aureus infection less likely. Other diagnoses on the differential included herpes simplex or herpes zoster, though it would be atypical for the rash to be pruritic and persist for months, and porphyria cutanea tarda since the lesions were photo-distributed. Suspicion was highest for a primary blistering process, and the elevated serum BP180 antibody level and biopsy results showing separation of the dermal-epidermal junction with eosinophilic infiltrate confirmed a diagnosis of bullous pemphigoid (BP). The Common Terminology Criteria for Adverse Events (CTCAE) classification of the rash was grade 2 with limited body surface area involvement.

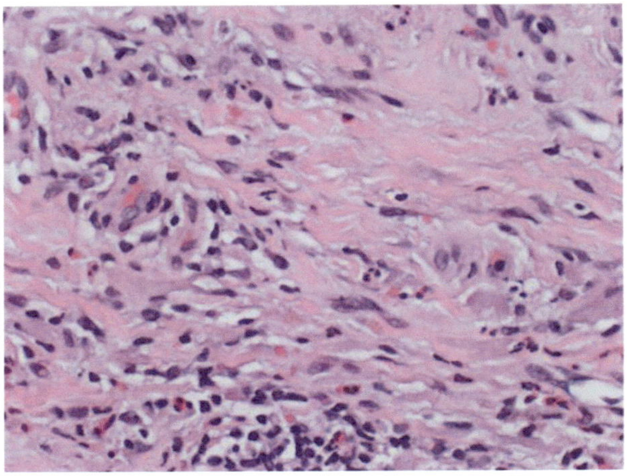

Fig. 2.3 H&E, 400×, Dermal infiltrate of lymphocytes, histiocytes, and eosinophils

Outcome

This patient had inadequate response to topical mometasone and was started on a prednisone taper followed by dupilumab for long-term steroid-sparing management. The dosing regimen of dupilumab followed the schedule used to treat atopic dermatitis: 600 mg subcutaneously for a loading dose followed by 300 mg every other week. Other treatment options considered include omalizumab 300 mg subcutaneously every 4 weeks following the prednisone taper, though patients need to go to a hospital or clinic to receive the injection to monitor for anaphylaxis, which may not be compatible with their schedules [1].

The patient reported significant improvement after the steroid taper, which started with 60 mg of prednisone daily and decreased by 20 mg per week, with additional improvement after two doses of dupilumab. The pruritus became minimal, and the lesions crusted over without development of new lesions (Fig. 2.4). Two months after initiating dupilumab, the patient continued to have some residual disease on the cheeks, though without blisters. In addition to the dupilumab, the patient was started on mometasone 0.1% cream applied twice a day for 7 days to the affected areas on the face, followed by hydrocortisone 2.5% cream daily for up to 10 days per month for flares, which allowed the patient to achieve disease clearance. Other options considered were switching to omalizumab or increasing the frequency of dupilumab injections, the latter of which has been shown to further improve treatment outcomes with BP for those who fail to achieve complete disease clearance with dupilumab every 2 weeks [2]. Two years after diagnosis, the patient tapered the dupilumab dosing to every 4 weeks. At the last follow up more than 2 years after starting dupilumab therapy, the patient continued to experience clearance of disease with dupilumab management. Discontinuation of dupilumab was attempted, but patient pruritus and small vesicles began to return and patient self-resumed his dupilumab. Future plans include gradually increasing the spacing of dupilumab administration.

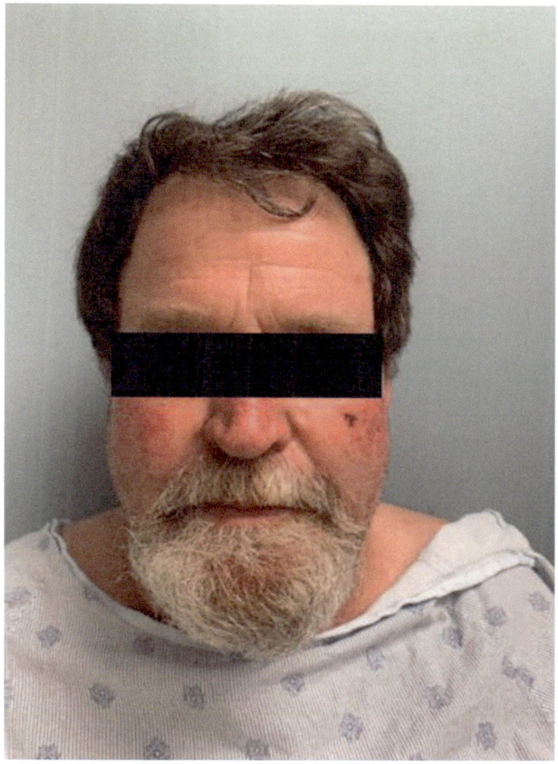

Fig. 2.4 After treatment with a prednisone taper and two doses of dupilumab, the patient had few crusted lesions on the cheeks without development of new lesions

Summary

We present a case of a Caucasian male in 50s with metastatic melanoma who developed immune checkpoint inhibitor (ICI)-induced BP. The case timeline is summarized in Fig. 2.5. This uncommon immune-related adverse event can be diagnosed by evaluating the patient's history and clinical findings in combination with biopsy and serologic testing. Classic biopsy results will reveal subepidermal separation with lymphocytic and/or eosinophilic infiltrate, and positive serologic testing for BP180 and/or BP230 antibodies further support the diagnosis. Topical corticosteroids are a mainstay for mild disease, but severe disease may require a course of systemic corticosteroids with a steroid-sparing agent for long-term management. Salient points demonstrated by the case above include:

- ICI-induced BP may have a delayed onset or occur even after ICI treatment has been stopped.
- ICI-induced BP may persist for prolonged periods of time. This patient has been receiving BP treatment for almost 3 years and still has active BP.
- Dupilumab is an effective and safe treatment for ICI-induced BP. Long-term treatment with dupilumab allows the patient to avoid prolonged use of steroids

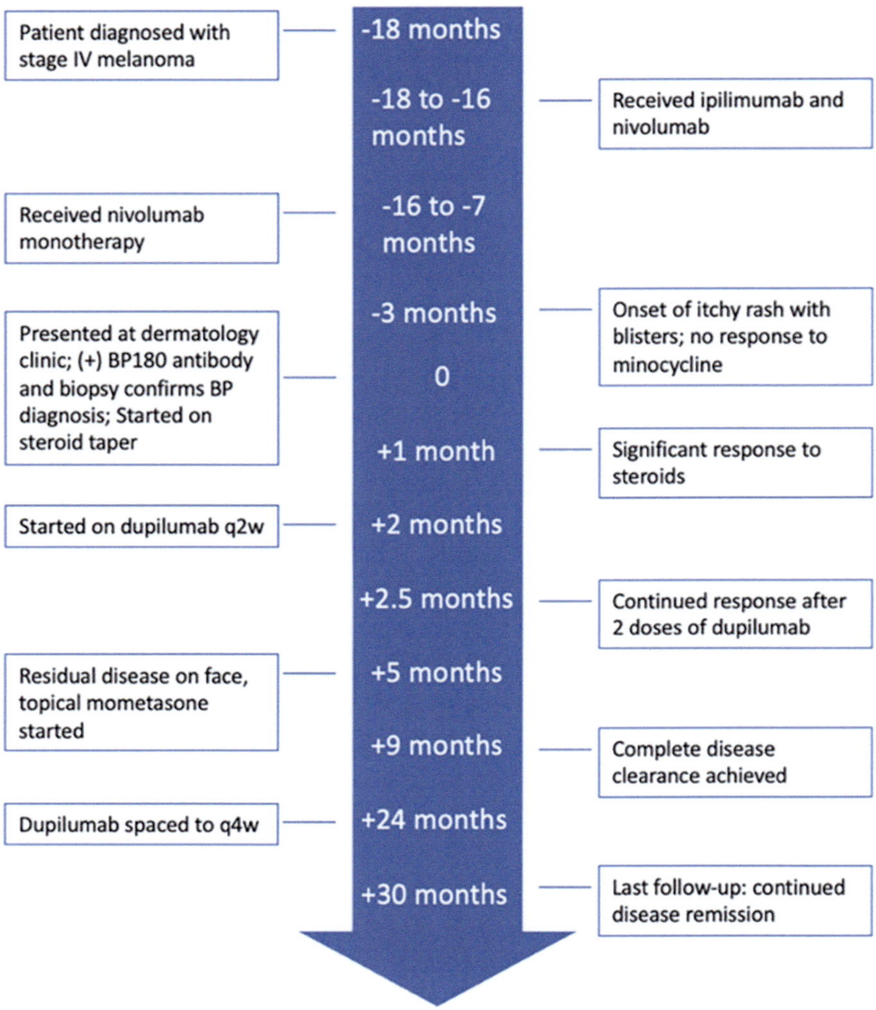

Fig. 2.5 Timeline of events. Timepoint of 0 is the diagnosis of BP

and lacks the safety concerns of other immunosuppressants and biologics. Early prescription may also help to minimize interruptions of ICI therapy. Omalizumab is an alternative biologic that offers a similar efficacy and safety profile, though there is an increased risk of anaphylaxis.

Discussion

BP is an autoimmune blistering dermatosis associated with antibodies directed against BP antigen 180 and BP antigen 230, two hemidesmosomal proteins that promote dermal-epidermal cohesion in the basement membrane. The disease classically presents as tense and pruritic blisters filled with serous or hemorrhagic fluid that spare the mucous membranes, primarily affecting elderly individuals [3]. Atypical presentations include localized eczema, urticarial lesions, erosions, and prurigo, and 10–30% of patients have oral mucosal involvement [3, 4]. The cutaneous lesions and pruritis can significantly disturb the quality of life in affected patients, especially those with other significant comorbidities.

Diagnosis requires integrating patient history and clinical findings with laboratory investigation. A detailed medical history should include the date of onset, evolution of signs and symptoms, comorbidities, and drug history. Immune checkpoint inhibitors have been recognized to induce BP, with associated malignancies including melanoma, non-small cell lung carcinoma, urothelial carcinoma, and head and neck squamous cell carcinomas [4]. Anti-programmed cell death protein-1 (PD-1) therapy is the most common culprit, though anti-programmed death-ligand 1 (PD-L1) and anti-cytotoxic T-lymphocyte-associated protein 4 (CTLA-4) therapy-induced BP has also been reported [5]. Immune checkpoint inhibitors have been noted to have a significant delay between drug initiation and drug-induced BP onset, even up to 1 year, which may be due to long-term activation of autoreactive T-cells by ICI [5–8]. As seen in this patient, BP onset may also occur after stopping the offending drug, highlighting the importance of considering prior ICI use when diagnosing drug-induced BP. ICI-induced BP is also more likely to present with a prolonged prodromal pruritic phase compared to idiopathic BP [9]. Clinicians should thus have a high suspicion for BP and pursue further workup in patients with ICI-induced pruritus that is refractory to topical steroids [4, 9].

Histopathology for BP demonstrates subepidermal bullae containing eosinophils and/or neutrophils. Findings for the non-bullous phase or atypical forms may be non-specific, such as the presence of eosinophilic spongiosis. Direct immunofluorescence testing should be performed on a sample of perilesional skin, which would demonstrate linear deposits of IgG and/or C3 along the dermal-epidermal junction [3]. Immune serological testing for antibodies to BP180 and BP230 further support a diagnosis of BP, though they may be undetectable in up to 20% of BP patients and present in 0.5% of healthy subjects [6].

Management Options

Treatment choice of BP depends on the severity of the disease as well as consideration of the patient's general health and comorbidities. Topical corticosteroids are the mainstay for treatment of mild or localized disease and maintenance of severe disease [10]. They can also be supplemented with adjuvant anti-inflammatories such as doxycycline, nicotinamide, dapsone, and low-dose systemic steroids for mild-to-moderate disease [11]. For patients with severe disease, 0.5–1 mg/kg/day of oral prednisone can be used for initial control with relatively rapid response, and the dosage should then be tapered down over several weeks to months to avoid long-term side effects from prolonged corticosteroid use [10]. Immunosuppressive therapy, such as methotrexate and mycophenolate mofetil, are often considered for patients who fail to respond to corticosteroids alone or those who need to be transitioned to a corticosteroid-sparing agent for long-term maintenance, but these drugs confer a significant risk of toxicity and require regular lab monitoring [10].

Recently, biologic agents such as dupilumab, omalizumab, and rituximab have been used to treat BP with great safety and efficacy. Dupilumab is a humanized IgG4 monoclonal antibody that targets the interleukin (IL)-4 receptor alpha chain and is FDA-approved for the treatment of atopic dermatitis and asthma. The sera and blister fluid of patients with BP have been shown to possess markedly elevated levels of IL-4 and IL-13, and dupilumab directly targets these disease biomarkers by inhibiting IL-4 and IL-13 signaling [12]. Omalizumab is a recombinant humanized anti-immunoglobulin E (IgE) monoclonal antibody that blocks binding of IgE to its receptor and is FDA-approved for the treatment of asthma, chronic spontaneous urticaria, and chronic rhinosinusitis. IgE autoantibodies have been implicated in the pathogenesis of BP through deposition in the epidermal basement membrane zone, suggesting a possible mechanism for omalizumab in the treatment of BP [13]. Rituximab is a human-mouse chimeric monoclonal antibody against B lymphocyte CD20 that is often used to treat chronic lymphocytic leukemia, non-Hodgkin lymphomas, and rheumatoid arthritis, but it can also decrease antibody production to treat bullous dermatoses [13]. Dupilumab and omalizumab are especially attractive options for treatment of ICI-induced BP because of their excellent safety profile in vulnerable populations. Unlike other biologic therapies, dupilumab and omalizumab do not significantly increase the risk of infection from immunosuppression and do not require regular lab monitoring. A systematic review comparing treatment outcomes for dupilumab, omalizumab, and rituximab in BP patients found that while the three biologics resulted in similar remission rates, rituximab resulted in higher BP recurrence rates, adverse events, and mortality rates, supporting the use of omalizumab and dupilumab over rituximab [13].

The decision to continue or stop immunotherapy with the onset of BP requires careful evaluation of the potential benefits and risks, and some recommend cessation of ICI until the BP is a CTCAE grade 0–1 [4]. However, a retrospective case-control study demonstrated an association between BP development and improved tumor response with anti-PD-1 therapy, which may signify the importance of continuing ICI therapy in patients who develop BP [14]. In a case series of 20 patients who developed immunotherapy-induced BP, the authors found that cessation or interruption of ICI therapy did not affect BP severity or need for a steroid-sparing agent, suggesting that patients can continue to receive ICI while managing their BP [7]. There is conflicting information on whether or not corticosteroids and other BP treatments attenuate the anti-tumor effect of ICI [15]. While steroid-sparing agents are often seen as second- or third-line therapies in the treatment of BP, the early introduction of steroid-sparing agents may minimize prolonged high-dose systemic corticosteroid use and minimize interruptions of ICI therapy.

References

1. Cox L, Platts-Mills TAE, Finegold I, Schwartz LB, Simons FER, Wallace DV, et al. American Academy of Allergy, Asthma & Immunology/American College of Allergy, Asthma and Immunology Joint Task Force Report on omalizumab-associated anaphylaxis. J Allergy Clin Immunol. 2007;120(6):1373–7.
2. Abdat R, Waldman RA, de Bedout V, Czernik A, Mcleod M, King B, et al. Dupilumab as a novel therapy for Bullous pemphigoid (BP): a multicenter case series. J Am Acad Dermatol [Internet]. 2020;83(1):46–52. [cited 2023 Jun 25]. Available from: https://www.sciencedirect.com/science/article/pii/S0190962220303996
3. Borradori L, Van Beek N, Feliciani C, Tedbirt B, Antiga E, Bergman R, et al. Updated S2 K guidelines for the management of bullous pemphigoid initiated by the European Academy of Dermatology and Venereology (EADV). J Eur Acad Dermatol Venereol [Internet]. 2022;36(10):1689–704. [cited 2023 Jun 18]. Available from: https://onlinelibrary.wiley.com/doi/abs/10.1111/jdv.18220
4. Geisler AN, Phillips GS, Barrios DM, Wu J, Leung DYM, Moy AP, et al. Immune checkpoint inhibitor—related dermatologic adverse events. J Am Acad Dermatol [Internet]. 2020;83(5):1255–68. [cited 2023 Jun 25]. Available from: https://www.ncbi.nlm.nih.gov/pmc/articles/PMC7572894/
5. Asdourian MS, Shah N, Jacoby TV, Reynolds KL, Chen ST. Association of bullous pemphigoid with immune checkpoint inhibitor therapy in patients with cancer: a systematic review. JAMA Dermatol [Internet]. 2022;158(8):933–41. [cited 2023 Jun 25]. Available from: https://doi.org/10.1001/jamadermatol.2022.1624
6. Sadik CD, Langan EA, Gutzmer R, Fleischer MI, Loquai C, Reinhardt L, et al. Retrospective analysis of checkpoint inhibitor therapy-associated cases of bullous pemphigoid from six German Dermatology Centers. Front Immunol [Internet]. 2021;11:588582. [cited 2023 Jun 25]. Available from: https://www.ncbi.nlm.nih.gov/pmc/articles/PMC7940359/
7. Bur D, Patel AB, Nelson K, Huen A, Pacha O, Phillips R, et al. A retrospective case series of 20 patients with immunotherapy-induced bullous pemphigoid with emphasis on management outcomes. J Am Acad Dermatol [Internet]. 2022;87(6):1394–5. [cited 2023 Jun 25]. Available from: https://www.jaad.org/article/S0190-9622(22)02427-6/fulltext
8. Naidoo J, Schindler K, Querfeld C, Busam K, Cunningham J, Page DB, et al. Autoimmune bullous skin disorders with immune checkpoint inhibitors targeting PD-1 and PD-L1. Cancer Immunol Res [Internet]. 2016;4(5):383–9. [cited 2023 Jun 25]. Available from: https://www.ncbi.nlm.nih.gov/pmc/articles/PMC5241697/
9. Molina GE, Reynolds KL, Chen ST. Diagnostic and therapeutic differences between immune checkpoint inhibitor-induced and idiopathic Bullous pemphigoid (BP): a cross-sectional study. Br J Dermatol [Internet]. 2020;183(6):1126–8. [cited 2023 Jun 27]. Available from: https://doi.org/10.1111/bjd.19313
10. Bernard P, Antonicelli F. Bullous pemphigoid (BP): a review of its diagnosis, associations and treatment. Am J Clin Dermatol [Internet]. 2017;18(4):513–28. [cited 2023 Jun 25]. Available from: https://doi.org/10.1007/s40257-017-0264-2
11. Patel PM, Jones VA, Murray TN, Amber KT. A review comparing international guidelines for the management of bullous pemphigoid, pemphigoid gestationis, mucous membrane pemphigoid, and epidermolysis bullosa acquisita. Am J Clin Dermatol. 2020;21(4):557–65.

12. Teraki Y, Hotta T, Shiohara T. Skin-homing Interleukin-4 and -13-producing cells contribute to Bullous pemphigoid (BP): remission of disease is associated with increased frequency of Interleukin-10-producing cells. J Invest Dermatol [Internet]. 2001;117(5):1097–102. [cited 2023 Jun 25]. Available from: https://www.sciencedirect.com/science/article/pii/S0022202X15414265
13. Cao P, Xu W, Zhang L. Rituximab, omalizumab, and dupilumab treatment outcomes in Bullous pemphigoid (BP): a systematic review. Front Immunol [Internet]. 2022;13:928621. [cited 2023 Jun 18]. Available from: https://www.ncbi.nlm.nih.gov/pmc/articles/PMC9235912/
14. Brahmer JR, Lacchetti C, Schneider BJ, Atkins MB, Brassil KJ, Caterino JM, et al. Management of immune-related adverse events in patients treated with immune checkpoint inhibitor therapy: American Society of Clinical Oncology Clinical Practice Guideline. J Clin Oncol Off J Am Soc Clin Oncol [Internet]. 2018;36(17):1714–68. [cited 2023 Jun 27]. Available from: https://www.ncbi.nlm.nih.gov/pmc/articles/PMC6481621/
15. Nelson CA, Singer S, Chen T, Puleo AE, Lian CG, Wei EX, et al. Bullous pemphigoid after anti–programmed death-1 therapy: a retrospective case-control study evaluating impact on tumor response and survival outcomes. J Am Acad Dermatol [Internet]. 2022;87(6):1400–2. [cited 2023 Jun 25]. Available from: https://www.jaad.org/article/S0190-9622(20)30048-7/fulltext

Chapter 3
Erosive Oral Lichen Planus with Pemphigus Vulgaris Post Immune Checkpoint Inhibitor Treatment

Hannah Y. Wang, Carlos A. Torres-Cabala, and Anisha B. Patel

Abbreviations

Ab	antibody
AGNA	antiglial nuclear antibody
AMPA	alpha-amino-3-hydroxy-5-methyl-4-isoxazole propionic acid
ANNA	antineuronal nuclear antibody
BID	twice daily
CASPR	contactin-associated protein-like
CBA	cell-binding assay
CCPQ	P/Q-type calcium channel
CRMP	collapsin response-mediator protein
CSF	cerebrospinal fluid
DPPX	dipeptidyl-peptidase-like protein-6
Dsg	desmoglein
GABA	gamma-aminobutyric acid
GAD	glutamic acid decarboxylase
GFAP	glial fibrillary acidic protein
ICI	immune checkpoint inhibitor
IFA	indirect immunofluorescence assay
IgG	immunoglobulin G

H. Y. Wang
Baylor College of Medicine, Houston, TX, USA
e-mail: hannah.wang@bcm.edu

C. A. Torres-Cabala
Department of Pathology, University of Texas MD Anderson Cancer Center, Houston, TX, USA
e-mail: ctcabala@mdanderson.org

A. B. Patel (✉)
Department of Dermatology, University of Texas MD Anderson Cancer Center, Houston, TX, USA
e-mail: apatel11@mdanderson.org

Y. Wang (ed.), *Challenging Cases in Immunotherapy Related Organ Toxicities*,
https://doi.org/10.1007/978-3-031-83533-9_3

LGI	leucine-rich glioma-inactivated
mGluR1	metabotropic glutamate receptor 1
MM	mycophenolate mofetil
MTX	methotrexate
NIF	neuronal intermediate filament
NMDA	N-methyl-D-aspartate
PCA	Purkinje cytoplasmic antibody
QW	weekly
R	receptor
VGKC	voltage-gated potassium channel

Clinical Presentation

A Caucasian male in his 70 s with a 30-pack-year smoking history presented to the dermatology clinic for a rash of 2 months' duration on the back and ankles. He was diagnosed with lung adenocarcinoma of the right lower lobe with pleural metastasis a year prior to his presentation and had received 6 cycles of combination therapy with ipilimumab and nivolumab alternating with 12 cycles of nivolumab monotherapy since then. His immunotherapy course had been complicated by immune checkpoint inhibitor (ICI)-associated adrenal insufficiency, requiring hydrocortisone replacement. His medication list also included atorvastatin, mirtazapine, and varenicline. The rash was pruritic and would bleed with scratching. On exam, the patient had mildly erythematous scaling papules and patches on the back and lower legs, with 5% of the total body surface area affected and no mucosal involvement. The patient was first managed with topical triamcinolone twice a day for 2 weeks for generalized dermatitis that was attributed to his immunotherapy. He was also prescribed 360 mg of fexofenadine every morning and 10 mg of cetirizine HCL every night for the pruritus.

One month later, the patient reported that the rash on his back and ankles improved with the triamcinolone cream. However, after some dental procedures, he experienced a new erosion on the lower lip that had been present for a month with associated dryness of the lip. He denied any preceding blisters or lesions elsewhere on the body. The lip lesion did not improve after he received 50 mg of prednisone for a recent course of bronchitis. On exam, the patient had a faint white lacy patch on the right lower lip with central erosion, and the right buccal mucosa had a faint white lacelike pattern. Since the site had improved within the last week, the patient opted to treat the lesion without a biopsy. After 2 weeks of applying fluocinonide 0.05% ointment twice a day, the original lesions persisted, and new erosions appeared on the left lower lip, the left posterior buccal mucosa, and the tongue [Fig. 3.1]. The patient was recommended to continue applying fluocinonide ointment twice a day to the oral erosions and to use a dexamethasone 0.5 mg/5 mL mouth wash while avoiding spicy, salty, acidic, and potentially mechanically traumatizing foods. His ICI treatment was also paused. One week later, he reported improvement

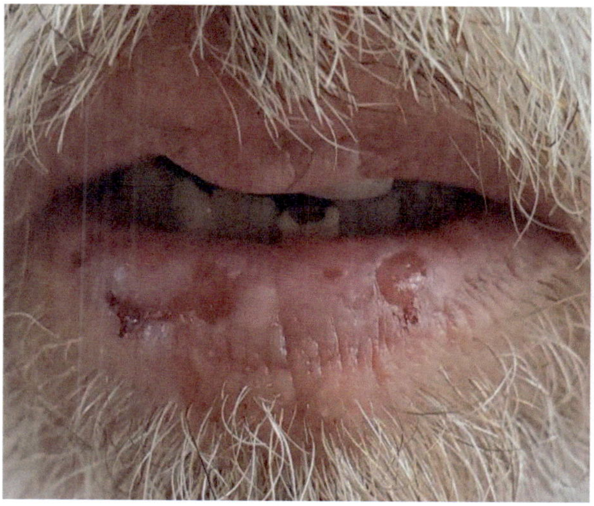

Fig. 3.1 Ulcerations on the left and right lower lip that persisted despite treatment with topical fluocinonide

with the topical steroids and no new lesions. Two weeks later, he developed a new lesion on the lower lip despite treatment with topical steroids.

A biopsy of the lower lip was performed, showing lichenoid dermatitis, which is described in detail below. The patient was started on a prednisone taper starting at 60 mg per day for 1 week, with taper by 20 mg each week. One week after starting the prednisone taper, the patient reported significant pain and discomfort of the oral mucosa and expressed desire to hold his ICI treatment for additional time, so it was recommended that he pause ICI treatment for 2 weeks until he finishes the steroid taper. After another 2 weeks, the patient's lip lesions were cleared, and he was resumed on ICI.

Three weeks later, he developed ICI-induced encephalopathy requiring additional treatment with prednisone taper starting at 80 mg and cessation of his ICI treatment. At this time, CT imaging of the chest, abdomen, and pelvis confirmed stable disease with regards to his lung adenocarcinoma. Two months later, he presented again to dermatology with persistent tongue ulcers, which he reports only improved when taking 80 mg of prednisone daily, though the lip lesions responded to lower prednisone doses. The oral ulcers continued to cause significant pain and limited his diet and speech, and he could only tolerate liquids. On exam, the patient had many erythematous superficial ulcerations of the tongue and oral mucosa with some white plaques of the tongue and buccal mucosa [Fig. 3.2].

Labs

The patient's testing for serum desmoglein (Dsg) antibodies yielded negative results [Table 3.1]. Similarly, the evaluation of the serum and cerebrospinal fluid for autoimmune and paraneoplastic encephalopathy was negative [Table 3.2].

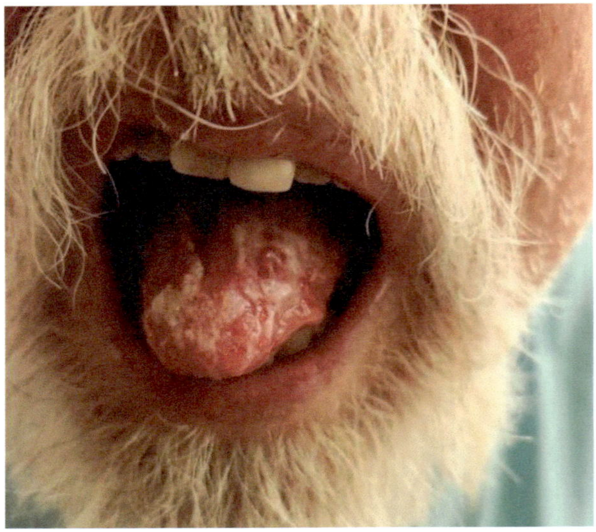

Fig. 3.2 After the patient started high dose prednisone, the lip erosions resolved, but superficial ulcerations and white plaques on the dorsal tongue persisted

Table 3.1 Results of serological desmoglein testing

Autoantibody (Serum)	Result
Dsg-1 Ab	Negative
Dsg-3 Ab	Negative

Abbreviations: *Dsg* desmoglein, *Ab* antibody

Pathology

Three biopsies were performed on the lower lip. Microscopy analysis revealed two samples with lichenoid dermatitis, one with focal ulceration and one with an area of complete squamous epithelial detachment. [Fig. 3.3] The third sample, taken for direct immunofluorescence (DIF), revealed abundant colloid bodies along a subepidermal split, which stained heavily with fibrin, C3, IgM, IgG, and less so with IgA. IgA and IgG stained the keratinocytes of the lower half of the epidermis in a chicken wire pattern. There was also diffuse staining of the dermis in a nonspecific pattern with fibrin, C3, IgG, and IgA.

Differential Diagnosis

The initial differential considered for this patient's lip erosions included lichen planus (LP) and autoimmune blistering disorders such as pemphigus vulgaris (PV) and paraneoplastic pemphigus (PNP). The white lacy patterns on the buccal mucosa were clinically suggestive of LP, resembling Wickham's striae. The biopsy results demonstrating an interface dermatitis and abundant colloid bodies along a

Table 3.2 Results of serological and cerebrospinal fluid (CSF) evaluation for autoimmune/paraneoplastic encephalopathy

Autoantibody (Serum and CSF)	Result
AMPA-R Ab CBA	Negative
Amphiphysin Ab	Negative
AGNA-1	Negative
ANNA-1	Negative
ANNA-2	Negative
ANNA-3	Negative
CASPR-2-IgG CBA	Negative
CRMP-5-IgG	Negative
DPPX Ab IFA	Negative
GABA-B-R Ab CBA	Negative
GAD 65 Ab assay	Negative
GFAP IFA	Negative
IgLON5 IFA	Negative
LGI1-IgG CBA	Negative
mGluR1 Ab IFA	Negative
NIF IFA	Negative
NMDA-R Ab CBA	Negative
PCA-1	Negative
PCA-2	Negative
PCA-Tr	Negative
Neuronal VGKC Ab	Negative
CCPQ Ab	Negative

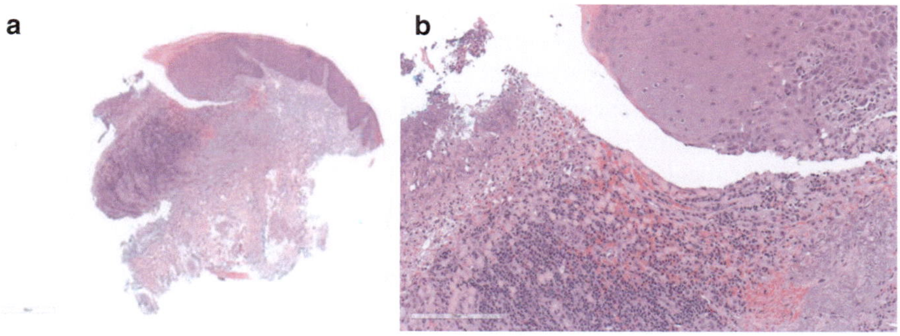

Fig. 3.3 (**a**) A punch biopsy from the lower lip shows a band-like lichenoid lymphoid infiltrate with ulceration. The adjacent epidermis is acanthotic and has areas of hyper-granulosis. (H&E, x20). (**b**) At higher magnification, numerous colloid (Civatte) bodies are seen, in association with dyskeratotic/apoptotic keratinocytes. The overall findings are those of a lichenoid dermatitis, consistent with lichen planus with erosion (H&E, x200)

subepidermal split was further supportive of a lichenoid dermatitis. However, the DIF demonstrating intraepidermal depositions of IgA and IgG was more consistent with pemphigus. Drug-induced PV and PNP can be difficult to differentiate in the setting of a malignancy. PNP is type of pemphigus associated with neoplasms and presents with erosive stomatitis and polymorphous skin lesions [1]. The pathophysiology involves the production of autoantibodies against various target antigens, primarily the plakin family proteins but also the desmogleins. The histopathology of PNP is varied but may include interface dermatitis and acantholytic blisters [2]. Eighty-four percent of PNP cases are related to hematologic neoplasms, making PNP associated with lung adenocarcinoma in this patient less likely [3]. While ICI may exacerbate subclinical PNP, patients with PNP should exhibit symptoms before initiating ICI treatment rather than many months afterwards, such as in our patient. Up to 50% of cases may even precede the diagnosis of the associated neoplasm [4]. PNP activity may also mirror the activity of the neoplastic disease [5]. This patient had worsening oral lesions while his lung adenocarcinoma was stable based on imaging results, further suggesting a drug-induced PV rather than PNP. Based on these clinicopathologic findings, we diagnosed the patient with ICI-induced oral LP with a component of PV.

Outcome

Since the patient had already received several courses of high-dose prednisone without resilient disease clearance, steroid-sparing agents were initiated for long-term management following a 7-day course of fluconazole 100 mg daily for oral candidiasis. The patient started on 15 mg of methotrexate weekly with daily folic acid supplementation. Four weeks later while receiving the treatment, he continued odynophagia with apparent candidiasis despite some improvement of ulcerations on the physical exam. Methotrexate treatment was held for 1 week to complete a second course of fluconazole. Afterwards, he resumed his methotrexate treatment with the addition of 500 mg mycophenolate mofetil twice daily and he reported significantly improved oral pain after 1 month of the combination treatment. Two months later, the patient denied any oral ulcers, and on exam the tongue had only residual atrophic plaques on the lateral edges and a fibrinous plaque on the dorsal surface, with normal buccal mucosa and gingiva. The mycophenolate mofetil dosing was subsequently increased to 1000 mg twice daily. After another 3 months, the patient had achieved disease clearance and his methotrexate was decreased to 12.5 mg weekly. The plan is to decrease methotrexate every 3 months if patient remains clear and completely taper off methotrexate. If necessary, we will continue disease maintenance with mycophenolate mofetil due to long-term potential liver toxicities with methotrexate. Future treatment considerations if the patient's disease worsens included rituximab or intravenous immunoglobulin G (IVIG).

Summary

We presented a case with metastatic lung adenocarcinoma who developed ICI-induced erosive oral LP with a component of PV. Biopsy results demonstrated a lichenoid dermatitis with abundant colloid bodies along a subepidermal split, while DIF staining revealed immunoglobulin deposition between the epidermal keratinocytes. The patient responded well to corticosteroid treatment initially but ultimately required methotrexate and mycophenolate mofetil for long-term clearance. The disease course with timeline are illustrated in Fig. 3.4.

Salient points demonstrated by the case above include:

- Though very rare, supra-basal acantholytic dermatoses such as PV may occur with ICI. PV and PNP within the setting of a concurrent malignancy may be differentiated based on the onset of disease with relation to the diagnosis of malignancy, type of malignancy, and timing relative to tumor response/progression of disease.
- Oral lichenoid dermatoses and PV can severely limit patients' quality of life and be recalcitrant to treatment.
- While corticosteroids are an effective initial treatment for controlling flares of LP and/or PV, patients should be transitioned to steroid sparing agents for long-term management with more favorable safety. There is no FDA-approved treatment for either of these diseases and methotrexate, mycophenolate mofetil, apremilast, acitretin, IVIG, rituximab, and TNF inhibitors are some of the many options which have been reported as efficacious.

Discussion

LP is a chronic inflammatory disease where autoreactive T-cells attack the basal keratinocytes, affecting the skin, hair, nails, and mucosa [6]. Oral LP is a variant of mucosal LP and can present in the classic reticular pattern with white lines, plaques, and papules; the atrophic or erythematous variant; and the erosive variant, including ulcerations and bullae [7]. The ulcerated presentation often causes pain and limitations in oral function, which can significantly affect patients' quality of life. White reticulations, often referred to as "Wickham's striae", are considered pathognomonic for LP. Acute flare-ups may be precipitated by factors such as stress, acidic and spicy foods, dental procedures, systemic illness, heavy alcohol consumption, and tobacco use. Histopathologic findings of LP include hypergranulosis of the epidermis with a "saw tooth" appearance of the rete ridges, a band of lymphocytic infiltration along the dermoepidermal junction, and apoptotic keratinocytes in the papillary dermis as eosinophilic colloid bodies. DIF staining usually reveals a band of fibrinogen along the dermoepidermal junction with colloid bodies staining with immunoglobulins and C3 [6].

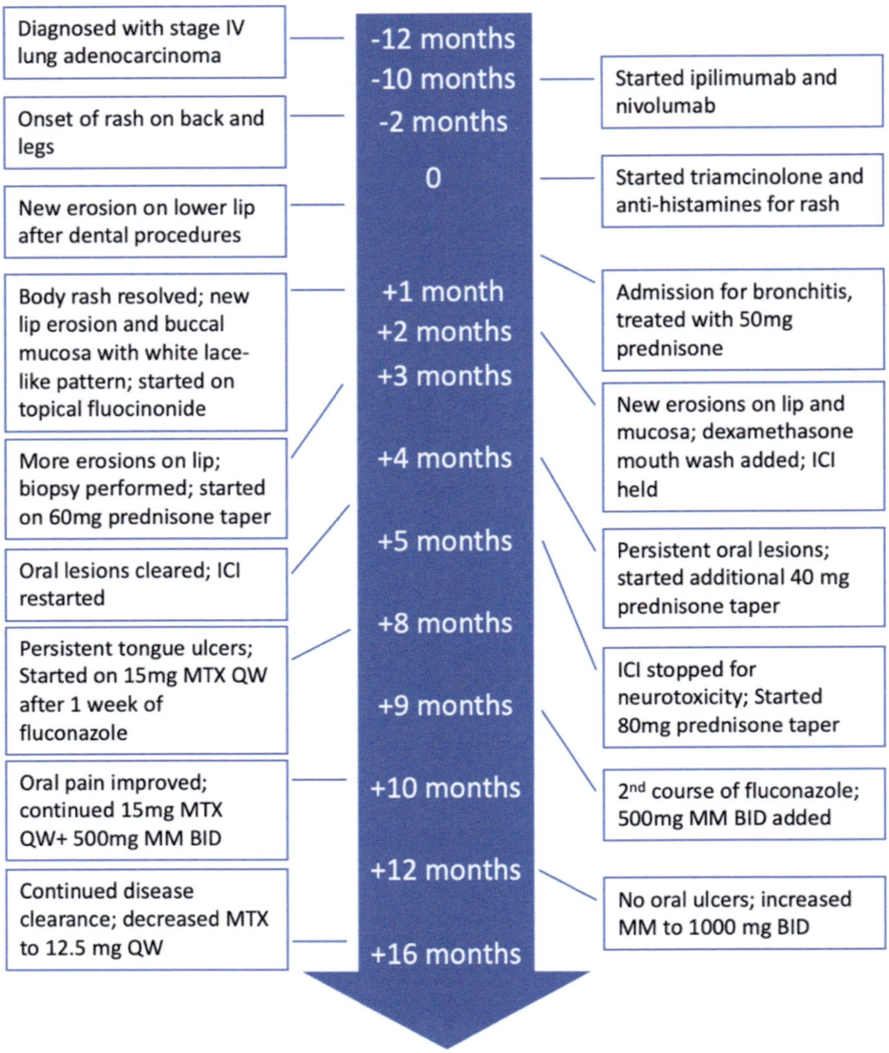

Fig. 3.4 Patient's disease course of erosive oral lichen planus with pemphigus vulgaris

PV is an intraepidermal blistering disease characterized by the production of autoantibodies directed against the intercellular adhesion molecules Dsg-1 and Dsg-3, inducing epidermal acantholysis [8]. The disease has a high mortality rate if not treated, with infection as the most frequent cause of death [9]. Clinically, patients may present with flaccid bullae or erosions on the skin and/or mucosa and minimal pruritus [10]. Diagnosis of PV requires correlation of the patient's history and physical exam findings with histopathology and antibody testing. Clinical evaluation of patients with suspected PV should clarify timing of symptoms, any loss of function from the disease, potential contraindications to treatment, and medication history.

Thiol and phenol drugs in particular are known triggers of drug-induced PV, though other drug types have also been described to trigger pemphigus, including ICIs [8, 10]. Histopathology would reveal intraepidermal suprabasal acantholysis, while direct immunofluorescence of a perilesional biopsy would reveal IgG and/or C3 deposits at the surface of the epidermal keratinocytes. IgA may be present in addition to IgG in some cases. Serologic detection of autoantibodies against the epithelial surface, detectable in 90% of patients, may be performed with indirect immunofluorescence or enzyme linked immunosorbent assay of Dsg1 and/or Dsg3 [8].

Interestingly, some cases of erosive oral LP have been associated with anti-Dsg-1 and -3 autoantibodies and anti-bullous pemphigoid 180 and 230 autoantibodies. While the pathogenicity of these autoantibodies in oral LP is unclear, they may represent the diversification of the immune response following the chronic inflammation of the skin disease and suggests a potential pathogenesis of a mixed LP and PV presentation, as seen in our patient [11]. While oral LP and PV may both present with ulcerations of the oral mucosa, LP alone will not demonstrate a "honeycomb" pattern of immunoglobulin or complement deposition on DIF, demonstrating the importance of considering DIF evaluation in a patient's workup of oral ulcers.

LP and PV have been identified as possible cutaneous immune-related adverse events (cirAEs) from immunotherapy. Both diseases have been associated with both anti-programmed cell death protein-1(PD-1)/programmed death-ligand 1 (PD-L1) and anti-cytotoxic T-lymphocyte-associated protein 4 (CTLA-4) treatment, though they seem to be more frequent with anti-PD-1/PD-L1 agents [10, 12]. While LP eruptions are one of the more common ICI-related cirAEs, lichenoid reactions are rarely observed in the oral mucosa [13]. Compared to cytotoxic chemotherapy, oral mucosal reactions are also less prevalent in patients on PD-1/PD-L1 inhibitors [14].

Autoimmune blistering disorders associated with ICIs typically exhibit subepidermal blistering with features of either bullous pemphigoid or dermatitis herpetiformis, while suprabasal acantholytic diseases secondary to ICI treatment, such as pemphigus, are significantly more rare and less understood [15]. In some patients, ICIs may "unmask" a genetic susceptibility for autoimmune stimulation and result in PV clinical expression. There are also cases of patients with pre-existing PV that experienced disease recurrence with immunotherapy [10]. ICI-induced PV has been linked with both PD-1/PD-L1 inhibitors and CTLA-4 inhibitors, and it can also occur with significant delay after the start of immunotherapy, with reports of time of onset ranging from 20 days to 5 months after ICI initiation [16, 17].

First line treatment for both PV and lichenoid mucositis includes topical corticosteroids, such as dexamethasone 0.5 mg/5 mL swish and spit solution and fluocinonide 0.05% gel, and oral steroids [8, 14, 18]. However, in a retrospective chart review of patients with ICI-associated lichenoid mucositis, only two-thirds of patients were successfully treated with either topical or oral steroids, with others requiring non-steroidal treatment [18]. Management for severe or refractory cases of lichenoid reactions may include acitretin, methotrexate, and other immune modulators. Systemic therapy for PV includes systemic corticosteroids, rituximab, azathioprine, or mycophenolate mofetil [8]. While methotrexate is not recommended for PV based on treatment guidelines issued by the International Bullous Diseases Consensus Group, there is a case of a patient with recurrence of PV after initiating immunotherapy who had complete clearance with prednisolone and methotrexate [8, 19]. Another case of PV in the setting of concomitant immunotherapy was treated with rituximab, though the patient died shortly after due to cancer progression [20]. Topicals with local anesthetics and analgesics should be considered for those with significant accompanying pain, especially for mucosal involvement. Patients receiving prolonged steroid therapy should also receive the appropriate prophylaxis and/or treatment against side effects, such as anti-fungals for steroid-associated candidiasis described in this case.

While systemic corticosteroids may provide excellent initial disease control and sometimes disease clearance, patients with recalcitrant or recurring disease should optimally be transitioned to a steroid-sparing agent for long-term management. Oral LP and PV can be difficult to control with a single course of corticosteroids. Cutaneous LP tends to be self-limiting with pruritus, while oral lesions rarely undergo spontaneous remission and can significantly hinder quality of life [7]. This pattern seems to persist within ICI-associated lichenoid eruptions, as lichenoid mucositis is more likely than lichenoid dermatitis to not respond to treatment [18]. As seen in our patient, lichenoid reactions may also even persist after immunotherapy is ceased [14]. While increasing the dose and frequency of corticosteroid treatments may help to control symptoms, there are also concerns that high dose corticosteroid therapy may dampen the anti-tumor effect of ICI [21]. Steroid-sparing agents are thus particularly important to implement for patients with recalcitrant and/or recurring disease to avoid the side effects of prolonged steroid therapy and optimize the effects of the immunotherapy.

Treatment of ICI-induced cirAEs requires consideration of the patient's comorbidities, the cirAE severity, and the cancer treatment status to optimize limiting cancer progression while controlling symptoms. Several consensus guidelines recommend the cessation of immunotherapy for grade 2 or higher cirAEs that are immunobullous or have mucosal involvement [22]. However, a balance between receiving immunotherapy and managing toxicities may benefit patient survival. Some studies have suggested that presence of cirAEs, including lichenoid reactions, may indicate a better anti-tumor effect of ICIs, highlighting the importance of continuing immunotherapy when possible [23].

References

1. Gallo E, García-Martín P, Fraga J, Teye K, Koga H, Hashimoto T, et al. Paraneoplastic pemphigus with eosinophilic spongiosis and autoantibodies against desmocollins 2 and 3. Clin Exp Dermatol [Internet]. 2014;39(3):323–6. [cited 2023 Aug 6]. https://doi.org/10.1111/ced.12296.
2. Anhalt GJ. Paraneoplastic pemphigus. J Investig Dermatol Symp Proc [Internet]. 2004;9(1):29–33. [cited 2023 Aug 6]. Available from: https://www.jidsponline.org/article/S0022-202X(15)52978-3/fulltext

3. Kaplan I, Hodak E, Ackerman L, Mimouni D, Anhalt GJ, Calderon S. Neoplasms associated with paraneoplastic pemphigus: a review with emphasis on non-hematologic malignancy and oral mucosal manifestations. Oral Oncol. 2004 Jul;40(6):553–62.
4. Anderson HJ, Huang S, Lee JB. Paraneoplastic pemphigus/paraneoplastic autoimmune multiorgan syndrome: part I. Clinical overview and pathophysiology. J Am Acad Dermatol. 2023;S0190-9622(23):02512–4.
5. Antiga E, Bech R, Maglie R, Genovese G, Borradori L, Bockle B, et al. S2k guidelines on the management of paraneoplastic pemphigus/paraneoplastic autoimmune multiorgan syndrome initiated by the European Academy of Dermatology and Venereology (EADV). J Eur Acad Dermatol Venereol [Internet]. 2023;37(6):1118–34. [cited 2023 Sep 6]. Available from: https://onlinelibrary.wiley.com/doi/abs/10.1111/jdv.18931
6. Tziotzios C, Lee JYW, Brier T, Saito R, Hsu CK, Bhargava K, et al. Lichen planus and lichenoid dermatoses: clinical overview and molecular basis. J Am Acad Dermatol. 2018;79(5):789–804.
7. Eisen D. The clinical features, malignant potential, and systemic associations of oral lichen planus: a study of 723 patients. J Am Acad Dermatol [Internet]. 2002;46(2):207–14. [cited 2023 Aug 25]. Available from: https://www.sciencedirect.com/science/article/pii/S0190962202632244
8. Murrell DF, Peña S, Joly P, Marinovic B, Hashimoto T, Diaz LA, et al. Diagnosis and management of pemphigus: recommendations of an international panel of experts. J Am Acad Dermatol [Internet]. 2020;82(3):575–585.e1. [cited 2023 Aug 28]. Available from: https://www.ncbi.nlm.nih.gov/pmc/articles/PMC7313440/
9. Kridin K. Pemphigus group: overview, epidemiology, mortality, and comorbidities. Immunol Res [Internet]. 2018;66(2):255–70. [cited 2023 Aug 30]. https://doi.org/10.1007/s12026-018-8986-7.
10. Merli M, Accorinti M, Romagnuolo M, Marzano A, Di Zenzo G, Moro F, et al. Autoimmune bullous dermatoses in cancer patients treated by immunotherapy: a literature review and Italian multicentric experience. Front Med (Lausanne) [Internet]. 2023;10:1208418. [cited 2023 Aug 25]. Available from: https://www.ncbi.nlm.nih.gov/pmc/articles/PMC10400335/
11. Didona D, Hertl M. Detection of anti-desmoglein antibodies in oral lichen planus: what do we know so far. Front Immunol [Internet]. 2022;13:1001970. [cited 2023 Aug 23]. Available from: https://www.ncbi.nlm.nih.gov/pmc/articles/PMC9575987/
12. Curry JL, Tetzlaff MT, Nagarajan P, Drucker C, Diab A, Hymes SR, et al. Diverse types of dermatologic toxicities from immune checkpoint blockade therapy. J Cutan Pathol [Internet]. 2017;44(2):158–76. [cited 2023 Aug 28]. Available from: https://onlinelibrary.wiley.com/doi/abs/10.1111/cup.12858
13. Watanabe T, Yamaguchi Y. Cutaneous manifestations associated with immune checkpoint inhibitors. Front Immunol [Internet]. 2023;14:1071983. [cited 2023 Aug 28]. Available from: https://www.ncbi.nlm.nih.gov/pmc/articles/PMC9986601/
14. Muhaj F, Karri PV, Moody W, Brown A, Patel AB. Mucocutaneous adverse events to immune checkpoint inhibitors. Front Allergy. 2023;4:1147513.
15. Chen WS, Tetzlaff MT, Diwan H, Jahan-Tigh R, Diab A, Nelson K, et al. Suprabasal acantholytic dermatologic toxicities associated checkpoint inhibitor therapy: a spectrum of immune reactions from paraneoplastic pemphigus-like to Grover-like lesions. J Cutan Pathol. 2018;45(10):764–73.
16. Ito M, Hoashi T, Endo Y, Kimura G, Kondo Y, Ishii N, et al. Atypical pemphigus developed in a patient with urothelial carcinoma treated with nivolumab. J Dermatol [Internet]. 2019;46(3):e90–2. [cited 2023 Aug 25]. Available from: https://onlinelibrary.wiley.com/doi/abs/10.1111/1346-8138.14601
17. Buquicchio R, Mastrandrea V, Strippoli S, Quaresmini D, Guida M, Filotico R. Case report: autoimmune Pemphigus vulgaris in a patient treated with Cemiplimab for multiple locally advanced cutaneous squamous cell carcinoma. Front Oncol. 2021;11:691980.
18. Masterson WM, Brown AM, Al Ameri MA, Patel AB. A retrospective chart review of management strategies for lichenoid eruptions associated with immune-checkpoint inhibitor

therapy from a single institution. Cancer Treat Res Commun [Internet]. 2022;30:100506. [cited 2023 Aug 23]. Available from: https://www.sciencedirect.com/science/article/pii/S2468294221002021
19. Krammer S, Krammer C, Salzer S, Bağci IS, French LE, Hartmann D. Recurrence of pemphigus vulgaris under nivolumab therapy. Front Med (Lausanne) [Internet]. 2019;6:262. [cited 2023 Aug 25]. Available from: https://www.ncbi.nlm.nih.gov/pmc/articles/PMC6861207/
20. Clawson RC, Tabata MM, Chen ST. Pemphigus vulgaris flare in a patient treated with nivolumab. Dermatol Ther [Internet]. 2021;34(2):e14871. [cited 2023 Aug 25]. Available from: https://onlinelibrary.wiley.com/doi/abs/10.1111/dth.14871
21. Goodman RS, Johnson DB, Balko JM. Corticosteroids and cancer immunotherapy. Clin Cancer Res [Internet]. 2023;29(14):2580–7. [cited 2023 Aug 30]. https://doi.org/10.1158/1078-0432.CCR-22-3181.
22. Park BC, Jung S, Chen ST, Dewan AK, Johnson DB. Challenging dermatologic considerations associated with immune checkpoint inhibitors. Am J Clin Dermatol [Internet]. 2022;23(5):707–17. [cited 2023 Aug 28]. https://doi.org/10.1007/s40257-022-00706-y.
23. Zhang S, Tang K, Wan G, Nguyen N, Lu C, Ugwu-Dike P, et al. Cutaneous immune-related adverse events are associated with longer overall survival in advanced cancer patients on immune checkpoint inhibitors: a multi-institutional cohort study. J Am Acad Dermatol [Internet]. 2023;88(5):1024–32. [cited 2023 Aug 28]. Available from: https://www.ncbi.nlm.nih.gov/pmc/articles/PMC10283025/

Chapter 4
Dermatomyositis Post Immune Checkpoint Inhibitor Therapy

Rishabh Lohray and Anisha B. Patel

Abbreviations

ANA	Anti-nuclear antibodies
CK	Creatine kinase
CKMB	Creatine kinase myoglobin binding
CR	Complete response
CTCAE	Common Terminology Criteria for Adverse Events
CTLA	Cytotoxic T-lymphocyte-associated protein
DM	Dermatomyositis
DM dx	Dermatomyositis diagnosis
HCQ	Hydroxychloroquine
HLA	Human leukocyte antigen
ICI	immune checkpoint inhibitors
ILD	Interstitial lung disease
irAEs	Immune related adverse events
IVIG	Intravenous immunoglobulin
MCC	Merkel cell carcinoma
MDA	Melanoma differentiation-associated gene
MDACC	MD Anderson Cancer Center
MM	Malignant melanoma
MMF	Mycophenolate mofetil
MTX	Methotrexate
MSA	Myositis-specific antibodies

R. Lohray
Baylor College of Medicine, Houston, TX, USA
e-mail: rishabh.lohray@bcm.edu

A. B. Patel (✉)
Department of Dermatology, University of Texas MD Anderson Cancer Center, Houston, TX, USA
e-mail: apatel11@mdanderson.org

Y. Wang (ed.), *Challenging Cases in Immunotherapy Related Organ Toxicities*,
https://doi.org/10.1007/978-3-031-83533-9_4

NXP	Nuclear matrix protein
PD	Programmed cell death protein
PR	Partial response
PRG	Progression
RCC	Renal cell carcinoma
SAE	Small ubiquitin-like modifier activating enzyme
SCC	Squamous Cell Carcinoma
SD	Stable disease
SPF	Sun protection factor
TIF	Transcription intermediary factor
UCC	Urothelial carcinoma

Patient Presentation

Five patients were identified with dermatomyositis (DM) while on immune checkpoint inhibitors (ICI) at our institution. Three were female and four were Caucasian. The median age at DM diagnosis was 68 years and the median time from ICI initiation to DM diagnosis, where applicable, was 8 months. Two patients had preexisting DM which worsened while on ICI, while the remaining 3 patients were diagnosed with DM after ICI initiation. All patients presented with a combination of subjective muscle weakness, photodistributed rash, and Gottron's papules. The implicated ICIs were nivolumab, pembrolizumab, and avelumab. Case presentation details are summarized in Table 4.1.

Lab Evaluations

Elevated muscle enzymes (including aldolase, CK, CKMB, and Troponin T) were observed in 4 out of 5 patients. Four patients also had myositis-associated antibodies. Anti-TIF1γ antibody was negative in all but one of the tested patients. One patient was positive for anti-Jo1 antibody, and one was positive for anti-SAE antibody. Electromyography was performed in two patients and revealed muscle membrane instability indicative of myositis.

The patients' complete blood count and complete metabolic panel were largely unremarkable. Two patients had mild to moderate transaminitis.

Pathology

Three out of five patients had skin biopsies showing interface dermatitis.

Table 4.1 Patient characteristics and outcomes

Median age at DM diagnosis in years (Range)		68 (41–73)
Sex	Female	3
	Male	2
Ethnicity	Caucasian	4
	African American	1
Primary malignancy (cancer stage)		MCC (III)
		SCC lung (III)
		RCC (IV)
		MM (IV)
		UCC (IV)
ICI type	Pembrolizumab	4
	Nivolumab	2
	Avelumab	1
Median time from ICI initiation to DM in months (range)[a] N = 3		8 (5–10)
DM presentation[b]	Gottron's papules	5
	Photo-distributed rash	5
	Subjective muscle weakness	5
	Elevated muscle enzymes	3
	DM at presentation	2
DM management	Topical steroids	3
	Oral steroids	4
	HCQ	3
	IVIG	3
	MMF	1
	PLEX	1
	MTX	1
Re-challenged ICI	Yes	4
	No	1
Attribution of DM	Paraneoplastic	2
	ICI-induced	1
	Combination	2
Rash outcome	Resolved	3
	Improved	2
	Worsened	0
Tumor response to ICI	CR	3
	PR	0
	SD	1
	PRG	3

[a]Two out of five patients were diagnosed with DM before ICI initiation
[b]Biopsies done in 3 out of 5 patients revealed interface dermatitis

Diagnosis

In applicable cases, the diagnosis of DM was made with a combination of patient history, physical exam, skin biopsy, muscle injury markers, myositis antibody panel, and electromyography. It could be secondary to paraneoplastic phenomenon, ICI related adverse event or combined effect of both. The details are included in the description of individual patient below. Among them, two were deemed to have paraneoplastic DM in the context of ICI treatment, two had presumed DM related to combination effect of ICI and paraneoplastic phenomenon, and one had ICI related DM.

Management

Four out of five patients were managed with a course of oral high dose steroids due to the severity of the disease. Skin disease was managed with a combination of topical steroids and when needed oral hydroxychloroquine and methotrexate. IVIG, plasma exchange, and mycophenolate mofetil were used in treatment refractory cases for myositis. Details of the treatment regimen and disease course are listed in the section below.

Timeline and Outcomes of Each Individual

A timeline of key events is delineated in Fig. 4.1.

Patient 1 presented with proximal muscle weakness and transaminitis 2 weeks after his first dose of ICI but was not diagnosed with DM until 10 months later. On myositis antibody panel, he was positive for anti-SSA and anti-Jo1 antibodies. Despite ICI discontinuation, his DM continued to flare with cardiac involvement also in the setting of tumor progression, which suggests a paraneoplastic mechanism of DM. DM was managed successfully with topical corticosteroids, prednisone, budesonide, HCQ, MMF, IVIG, and physical therapy with almost complete functional recovery noted at last visit. He was never re-challenged with ICI after the first dose and his cancer is now stable for 22 months of follow up from the initial ICI treatment.

Patient 2 already had a diagnosis of paraneoplastic DM (photo-distributed rash on trunk and extremities with proximal muscle weakness initially) at the time of her malignancy diagnosis. On myositis antibody panel, she was positive for anti-SSA antibody. Her DM was noted to worsen with ICI initiation. The patient achieved cancer remission while on ICI, but her DM continued to flare and had to be managed with high-dose oral steroids with good response. Eight months after ICI conclusion, her cancer recurred but this was not accompanied by a concurrent flare of

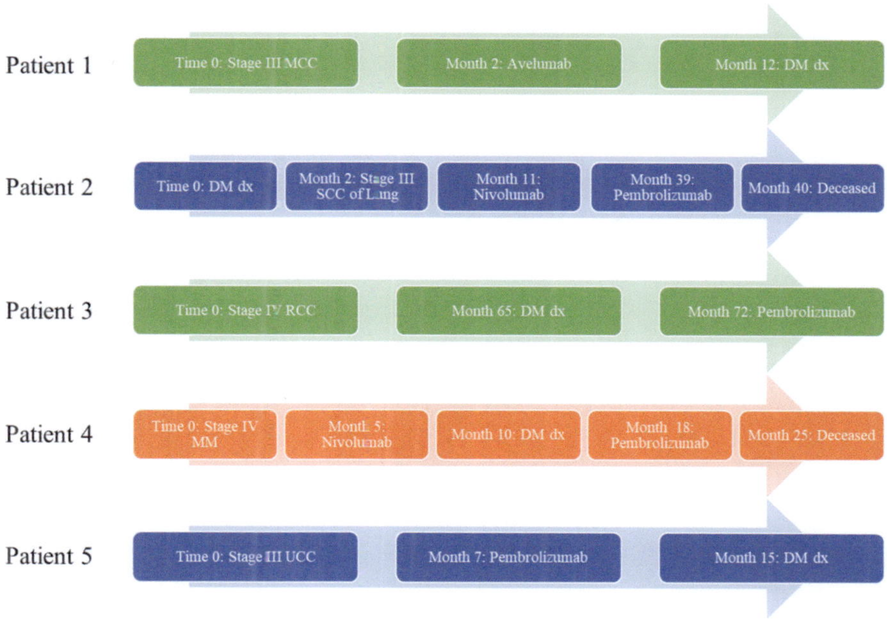

Fig. 4.1 Overview of key events; color scheme reflects the primary proposed mechanism of DM: paraneoplastic (patient 1 and 3 in green), combination (patients 2 and 5 in blue), and ICI-induced (patient 4 in orange)

her DM. This suggests that the patient might have had a combination of paraneoplastic and ICI-induced DM. Of note, the patient was subsequently started on a different ICI but no DM flare occurred. Her cancer was refractory to therapy, and she died a few months later.

Patient 3 primarily had paraneoplastic DM (photo-distributed rash on trunk and extremities and Gottron's papules initially) (Fig. 4.2). DM was managed successfully with prednisone and topical corticosteroids before ICI initiation. On myositis antibody panel, she was positive for anti-SAE, anti-SSA, anti- TIF1γ antibodies. She only had mild worsening of her muscle weakness on ICI and did not require any additional DM management. She finished her ICI course successfully and is currently in complete cancer remission for 18 months after first ICI treatment.

Patient 4 had ICI-induced dermatomyositis (symmetric photo-distributed rash on the face and upper extremities with muscle weakness and joint pains initially) (Fig. 4.3) 1 week after the seventh cycle of ICI. On myositis antibody panel, he was positive for anti-SSA antibody. His DM flared in the absence of his cancer while on ICI, and it also flared right after ICI rechallenge in the setting of cancer relapse. His DM was successfully managed with prednisone, MTX, HCQ, and IVIG. However, when DM recurred the second time in the setting of ICI rechallenge (due to cancer progression), it was poorly controlled despite IVIG therapy. He eventually passed away 2 years after his cancer diagnosis due to poor response to ICI and inability to tolerate traditional chemotherapy.

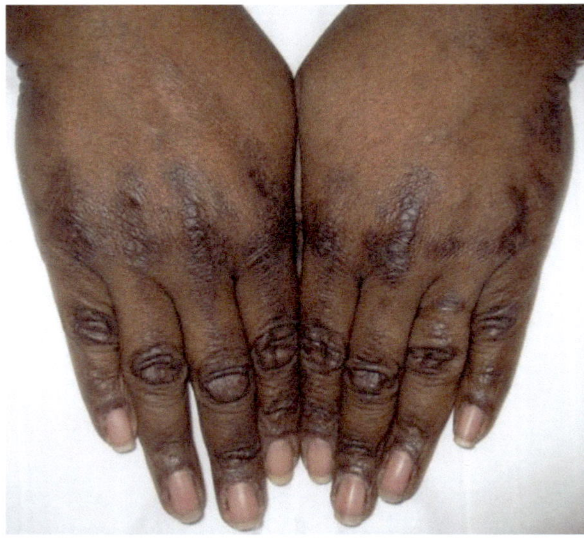

Fig. 4.2 Gottron's papules of the dorsal hand

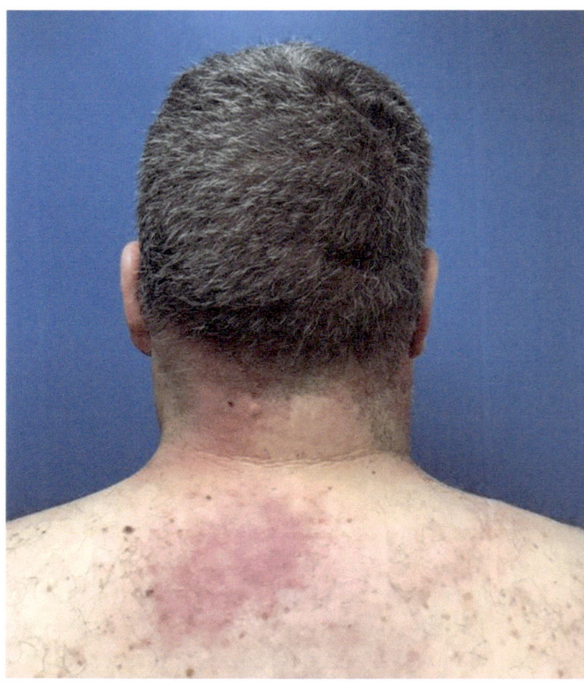

Fig. 4.3 Erythematous to violaceous patch of the upper back "shawl sign"

Patient 5 developed DM (photo-distributed rash and muscle weakness initially) right after finishing her 6-month treatment course of ICI (anti-SSA antibody positive on myositis panel). While this suggests an ICI-induced mechanism of DM, her DM recurred in the setting of cancer recurrence a few months after achieving complete remission, hence suggesting a combination of paraneoplastic and ICI-induced mechanism of DM in this patient. DM was managed successfully with topical corticosteroids, prednisone, HCQ, IVIG, and PLEX. Cancer relapse was poorly managed with ICI, so the patient received chemotherapy. The patient responded well to the treatment and her cancer is in complete remission at this time 1 year after relapse.

Of note, all patients reported that their rash had completely resolved or significantly improved since initiation of DM treatment.

Discussion

In general, dermatomyositis is an inflammatory myopathy with cutaneous manifestations that may have multi-organ systemic involvement. Cutaneous signs can be pathognomonic such as Gottron's papules, heliotrope rash, and Gottron's sign [1]. It can also present in a variety of ways including photodistributed erythema and poikiloderma of the back and upper shoulders (shawl sign) or anterior neck and upper shoulders (V-sign), periungual erythema and telangiectasias, hemorrhagic nail bed infarcts, dystrophic cuticles, periorbital edema, holster sign, scaly plaques on the scalp, calcinosis cutis, and vesiculobullous ulcerative lesions [1–3]. Skin disease tends not to mimic the course of muscle disease and can precede or follow myositis [1]. Photosensitivity, burning, and pruritus in the skin can significantly impact patient quality of life [4]. Eighty percent of patients have muscle involvement, and commonly accompanied by elevations in muscle enzymes such as creatine kinase, aldolase, aspartate aminotransferase, and alanine aminotransferase [1, 5]. Muscles of the pharynx and esophagus can also be affected and cause dysphonia and aspiration [1, 6]. Finally, systemic disease may present as interstitial lung disease, myocarditis, gastrointestinal dysmotility, and vasculitis [7–10].

These varied presentations of DM can make it a diagnostic challenge. A skin biopsy, blood testing for muscle enzymes and DM-associated antibodies, and electromyography may facilitate the confirmation of diagnosis which will warrant a thorough screening for malignancy subsequently [11]. Paraneoplastic DM is well documented in the setting of ovarian, gastric, lung, urothelial, and breast cancers as well as melanoma [12–14]. DM is rare on sequence of ICIs and a recent article by Guerra et al. identified 22 cases in the literature [15]. The mechanism behind ICI-induced DM remains unclear. Some tumors express TIF1γ which is a protein that is also found in muscles [16]. Upon initiation of ICI, the immune system can misidentify TIF1γ as a cancer associated antigen and hence trigger myositis and DM [16]. This is more in line with a paraneoplastic process which is unmasked or worsened by ICIs. However, not all such cases are anti-TIF1γ positive and in fact most cases are negative for currently tested antibodies [11].

Histopathology reveals vacuolar interface dermatitis with dermal mucin deposition, both of which may also be seen in lupus [11]. Hence clinicopathologic correlation is essential to confirm the diagnosis. A myositis panel checking for common myositis-specific antibodies (MSA) can further help support the diagnosis [11]. Certain MSAs have been correlated with specific manifestations of DM. MSAs include anti-Mi2 (classic photodistributed rash with highly elevated muscle enzymes), anti-TIF1γ (more severe cutaneous disease and associated with malignancy and GI disorders), anti-melanoma differentiation associated protein-5 or anti-MDA5 (no clinical muscle involvement, and interstitial lung disease), anti-nuclear matrix protein 2 or anti-NXP2 (classic photodistributed rash and increased risk of malignancy), and anti-SAE (strong HLA association, severe cutaneous disease, and GI involvement) [1, 11]. However only 20% of DM cases have the mentioned MSAs which lowers the diagnostic utility of these tests [17].

DM with significant muscle and skin involvement is treated with high dose corticosteroids which are eventually tapered over many months after muscle disease is fully controlled. The initial oral dose may be 0.5–1 mg/kg/day but in severe cases IV methylprednisolone may be indicated [18]. Once the initial flare is controlled, a steroid-sparing agent like methotrexate may be added to reduce the risk of steroid-related adverse events such as osteoporosis and metabolic syndrome.

Cutaneous manifestations are not as well controlled on oral steroids and may need additional therapy. Topical glucocorticoids and calcineurin inhibitors are first-line options for controlling erythema and pruritus [11]. However, in most cases, topical agents are inadequate and oral therapies may need to be added. Hydroxychloroquine has anti-inflammatory and photoprotective properties which makes it ideal for use in DM [11]. To avoid ocular toxicity the daily HCQ dose should not exceed 5 mg/kg/day [19]. Response to HCQ may be delayed by up to 6–12 weeks and its benefits are largely limited to skin disease [11]. Methotrexate is another option with anti-inflammatory properties, and it can treat both skin and muscle disease, making it the ideal steroid-sparing agent. It is usually dosed at 25 mg weekly [11]. Sun avoidance, sun protective clothing, wide-brimmed hats, and sunscreen with an SPF over 30 are also essential at preventing flares [6, 11]. Pruritus in DM may have a significant impact on patient sleep, activities of daily living and overall quality of life. It can be managed with emollients for xerosis, oral antihistamines, and oral gabapentin [11]. Additionally, patients at risk of developing contractures should start physical therapy early to maintain flexibility and functionality for their activities of daily living [6].

In treatment resistant cases, IVIG or plasma exchange and mycophenolate may be considered. Mycophenolate's lymphocyte-specific anti-inflammatory properties make it ideal for managing DM [11]. It has shown efficacy in treating cutaneous disease, myositis, and DM-associated ILD, however therapeutic response is not fully apparent until 6–12 weeks of therapy. Doses reported in literature include a starting dose of 500 mg twice a day which may be up titrated to 1.5 g twice a day [11]. IVIG is another option for refractory cutaneous and muscle disease. The mechanism of its efficacy is unclear, but it may act by neutralizing DM-associated antibodies [11]. It can be an effective steroid-sparing agent and may allow for the discontinuation of immunosuppressive regimens [20]. It can be started as 2 g/kg divided over 2 days every 4 weeks and can be spaced out to every 5 or 6 weeks once expected clinical response is achieved [11].

Management of DM in the setting of cancer treated with checkpoint inhibitors must also consider the role of the ICIs in exacerbating DM, and the implications of longer-term immunosuppression on cancer remission and progression [21]. Treatment cessation is recommended when a drug therapy is identified as the cause or exacerbator of DM [13]. Based on the CTCAE criteria, grade 1 and 2 reactions are managed with temporary suspension of therapy, grade 3 with suspension followed by a discussion of risks and benefits of rechallenging, and grade 4 reactions are managed by permanently discontinuing the agent [22]. However, when the offending agent is an ICI being used to manage a life-threatening malignancy, this decision is not easily made. Additionally, iRAEs with ICIs are associated with a better tumor response, which further argues against treatment cessation [22]. Currently there are no standardized guidelines for managing ICI-associated DM. Hence, multidisciplinary teams consisting of dermatologists, rheumatologists and medical oncologists must work together to manage these patients and balance the adverse events associated with ICI with their benefits in prolonging survival.

Summary

In summary, we present 5 patients with DM who received ICI. In this series, avelumab, nivolumab, and pembrolizumab were identified as potential inducers or exacerbators of DM. Patients were managed with a combination of corticosteroids and steroid-sparing agents by multidisciplinary teams of dermatologists, oncologists, and rheumatologists. DM treatment was balanced with the need to discontinue or temporarily pause ICI. Patient outcomes for their cancer varied in our series, with some attaining remission while others progressing and eventually passing away. Cancer outcomes related to ICI-cessation or long-term impact of immunosuppressive agents and systemic corticosteroids for DM management in those with malignancy remain to be further investigated.

References

1. DeWane ME, Waldman R, Lu J. Dermatomyositis: clinical features and pathogenesis. J Am Acad Dermatol. 2020;82(2):267–81. https://doi.org/10.1016/j.jaad.2019.06.1309.
2. Mainetti C, Terziroli Beretta-Piccoli B, Selmi C. Cutaneous manifestations of dermatomyositis: a comprehensive review. Clin Rev Allergy Immunol. 2017;53(3):337–56. https://doi.org/10.1007/s12016-017-8652-1.
3. Bogdanov I, Kazandjieva J, Darlenski R, Tsankov N. Dermatomyositis: current concepts. Clin Dermatol. 2018;36(4):450–8. https://doi.org/10.1016/j.clindermatol.2018.04.003.
4. Hundley JL, Carroll CL, Lang W, et al. Cutaneous symptoms of dermatomyositis significantly impact patients' quality of life. J Am Acad Dermatol. 2006;54(2):217–20. https://doi.org/10.1016/j.jaad.2004.12.015.
5. Dalakas MC. Inflammatory muscle diseases. N Engl J Med. 2015;372(18):1734–47. https://doi.org/10.1056/NEJMra1402225.

6. Qudsiya Z, Waseem M. Dermatomyositis. [Updated 2023 Aug 7]. In: StatPearls [Internet]. Treasure Island, StatPearls Publishing; 2023. Available from: https://www.ncbi.nlm.nih.gov/books/NBK558917/.
7. Schmidt J. Current classification and management of inflammatory myopathies. J Neuromuscul Dis. 2018;5(2):109–29. https://doi.org/10.3233/JND-180308.
8. Schwartz T, Diederichsen LP, Lundberg IE, Sjaastad I, Sanner H. Cardiac involvement in adult and juvenile idiopathic inflammatory myopathies. RMD Open. 2016;2(2):e000291. Published 2016 Sep 27. https://doi.org/10.1136/rmdopen-2016-000291.
9. Gadiparthi C, Hans A, Potts K, Ismail MK. Gastrointestinal and hepatic disease in the inflammatory myopathies. Rheum Dis Clin N Am. 2018;44(1):113–29. https://doi.org/10.1016/j.rdc.2017.09.006.
10. Ono N, Kai K, Maruyama A, et al. The relationship between type 1 IFN and vasculopathy in anti-MDA5 antibody-positive dermatomyositis patients [published correction appears in Rheumatology (Oxford). 2020;59(4):918]. Rheumatology (Oxford). 2019;58(5):786–91. https://doi.org/10.1093/rheumatology/key386.
11. Cobos GA, Femia A, Vleugels RA. Dermatomyositis: an update on diagnosis and treatment. Am J Clin Dermatol. 2020;21(3):339–53. https://doi.org/10.1007/s40257-020-00502-6.
12. Requena C, Alfaro A, Traves V, et al. Paraneoplastic dermatomyositis: a study of 12 cases. Actas Dermosifiliogr. 2014;105(7):675–82. https://doi.org/10.1016/j.ad.2013.11.007.
13. Messer A, Drozd B, Glitza IC, Lu H, Patel AB. Dermatomyositis associated with nivolumab therapy for melanoma: a case report and review of the literature. Dermatol Online J. 2020;26(8):13030/qt4c21b068. Published 2020 Aug 15
14. Shorr AF, Yacavone M, Seguin S, Jackson LW, Dennis GJ. Dermatomyositis and malignant melanoma. Am J Med Sci. 1997;313(4):249–51. https://doi.org/10.1097/00000441-199704000-00011.
15. Guerra NL, Matas-García A, Serra-García L, et al. Dermatomyositis unleashed by immune checkpoint inhibitors. Three additional cases and a review of the literature. Autoimmun Rev. 2023;22(8):103375. https://doi.org/10.1016/j.autrev.2023.103375.
16. Sakurai T, Takahashi J, Komatsu T, Mitsumura H, Iguchi Y. Anti-TIF1γ antibody-positive dermatomyositis associated with nivolumab administration in a patient with advanced oesophageal squamous cell carcinoma: a case report and literature review. Mod Rheumatol Case Rep. 2023;7(2):416–21. https://doi.org/10.1093/mrcr/rxad007.
17. Hamaguchi Y, Kuwana M, Hoshino K, et al. Clinical correlations with dermatomyositis-specific autoantibodies in adult Japanese patients with dermatomyositis: a multicenter cross-sectional study. Arch Dermatol. 2011;147(4):391–8. https://doi.org/10.1001/archdermatol.2011.52.
18. Drake LA, Dinehart SM, Farmer ER, et al. Guidelines of care for dermatomyositis. American Academy of Dermatology. J Am Acad Dermatol. 1996;34(5 Pt 1):824–9.
19. Marmor MF, Kellner U, Lai TY, Melles RB, Mieler WF, Academy A, of Ophthalmology. Recommendations on screening for chloroquine and hydroxychloroquine retinopathy (2016 revision). Ophthalmology. 2016;123(6):1386–94. https://doi.org/10.1016/j.ophtha.2016.01.058.
20. Femia AN, Eastham AB, Lam C, Merola JF, Qureshi AA, Vleugels RA. Intravenous immunoglobulin for refractory cutaneous dermatomyositis: a retrospective analysis from an academic medical center. J Am Acad Dermatol. 2013;69(4):654–7. https://doi.org/10.1016/j.jaad.2013.06.007.
21. Selva-O'Callaghan A, Trallero-Araguás E, Ros J, et al. Management of cancer-associated myositis. Curr Treatm Opt Rheumatol. 2022;8(4):91–104. https://doi.org/10.1007/s40674-022-00197-2.
22. Michot JM, Bigenwald C, Champiat S, et al. Immune-related adverse events with immune checkpoint blockade: a comprehensive review. Eur J Cancer. 2016;54:139–48. https://doi.org/10.1016/j.ejca.2015.11.016.

Chapter 5
Rapid Resolution of Refractory Immunotherapy-Related Transient Acantholytic Dermatosis with Dupilumab

Melissa R. Laughter and Ata S. Moshiri

Abbreviations

CTLA-4	cytotoxic T-lymphocyte-associated protein 4
IL	interleukin
IRAE	immune related adverse event
PD-1	programmed cell death protein 1
TAD	transient acantholytic dermatosis; Grover disease
UVB	ultraviolet-B

Case Presentation

This is a male in 70 s with metastatic renal cell carcinoma presented with a highly pruritic rash over his chest, arms and back resulting in sleep disturbance 2 months following four doses of ipilimumab and nivolumab. He was initially treated with topical steroids and antihistamines, with worsening of symptoms, at which point he was placed on an oral 60 mg prednisone taper for 8 days. When this failed, he was referred for dermatologic evaluation.

Physical exam at his initial evaluation was notable for scattered eroded, erythematous macules and papules on the trunk and arms (Fig. 5.1). The clinical differential diagnosis included folliculitis, miliaria, lichenoid dermatitis, transient acantholytic dermatosis (TAD; Grover disease), incipient bullous pemphigoid, or pemphigus. Histology from a punch biopsy of the left arm showed suprabasilar acantholysis, perivascular lymphocytic inflammation with eosinophils (Fig. 5.2).

M. R. Laughter (✉) · A. S. Moshiri
Ronald O. Perelman Department of Dermatology, New York University, School of Medicine, New York, NY, USA
e-mail: melissa.laughter@nyulangone.org; ata.moshiri@nyulangone.org

Y. Wang (ed.), *Challenging Cases in Immunotherapy Related Organ Toxicities*,
https://doi.org/10.1007/978-3-031-83533-9_5

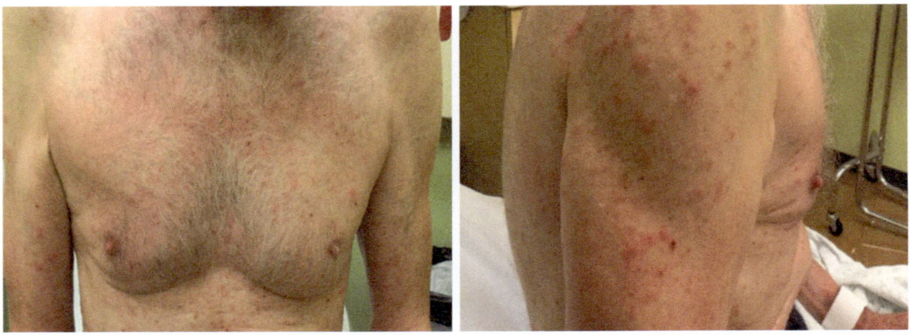

Fig. 5.1 Highly pruritic scattered, erythematous papules with overlying erosions on the torso and arms

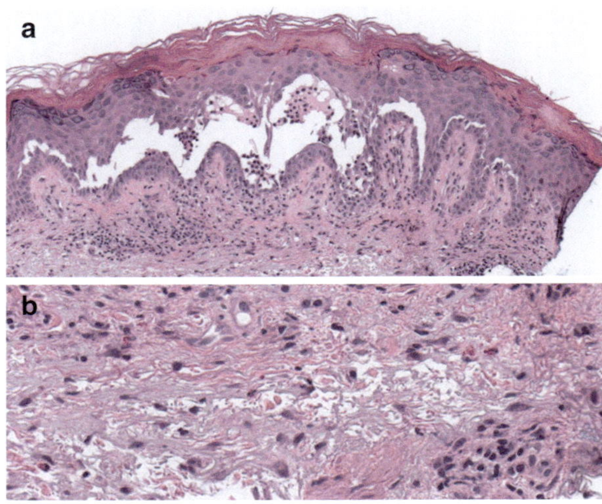

Fig. 5.2 (**a**) Medium power view of the epidermis shows intraepidermal acantholysis with dyskeratosis. (**b**) High power view of the dermis shows numerous perivascular and interstitial eosinophils

Direct immunofluorescence studies were negative. A diagnosis of immunotherapy-induced TAD was made.

Treatment and Outcome

He was subsequently trialed on a variety of therapies, including 0.1% triamcinolone ointment under occlusion with a sauna suit, gabapentin, longer courses of prednisone, aprepitant, hydroxyzine, diphenhydramine, cetirizine, and eventually 16 sessions of narrow-band Ultraviolet B (UVB) phototherapy, none of which provided any relief which was subsequently stopped. Nivolumab monotherapy was discontinued 4 months after symptom onset due to the severity of his cutaneous reaction. Approximately 8 months following rash onset, he was transitioned to dupilimab

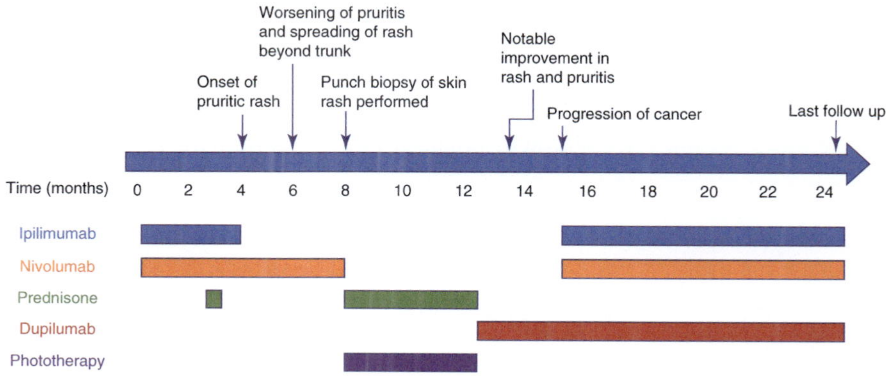

Fig. 5.3 Timeline of patient's disease course with timepoint of 0 referring to symptom onset

(IL-4 receptor antagonist) at standard dosing, and within a week of his first injection, he noticed a significant reduction in the itch and near total resolution of his rash, with complete resolution of itch and rash noted at his three-month follow-up. To date, he remains in remission of his TAD despite having restarted on ipilimumab and nivolumab for progression of his metastatic disease. Given the severity of symptoms in the past and likely need for continued treatment, dupilumab was continued as concurrent therapy. His cancer remained stable at the last follow up. The timeline of this patient's disease course and treatment can be found in Fig. 5.3 above.

Summary

This case demonstrates a patient with metastatic renal cell carcinoma who developed a severe, pruritic rash diagnosed as transient acantholytic dermatosis (TAD) following immunotherapy. Despite several unsuccessful treatments, dupilumab therapy provided substantial relief, resulting in complete resolution of the TAD symptoms and has sustained effect even after resuming immunotherapy for his cancer.

Discussion

Transient acantholytic dermatosis (TAD), also known as Grover's disease, is an inflammatory immune condition characterized by small, erythematous papules most commonly affecting the trunk and extremities of middle-aged males with a history of sun-exposure. Skin pathology often demonstrates acantholytic dyskeratosis within the epidermis with varying degrees of associated dermal inflammation, often with eosinophils. Lesions typically last for weeks to months, though there is a propensity for recurrence. In some cases, the course can be prolonged and can last for years (such cases are often labeled "persistent acantholytic dermatosis"). Common treatments include pramoxine, topical vitamin D analogues, topical corticosteroids, tetracycline antibiotics and antihistamines for mild cases, while oral corticosteroids, oral retinoids, narrow-band ultraviolet B and psoralen plus ultraviolet A are usually reserved for more severe, refractory disease [1].

The pathophysiology of TAD has yet to be elucidated, though some recent evidence suggests that overexpression of IL-4 may play a role [2, 3]. IL-4 has also been identified as having a significant role in various other inflammatory skin conditions, including atopic dermatitis and bullous disorders [4–6]. Consequently, as a medication that inhibits IL-4, dupilumab represents a promising therapeutic option for these conditions [7–9].

TAD has been reported in a variety of different settings involving various conventional chemotherapies as well as ICI therapies [10–13]. Patients receiving checkpoint inhibitor therapies have been found to have higher serum levels of IL-4 [14, 15], it is plausible that IL-4 upregulation plays a part in the pathogenesis of TAD in this setting. Dupilumab is an attractive choice for treatment of many IRAEs in the setting of immunotherapy for cancer due to its infrequency of dosing, quick onset of action, lack of need for lab monitoring, low side effect profile, and minimal immune suppression.

Conclusion

ICI-related TAD is rare and long-lasting that may benefit from dupilumab treatment in refractory condition. The upregulation of IL-4 in the setting of various immunotherapies, supports our treatment success of dupilumab for both idiopathic TAD [16], TAD in the setting of immunotherapy, and possibly other skin IRAEs related to checkpoint inhibitor therapy.

References

1. Aldana PC, Khachemoune A. Grover disease: review of subtypes with a focus on management options. Int J Dermatol. Published online. 2020;59:543–50. https://doi.org/10.1111/ijd.14700.
2. Sehra S, Yao Y, Howell MD, et al. IL-4 regulates skin homeostasis and the predisposition toward allergic skin inflammation. J Immunol. Published online. 2010;184:3186–90. https://doi.org/10.4049/jimmunol.0901860.
3. Oh CK, Geba GP, Molfino N. Investigational therapeutics targeting the IL-4/IL-13/STAT-6 pathway for the treatment of asthma. Eur Respir Rev. Published online. 2010;19:46–54. https://doi.org/10.1183/09059180.00007609.
4. Maloney NJ, Tegtmeyer K, Zhao J, Worswick S. Dupilumab in dermatology: potential for uses beyond atopic dermatitis. J Drug Dermatol. Published online. 2019;18:S1545961619P1053X.

5. Russo R, Cozzani E, Gasparini G, Parodi A. Targeting interleukin 4 receptor α: a new approach to the treatment of cutaneous autoimmune bullous diseases? Dermatol Ther. Published online. 2020;33:e13190. https://doi.org/10.1111/dth.13190.
6. Cozzani E, Gasparini G, Di Zenzo G, Parodi A. Immunoglobulin E and bullous pemphigoid. Eur J Dermatol. Published online. 2018;28:440–8. https://doi.org/10.1684/ejd.2018.3366.
7. Fishbein AB, Silverberg JI, Wilson EJ, Ong PY. Update on atopic dermatitis: diagnosis, severity assessment, and treatment selection. J Allergy Clin Immunol Pract. Published online. 2020;8:91–101. https://doi.org/10.1016/j.jaip.2019.06.044.
8. Darrigade AS, Legrand A, Andreu N, et al. Dual efficacy of dupilumab in a patient with concomitant atopic dermatitis and alopecia areata. Br J Dermatol. Published online. 2018;179:534–6. https://doi.org/10.1111/bjd.16711.
9. Kaye A, Gordon SC, Deverapalli SC, Her MJ, Rosmarin D. Dupilumab for the treatment of recalcitrant bullous pemphigoid. JAMA Dermatol. Published online. 2018;154:1225–6. https://doi.org/10.1001/jamadermatol.2018.2526.
10. Beer J, Rosenbach M. Grover disease associated with chemotherapy: review of potential pathophysiology, current treatments, and future directions. J Drugs Dermatol. Published online. 2020;19:1056–64. https://doi.org/10.36849/JDD.2020.5648.
11. Khan MS, Khan M, Aivaz O. Transient acantholytic dermatosis in a patient with prostate cancer. Dermatol Online J. Published online. 2020;26 https://doi.org/10.5070/d3262047431.
12. Chen WS, Tetzlaff MT, Diwan H, et al. Suprabasal acantholytic dermatologic toxicities associated checkpoint inhibitor therapy: a spectrum of immune reactions from paraneoplastic pemphigus-like to Grover-like lesions. J Cutan Pathol. Published online. 2018;45:764–73. https://doi.org/10.1111/cup.13312.
13. Munoz J, Guillot B, Girard C, Dereure O, Du-Thanh A. First report of ipilimumab-induced Grover disease. Br J Dermatol. Published online. 2014;171:1236–7. https://doi.org/10.1111/bjd.13058.
14. Hardy-Werbin M, Rocha P, Arpi O, et al. Serum cytokine levels as predictive biomarkers of benefit from ipilimumab in small cell lung cancer. Oncoimmunology. Published online. 2019;8:e1593810. https://doi.org/10.1080/2162402X.2019.1593810.
15. Myklebust JH, Irish JM, Brody J, et al. High PD-1 expression and suppressed cytokine signaling distinguish T cells infiltrating follicular lymphoma tumors from peripheral T cells. Blood. Published online. 2013;121:1367–76. https://doi.org/10.1182/blood-2012-04-421826.
16. Butler DC, Kollhoff A, Berger T. Treatment of Grover disease with Dupilumab. JAMA Dermatol. Published online. 2021;157:353–6. https://doi.org/10.1001/jamadermatol.2020.5097.

Part III
Endocrinology

Chapter 6
Hypophysitis Post Immune Checkpoint Inhibitor Therapy

Sean Ngo and Jeena Varghese

Abbreviations

ACTH	Adrenocorticotropic hormone
CT	computed tomography
ICI	immune checkpoint inhibitor
IV	intravenous
PET	positron emission tomography
T4	Thyroxine
TSH	Thyroid stimulating hormone

Clinical Presentation

This is a male in his 70 s with presentation of abnormal, incidental imaging findings about 1 month after receiving immunotherapy. He has a history of high-grade sarcoma of the left foot diagnosed 15 years ago treated with surgical resection and brachytherapy. 11 years later he was diagnosed with stage IIIC acral melanoma of the right first toe with metastasis to the right inguinal lymph node. He was started on neoadjuvant combination immunotherapy with ipilimumab and nivolumab. Surgery was planned for 6 weeks after receiving two cycles of ipilimumab/nivolumab. Restaging imaging with PET/CT showed abnormal activity in the region of the pituitary gland suspicious for metastasis versus hypophysitis (Fig. 6.1a,b).

S. Ngo
McGovern Medical School at The University of Texas Health Science Center at Houston, Houston, TX, USA
e-mail: sean.b.ngo@uth.tmc.edu

J. Varghese (✉)
Department of Endocrine Neoplasia and Hormonal Disorders, The University of Texas MD Anderson Cancer Center, Houston, TX, USA
e-mail: jvarghese@mdanderson.org

Y. Wang (ed.), *Challenging Cases in Immunotherapy Related Organ Toxicities*,
https://doi.org/10.1007/978-3-031-83533-9_6

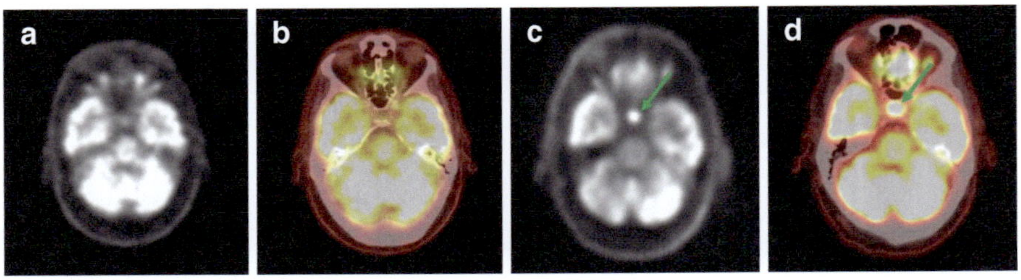

Fig. 6.1 (**a & b**) PET/CT images of the brain 36 days prior to the onset of immunotherapy. (**c & d**) PET/CT images with contrast of the brain 43 days after the first dose of immunotherapy showed elevated ^{18}F-fluorodeoxyglucose (^{18}FDG) metabolic activity (green arrows) with a max standardized uptake value (SUVmax) of 13.1 in the region of the pituitary gland

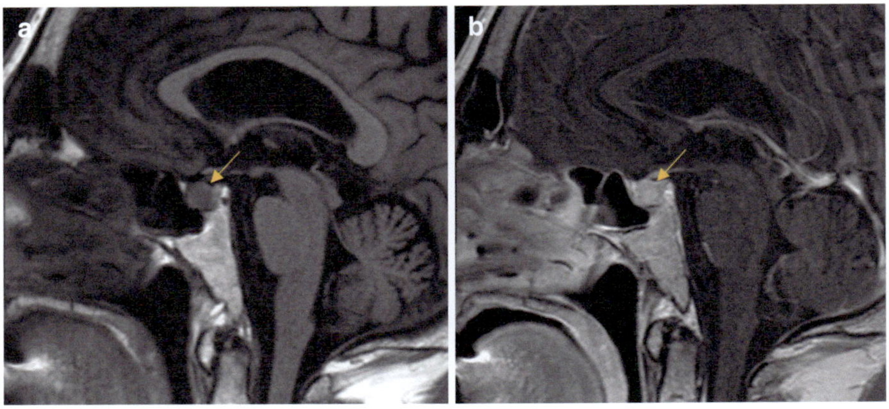

Fig. 6.2 MRI findings used to differentiate between malignancy and hypophysitis in the setting of positive ^{18}FDG uptake on PET/CT. (**a**) Sagittal T1 Flair showing a homogenous hypointense signal on T1. (**b**) Sagittal T1 with contrast demonstrating intense homogenous enhancement after administration of IV contrast

Subsequent MRI of the pituitary gland demonstrated increased size of the pituitary gland compared to the patient's previous imaging and had a homogenous hypointense signal on T1 with intense homogenous enhancement after IV contrast (Fig. 6.2). He denied any fatigue, appetite loss, nausea, vomiting, malaise, dizziness, or visual defects. Lab results at the time revealed mild hyponatremia, low thyroid stimulating hormone (TSH), normal free thyroxine (T4), normal cortisol, and normal adrenocorticotropic hormone (ACTH) (Table 6.1). He was scheduled to have surgery as his laboratory testing was within normal limits and the imaging findings were not suggestive of malignancy.

He underwent surgery without any complications. Stress dose steroids were not given as his ACTH and cortisol levels were normal on the day of surgery. However, it is to be noted that he received 4 mg of dexamethasone intraoperatively as a part of anesthesia protocol. The patient did well during post-operative monitoring without any significant complications besides a mild hyponatremia that improved with

Table 6.1 Pertinent Lab Values

Test	Value at time of first positive imaging (day 43[a])	Value at time of first symptoms (day 56[a])	Value at latest visit after treatment (day 196[a])
Cortisol, total (ref: 2.0–14.0 μg/dL)	14.05 μg/dL	**1.8 μg/dL**	N/A
ACTH (ref: 7.2–63.3 pg/mL)	59 pg/mL	**2.3 pg/mL**	N/A
TSH (ref: 0.36–3.74 μ [IU]/mL)	**0.06 μ [IU]/mL**	**0.03 μ [IU]/mL**	1.02 μ [IU]/mL
Free T4 (ref: 0.76–1.46 ng/dL)	1.14 ng/dL	0.99 ng/dL	1.22 ng/dL

Abnormal values are bolded in the table

mcg microgram, *dL* deciliter, *ref.* normal reference range, *ACTH* adrenocorticotropic hormone, *pcg* picogram, *mL* milliliter, *mc [IU]* micro-international units, *TSH* thyroid-stimulating hormone, *ng* nanogram

[a]Days after ICI initiation

intravenous (IV) fluids. Two days after discharge from the hospital, more blood work came back and showed further decrease in TSH and cortisol levels, but again, normal ACTH and free T4 levels (Table 6.1). The patient remained asymptomatic and recovered well. Close monitoring of labs and symptoms was initiated, with particular attention put towards recognizing any developing fatigue, hypotension, dizziness, nausea, or vomiting.

On post-operative day 10, the patient presented to the emergency department for extreme weakness. He had low blood pressure, hyponatremia, and elevated white blood cell count. His cortisol, ACTH, and TSH levels were all abnormally decreased, and free T4 was still within reference range but down trending (Table 6.1). Given these findings the patient was diagnosed with adrenal insufficiency and hypothyroidism secondary to ipilimumab/nivolumab. He was admitted and treated with 100 mg of IV hydrocortisone, started on levothyroxine, and given fluids with clinical improvement. After the patient was discharged, the patient was prescribed hydrocortisone 15 mg in the morning and 10 mg in the evening and levothyroxine 88mcg every day.

Clinical Outcome

Three weeks after this last hospital admission, the patient followed up with the endocrinology clinic and was found to be doing well on his current steroid and levothyroxine dosages without any symptoms. The patient's most recent imaging 5 months after his first dose of immune checkpoint inhibitor (ICI) therapy has come back without any evidence of disease. His disease is currently being monitored with active surveillance for any cancer recurrence, and he continues to follow up with the endocrinology clinic.

Summary of the Case

This is a case of melanoma treated with ipilimumab/nivolumab and surgical resection. During pre-operative evaluation, imaging findings on PET/CT and MRI were suggestive of hypophysitis despite a lack of symptoms and normal hormone levels. The patient became symptomatic 2 weeks after MRI findings were reported with an abnormality of cortisol, ACTH, TSH, and T4 laboratory values confirming adrenal insufficiency and hypothyroidism, which has since been managed with steroids and levothyroxine effectively. His cancer also achieved remission. Summary of the timeline events is shown in Fig. 6.3.

Discussion

The diagnosis of ICI hypophysitis is often made through clinical presentation, laboratory testing, and radiological findings. Relying on imaging for ICI hypophysitis can be challenging as only a third of patients with ICI hypophysitis may show MRI abnormalities (compared to nearly 97% of patients with primary hypophysitis) and the specific imaging findings are often subtle and transient [1]. In a study examining the diagnosis of ICI hypophysitis, 70% of the patients with positive MRI findings were already symptomatic [2]. Furthermore, 55% of these positive imaging findings were detected after or on the day the patient was diagnosed, rather than before [2]. In contrast, this study presents a case of PET/CT and MRI findings being the first sign of ICI hypophysitis, preceding any symptoms, lab abnormalities, or formal diagnosis by nearly 2 weeks. Detecting these imaging findings early on should prompt continued, close monitoring for worsening pituitary deficiencies.

On ^{18}F-FDG PET/CT, ICI hypophysitis reveals focal increases of FDG metabolic activity in the pituitary gland [3]. In differentiating between malignancy and hypophysitis with MRI, one study employing machine learning found that in ICI hypophysitis, pituitary height did not surpass 2 cm, the enhancement was homogenous, the pituitary stalk was more commonly thickened, and extension above the sellar diaphragm or into the cavernous sinus was less common [4]. As this case demonstrates, increased FDG uptake during immunotherapy might signal ICI hypophysitis, even before the development of any symptoms or hormonal deficiencies. MRI findings can then be used to rule out malignancy.

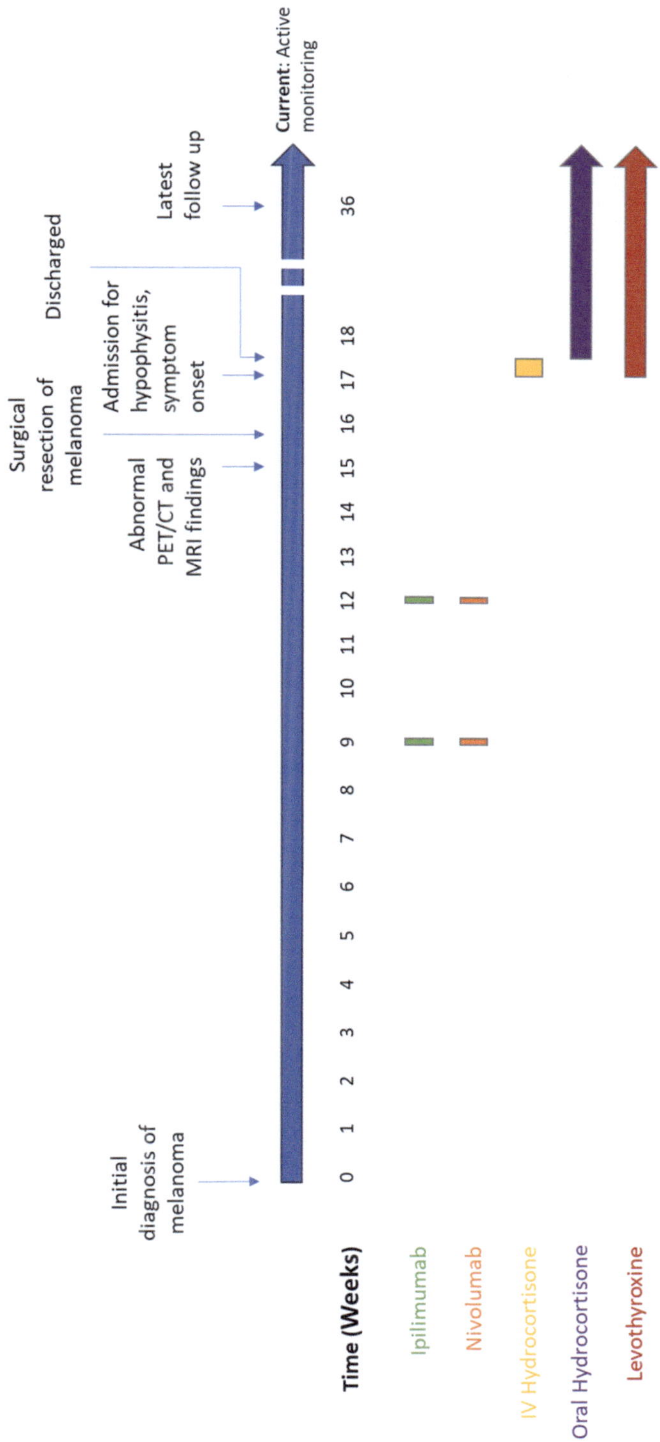

Fig. 6.3 Clinical course and timeline of events. (Timepoint 0 is the initial diagnosis of melanoma)

Conclusion

Imaging findings may not be present in all cases of ICI hypophysitis, but when present, can be an early indicator of organ toxicity. Following positive imaging, close monitoring of lab values such as ATCH, cortisol, TSH, and free T4 may allow for early initiation of appropriate treatment and management of secondary hypophysitis.

References

1. Di Dalmazi G, Ippolito S, Lupi I, Caturegli P. Hypophysitis induced by immune checkpoint inhibitors: a 10-year assessment. Expert Rev Endocrinol Metab. 2019;14(6):381–98. https://doi.org/10.1080/17446651.2019.1701434.
2. Jessel S, Weiss SA, Austin M, et al. Immune checkpoint inhibitor-induced hypophysitis and patterns of loss of pituitary function. Front Oncol. 2022;12:836859. https://doi.org/10.3389/fonc.2022.836859.
3. Cherk MH, Nadebaum DP, Barber TW, Beech P, Haydon A, Yap KS. 18F-FDG PET/CT features of immune-related adverse events and pitfalls following immunotherapy. J Med Imaging Radiat Oncol. 2022;66(4):483–94. https://doi.org/10.1111/1754-9485.13390.
4. Mekki A, Dercle L, Lichtenstein P, et al. Machine learning defined diagnostic criteria for differentiating pituitary metastasis from autoimmune hypophysitis in patients undergoing immune checkpoint blockade therapy. Eur J Cancer. 2019;119:44–56. https://doi.org/10.1016/j.ejca.2019.06.020.

Chapter 7
Graves' Disease After Prolonged Immune Checkpoint Inhibitor Therapy

Janki Patel and Conor Best

Abbreviations

ICI	Immune Checkpoint Inhibitors
IU	International Units
TSH	Thyroid Stimulating Hormone
T4	Thyroxine
T3	Triiodothyronine
TSI	Thyroid Stimulating Immunoglobulins
PTU	Propylthiouracil

Clinical Presentation

This is a woman in her 40s with a history of adenocarcinoma of the lung that had metastasized to regional lymph nodes was initially treated with carboplatin and pemetrexed. After completing 6 cycles of this treatment, pembrolizumab was added to her therapy. Carboplatin and pemetrexed were discontinued at cycle 9 due to hypersensitivity and myelosuppression. She transitioned to single agent pembrolizumab every 3 weeks for maintenance and received a total of 30 cycles. During her treatment, she also received radiation therapy to her chest.

She had a preexisting history of hypothyroidism and was taking levothyroxine at a daily dose of 50 μg daily when she was diagnosed with lung cancer. She also had

J. Patel
Department of Endocrinology, University of Texas Health Science Center, Houston, TX, USA
e-mail: Janki.M.Patel@uth.tmc.edu

C. Best (✉)
Department of Endocrine Neoplasia and Hormonal Disorders, The University of Texas MD Anderson Cancer Center, Houston, TX, USA
e-mail: cjbest@mdanderson.org

Y. Wang (ed.), *Challenging Cases in Immunotherapy Related Organ Toxicities*,
https://doi.org/10.1007/978-3-031-83533-9_7

Table 7.1 Lab values

Test	Value prior to cycle 29 of pembrolizumab	Value prior to cycle 30	3 weeks later	3 months later
TSH (0.27–4.2)	1.5 μIU/mL	**0.02 μIU/mL**	**<0.01 μIU/mL**	**<0.01 μIU/mL**
Free T4 (0.93–1.7)	1.9 ng/dL	**2.69 ng/dL**	**2.83 ng/dL**	**3.57 ng/dL**
Total T3 (80–200)	–	–	**369 ng/dL**	**360 ng/dL**
TSH receptor ab (< 1.75)	–	–		**33.3 IU/L**

mcIU micro international units, *ng* nanogram, *mL* milliliter, *dL* deciliter, *IU* international units, *L* liter
Abnormal values are bolded in the table

a family history of Graves' disease in her mother, treated with radioactive iodine. During her cancer therapy, her levothyroxine dose was increased to 112 μg daily, which approximately matched her weight-based dose of 1.6 μg/kg/day. Her thyroid-stimulating hormone (TSH) and free T4 levels remained stable.

Prior to her 30th cycle of pembrolizumab, she reported new-onset fatigue and palpitations. Laboratory tests showed evidence of thyrotoxicosis, with a free T4 level of 2.69 ng/dL (ref range: 0.93–1.70) and a TSH level of 0.02 ng/mL (ref range: 0.27–4.20). Follow-up labs performed 3 weeks later showed a progression of her condition, with a free T4 level of 2.83, a TSH level below 0.01, and a Total T3 level of 369 ng/dL (ref range: 80–200) (Table 7.1). Consequently, levothyroxine treatment was discontinued. At this juncture, it was suspected that she had onset of thyroiditis induced by immune checkpoint inhibitors (ICI), and her thyroid hormone levels were closely monitored. Propranolol was prescribed to manage her symptomatic discomfort.

Despite discontinuation of levothyroxine, her hyperthyroidism persisted and worsened over the course of an additional 3 months and Graves' disease was suspected. An iodine-123 thyroid uptake and scan was considered but deferred due to frequent intravenous (IV) iodinated contrast administration. A thyrotropin receptor antibody test revealed elevated levels at 33.3 international units/L (ref range: 0.0–1.75), which was suggestive of Graves' disease. Consequently, methimazole was initiated to treat her hyperthyroidism.

Differential Diagnosis

When clinical and biochemical hyperthyroidism occurs at or below the expected weight-based dose of 1.6 μg/kg/day of levothyroxine, endogenous release of thyroid hormone should be considered. This release may be due to thyroid cell damage, such as in thyroiditis, or the overproduction of thyroid hormone as seen in Graves' disease or an autonomous nodule.

In Graves' disease, there is persistent stimulation of the thyroid gland through the TSH receptor due to autoantibodies. This constant stimulation leads to heightened thyroid cell activity, resulting in the production of a proportionately larger amount of triiodothyronine (T3). Consequently, individuals with Graves' disease often have higher T3 levels, which can lead to more pronounced symptoms.

In this case, the persistence of thyrotoxicosis for several months suggested ongoing thyroid hormone production. Furthermore, the presence of significant symptoms, proportional T3 elevation, and progressive goiter were suggestive of Graves' disease. While elevated and diffuse uptake of iodine-123 is typically diagnostic of Graves' disease, excess iodine exposure through iodinated contrast can lead to false negative results if thyroid cells are already saturated with iodine. Therefore, the presence of TSH receptor antibodies or thyroid-stimulating immunoglobulins (TSI) in conjunction with endogenous thyrotoxicosis is generally sufficient for diagnosis.

Treatment Course

At her follow-up, methimazole had achieved initial response for her thyroid hormone levels. During the examination, it was observed that she had developed a goiter, mild Graves' ophthalmopathy without proptosis, and pretibial myxedema. During the following disease course, despite treatment with methimazole, she continued to experience fluctuating thyroid hormone levels which were symptomatic. Ultimately, she opted for a surgical total thyroidectomy due to concern that radioactive iodine treatment could exacerbate her ophthalmopathy. Her cancer remains in remission over 3 years following the completion of pembrolizumab.

Summary

This is a case with preexisting hypothyroidism, who developed new-onset thyrotoxicosis after an extended period of receiving pembrolizumab for her cancer. This was associated with development of a goiter, worsening hyperthyroidism, and positive TSH receptor antibodies, all consistent with a diagnosis of Graves' disease. Despite an extended course of methimazole therapy, her Graves' disease remained suboptimally controlled, prompting her surgical thyroidectomy as definitive treatment. Summary of timeline events is shown in Fig. 7.1.

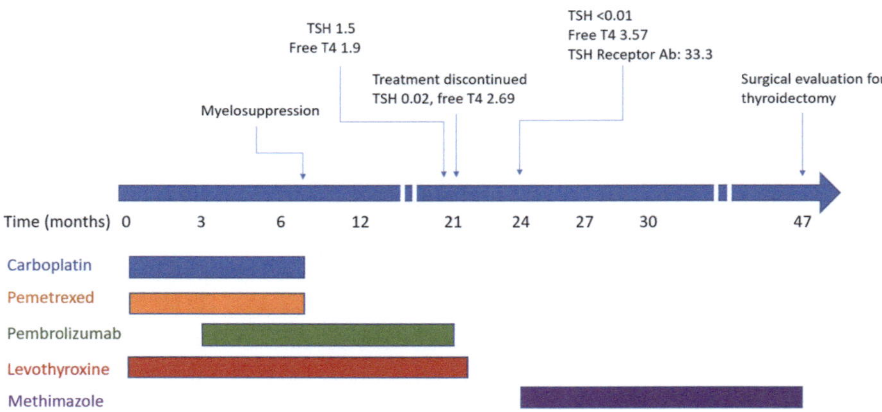

Fig. 7.1 Summary of timeline events (timepoint of 0 is starting time of cancer treatment)

Discussion

Thyroid disorders are highly prevalent, and many patients are already on levothyroxine supplementation before undergoing cancer therapy. Adjustments to levothyroxine doses are often necessary, particularly in response to changes in body weight, medication absorption, and medication adherence.

Immune checkpoint inhibitor (ICI)-associated thyroiditis typically manifests as a mild condition affecting over 10% of treated patients, and many patients remain asymptomatic (1, 2). Usually, this process is self-limited and most commonly resolves into hypothyroidism, necessitating levothyroxine supplementation at relatively higher doses, more than are often required in Hashimoto's thyroiditis (3).

ICI induced Graves' disease is rare and largely isolated to a few reports. Both long-term treatment with methimazole and definitive therapy with surgical thyroidectomy have been performed in these studies (4, 5). It is not known whether family history of Graves' disease increases risk.

Treatment with thioamides, such as methimazole or propylthiouracil (PTU), can effectively control excess thyroid hormone production but does not address the underlying immune disorder. During the initial therapy with thioamides, close monitoring is essential to watch for potential side effects such as agranulocytosis and hepatotoxicity. While some patients are well controlled on chronic thioamides, others have fluctuating thyroid hormone production which can be symptomatic. Many patients eventually opt for definitive therapy, with radioactive iodine ablation or surgical thyroidectomy.

Conclusions

Although thyroid disorders related to ICI therapy are frequently encountered, the occurrence of Graves' disease is rare. It should be considered when dealing with patients who present with symptomatic thyrotoxicosis that doesn't resolve after 6 weeks or is associated with symptoms such as goiter, ophthalmopathy, or pretibial myxedema. Delayed onset of endocrine toxicities should be considered even patient tolerates prolonged course of ICI therapy prior.

References

1. Iyer PC, Cabanillas ME, Waguespack SG, et al. Immune-related thyroiditis with immune checkpoint inhibitors. Thyroid. 2018;28(10):1243–51.
2. Muir CA, Menzies AM, Clifton-Bligh R, Tsang VHM. Thyroid toxicity following immune checkpoint inhibitor treatment in advanced cancer. Thyroid. 2020;30(10):1458–69.
3. Mosaferi T, Tsai K, Sovich S, et al. Optimal thyroid hormone replacement dose in immune checkpoint inhibitor-associated hypothyroidism is distinct from Hashimoto's thyroiditis. Thyroid. 2022;32(5):496–504.
4. Azmat U, Liebner D, et al. Treatment of ipilimumab induced graves' disease in a patient with metastatic melanoma. Case Rep Endocrinol. 2016;2016:2087525.
5. Min L, Vaidya A, Becker C. Thyroid autoimmunity and ophthalmopathy related to melanoma biological therapy. Eur J Endocrinol. 2011;164(2):303–7.

Chapter 8
Worsening Hyperglycemia During Immune Checkpoint Inhibitor Therapy

Irene J. Lee, Kei Takigawa, and Conor Best

Abbreviations

DKA	diabetic ketoacidosis.
ICI	immune checkpoint inhibitors.
IDO1	Indoleamine 2,3-dioxygenase 1.
LADA	latent autoimmune diabetes of adults.
PD-1/L1	Programmed death protein 1/ligand 1.
T1DM	type 1 diabetes mellitus.
T2DM	type 2 diabetes mellitus.

Clinical Presentation

This is a male in his 50 s with cutaneous melanoma on the right face that was resected. However, cancer recurred 1 year later, for which he was started on epacadostat 100 mg twice a day + durvalumab (immune checkpoint inhibitor: ICI) 10 mg/kg every 2 weeks and underwent a total of 24 cycles before transitioning to

I. J. Lee
Department of Internal Medicine, Baylor College of Medicine, Houston, TX, USA
e-mail: Irene.Lee@bcm.edu

K. Takigawa
Department of Medicine-Pediatrics, Baylor College of Medicine, Houston, TX, USA
e-mail: Kei.Takigawa@bcm.edu

C. Best (✉)
Department of Endocrine Neoplasia and Hormonal Disorders, The University of Texas MD Anderson Cancer Center, Houston, TX, USA
e-mail: CJBest@mdanderson.org

Y. Wang (ed.), *Challenging Cases in Immunotherapy Related Organ Toxicities*,
https://doi.org/10.1007/978-3-031-83533-9_8

epacadostat 100 mg BID for an additional 33 cycles. Otherwise, he had a medical history of type 2 diabetes mellitus, hyperlipidemia, and gastroesophageal reflux disease that were medically controlled with metformin, saxagliptin, atorvastatin, and ranitidine.

Prior to his third dose of durvalumab, the patient was referred to the Endocrinology clinic due to hyperglycemia with blood glucose of 422 mg/dL without acidosis and normal anion gap noted on pretreatment testing (Table 8.1). The patient reported he was diagnosed with Type 2 Diabetes Mellitus (T2DM) by his primary care provider approximately 8 months prior to Endocrinology referral and was started on combination metformin 1000 mg and saxagliptin 5 mg daily. He attributed his hyperglycemia to running out of his medication and a high carbohydrate meal. Testing performed later the same day showed spontaneous improvement in serum glucose to 260 mg/dL and a normal c-peptide level of 2.6 ng/mL (ref range 0.9–7.1). His medications were refilled, and he was provided precautions for development of worsening hyperglycemia and diabetic ketoacidosis (DKA). Given improvement he proceeded to his third dose of durvalumab after a 1 week hold. Critical labs are listed in Table 8.1.

Two days after his third dose of durvalumab the patient was presented to an outside emergency department with nausea and vomiting with testing demonstrating an anion gap acidosis consistent with DKA. He was discharged with metformin and glipizide without scheduled insulin and readmitted with recurrent acidosis after another 2 days. During the second admission he was hospitalized and discharged on insulin.

At follow-up 1 month after his initial presentation with hyperglycemia he had clear evidence of immune mediated pancreatic endocrine dysfunction with insulin deficiency with undetectable c-peptide of <0.01. Glutamic acid decarboxylase 65 (GAD-65) antibodies were positive at 0.12 nmol/L (≤0.02). He was placed on a regimen of short and long acting insulin which he has continued to require since then. ICI therapy was briefly held, but resumed after 1 month when his blood glucose levels were better controlled. Follow-up c-peptide levels drawn 7 months after

Table 8.1 Lab values

Test	Value prior to cycle 3 of treatment	Later that day	9 days later	3 weeks later
Glucose (70–110)	**422 mg/dL**	**260 mg/dL**	**402 mg/dL**	**269 mg/dL**
Bicarbonate (22–30)	24 mEq/L	–	**9 mEq/L**	24 mEq/L
Anion gap (4–14)	12 mEq/L	–	**35 mEq/L**	13 mEq/L
C-peptide (0.9–7.1)	–	2.6 ng/mL		**< 0.01 ng/mL**
GAD-65 antibodies (≤0.02)	–	–		**0.12 nmol/L**

Mg milligram, *mEq* milliequivalent, *mL* milliliter, *L* liter, *dL* deciliter, *ng* nanogram, *nmnol* nanomole
Abnormal values are bolded in the table

his initial diagnosis remained undetectable. He went on to complete 24 cycles of durvalumab over 1 year followed by an additional 14 months of monotherapy with epacadostat at which time both treatments were terminated.

Differential Diagnosis

Determining new onset insulin deficiency related to ICI therapy in a patient with preexisting T2DM is difficult. T2DM is characterized by insulin resistance, but many patients do experience progressive beta cell failure and many do eventually require insulin. However, the rate of beta cell death is greatly accelerated in ICI associated diabetes.

In this case, his normal c-peptide and declining glucose level were, incorrectly, felt to represent adequate insulin production. While insulin or c-peptide levels can provide an estimation of insulin production, there is not a cutoff that will distinguish ICI diabetes from progression of T2DM. Levels in the normal range may still represent inadequate or rapidly declining beta cell function in a hyperglycemic patient if detected early in the disease process. Progression from relatively mild hyperglycemia to DKA can be extremely rapid, occurring in only a few days.

Other features suggestive of developing insulin deficiency include poor response to oral medications (particularly sulfonylureas which require endogenous insulin stores) and disproportionate postprandial hyperglycemia due to inability to clear oral glucose from the bloodstream.

Clinical Outcome

The patient continued to follow with Endocrinology with adjustment of his subcutaneous insulin regimen until completion of his ICI therapy. He has since undergone routine surveillance examinations and imaging without recurrence of cutaneous findings or new metastatic disease. His diabetes has remained suboptimally controlled with most recent hemoglobin A1c at 8.4% related to noncompliance to a full insulin regimen.

Summary of the Case

This is a case with metastatic melanoma who developed insulin dependent T1DM with DKA upon treatment of epacadostat and durvalumab in the context of preexisting T2DM. The patient concluded cancer therapy with continued insulin requirement to maintain a stable hemoglobin A1c around 8%. He has since remained without recurrence of cutaneous disease until the last follow up for 7 years after

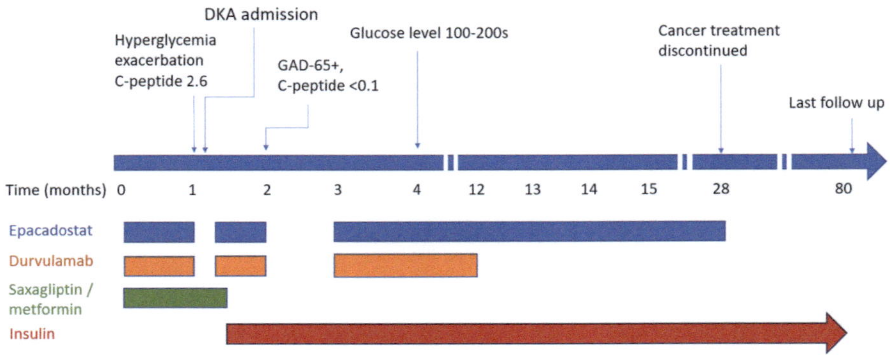

Fig. 8.1 Summary of timeline events (timepoint of 0 is starting time of cancer treatment)

pancreatic endocrine toxicity event. Timeline events have been summarized in Fig. 8.1.

Discussion

ICI related T1DM is a rare complication affecting ~1% of patients who receive ICIs (predominantly PD-1/L1) [1]. It is characterized by rapid, permanent damage to pancreatic beta cells and insulin deficiency leading to risk of DKA [2, 3]. Workups for previous cases of ICI related diabetes have shown that initial A1c in ICI-related T1DM are less than 10% with c-peptide relatively low for the degree of hyperglycemia or undetectable [4].

Because of the high risk of DKA, there should be a low threshold to start insulin in a patient on ICI therapy with new or worsening hyperglycemia. Serial c-peptide and glucose levels can be used to estimate endogenous insulin production and insulin can be discontinued if the patient's clinical picture is most consistent with T2DM. Patients with ICI induced diabetes typically progress to absolute insulin deficiency and with a lifelong insulin requirement, that does not change if ICI therapy is held.

GAD-65 antibodies are present in around 50% of patients with ICI diabetes [5]. Some patients with T2DM have positive autoantibodies that otherwise are associated with T1DM and are at increased risk of progression to low c-peptide levels and insulin dependence, termed latent autoimmune diabetes in adults (LADA) [6]. Both new onset and pre-existing antibodies have been reported in ICI related diabetes [7]. Patients with preexisting T2DM were at increased risk of developing ICI T1DM [5]. It is unknown if this is due to preexisting autoimmunity or a reduced beta cell reserve which is more likely to fail.

Conclusion

In conclusion, the diagnosis of ICI T1DM is challenging in a patient with a prior history of diabetes. With the increased use of ICIs as first-line therapies for a wide array of cancers, it is particularly important for clinicians and patients to be aware of new or worsening hyperglycemia, prompt recognition and treatment of hyperglycemia can reduce hospitalizations for DKA and interruptions to ICI therapy. Treatment of insulin should be considered for safety especially if the diagnosis is unclear. Further research is required to establish the pathophysiology and identify risk factors that could therefore minimize ICI-related toxicities. As ICI-related T1DM is typically irreversible, treatment can be continued if it is otherwise tolerated.

References

1. Akturk HK, Kahramangil D, Sarwal A, Hoffecker L, Murad MH, Michels AW. Immune checkpoint inhibitor-induced type 1 diabetes: a systematic review and meta-analysis. Diabet Med: J Br Diabet Assoc. 2019;36(9):1075–81. https://doi.org/10.1111/dme.14050.
2. de Filette JMK, Pen JJ, Decoster L, Vissers T, Bravenboer B, Van der Auwera BJ, Gorus FK, Roep BO, Aspeslagh S, Neyns B, Velkeniers B, Kharagjitsingh AV. Immune checkpoint inhibitors and type 1 diabetes mellitus: a case report and systematic review. Eur J Endocrinol. 2019;181(3):363–74. https://doi.org/10.1530/EJE-19-0291.
3. Hosokawa Y, Hanafusa T, Imagawa A. Pathogenesis of fulminant type 1 diabetes: genes, viruses and the immune mechanism, and usefulness of patient-derived induced pluripotent stem cells for future research. J Diabet Invest. 2019;10(5):1158–64. https://doi.org/10.1111/jdi.13091.
4. Elshimy G, Raj R, Akturk HK, Schriber A, Sisterna N, Ahmad I, Jacob A, Michels AW, Correa R. Immune checkpoint inhibitors related endocrine adverse events. In Feingold KR, et al., editors. Endotext. MDText.com, Inc.; 2022.
5. Chen X, Affinati AH, Lee Y, Turcu AF, Henry NL, Schiopu E, Qin A, Othus M, Clauw D, Ramnath N, Zhao L. Immune checkpoint inhibitors and risk of type 1 diabetes. Diabetes Care. 2022;45(5):1170–6. https://doi.org/10.2337/dc21-2213.
6. Maruyama T, et al. Heterogeneity among patients with latent autoimmune diabetes in adults. Diabetes Metab Res Rev. 2011;27:971–4. https://doi.org/10.1002/dmrr.1238.
7. Stamatouli A, et al. Collateral damage: insulin-dependent diabetes induced with checkpoint inhibitors. Diabetes. 2018;67:1471–80. https://doi.org/10.2337/dbi18-0002.

Chapter 9
Lipodystrophy after Receiving Immune Checkpoint Inhibitor Therapy

Nina Semsarzadeh, Pradnya D. Patil, Kord Honda, Joshua Arbesman, and Pauline Funchain

Abbreviations

ACTH	adrenocorticotropic hormone
ANA	antinuclear antibody
CT	computed tomography
ENA	extractable nuclear antigen
FSH	follicle stimulating hormone
HDL	high density lipoprotein
ICI	immune checkpoint inhibitor
LDL	low density lipoprotein
LH	luteinizing hormone
PD-L1	programmed death ligand-1
TSH	thyroid stimulating hormone

N. Semsarzadeh · J. Arbesman
Dermatology and Plastic Surgery Institute, Cleveland Clinic Foundation, Cleveland, OH, USA
e-mail: semsarn@ccf.org; arbesmj@ccf.org

P. D. Patil
Department of Hematology & Medical Oncology, Cleveland Clinic Foundation, Cleveland, OH, USA
e-mail: pradnya.patil@nuvancehealth.org

K. Honda
Department of Dermatology, University Hospitals Cleveland Medical Center, Cleveland, OH, USA
e-mail: kord.honda@UHhospitals.org

P. Funchain (✉)
Division of Oncology, Department of Medicine, Stanford Cancer Institute, Stanford University, Stanford, CA, USA
e-mail: funchap@stanford.edu

Y. Wang (ed.), *Challenging Cases in Immunotherapy Related Organ Toxicities*,
https://doi.org/10.1007/978-3-031-83533-9_9

Case Presentation

A female in her 40 s with history of stage IA malignant melanoma of the right back status post wide local excision presented with an enlarged right axillary lymph node on routine mammogram over 1 year after her original melanoma diagnosis. Subsequent lymph node biopsy confirmed recurrent metastatic melanoma. She underwent complete right axillary lymphadenectomy; metastatic melanoma was noted in one of fourteen lymph nodes. Molecular testing was positive for BRAF V600E and PD-L1 expression was 10%. She was started on biweekly infusions of nivolumab (240 mg) later that year as adjuvant therapy. The patient initially experienced mild and transient side effects including fatigue, headaches, grade 1 diarrhea, and grade 1 transaminitis that were managed conservatively.

Seven months after the initiation of nivolumab therapy, a generalized lipodystrophy was noted on physical exam. She had scattered, indurated nodules and depressed plaques without overlying surface change involving the bilateral upper extremities, lower extremities, and flank (Fig. 9.1). She was also noted to have increased truncal, dorsocervical, supraclavicular and facial adipose tissue typical of metabolic syndrome (Fig. 9.2). The subcutaneous adipose redistribution evident on physical exam was clinically consistent with a generalized acquired lipodystrophy.

She was simultaneously diagnosed with metabolic syndrome with elevations in total cholesterol (267 mg/dl), LDL cholesterol (164 mg/dl) and triglycerides (456 mg/dl), decreased HDL cholesterol (32 mg/dl) and impaired glucose tolerance with a hemoglobin A1C of 5.7%. A CT scan of the abdomen revealed imaging findings consistent with fatty liver. Prior to this, the patient had no history of elevated blood sugars or dyslipidemia. She had no history of prolonged systemic steroid use or autoimmune disease. Endocrine work up including growth hormone, insulin-like growth factor I, ACTH, cortisol, prolactin, estrogen, FSH, LH, TSH was unremarkable. Preliminary rheumatologic work up including ANA and ENA was within normal limits.

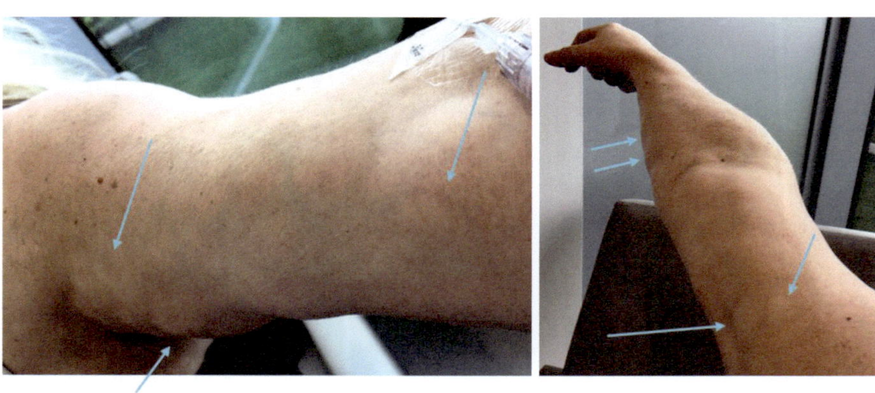

Fig. 9.1 Characteristic cobblestone appearance of lipodystrophy due to subcutaneous adipose redistribution

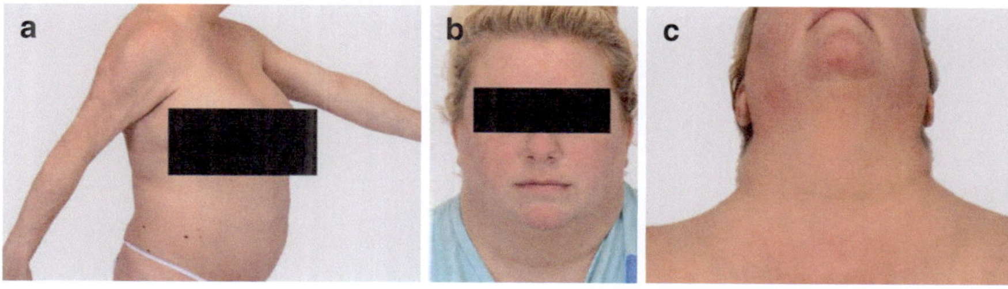

Fig. 9.2 Whole body photography showing adipose redistribution following typical lipodystrophy patterns. (**a**) Lateral truncal view; (**b**) Facial view; (**c**) Dorsocervical and supraclavicular view

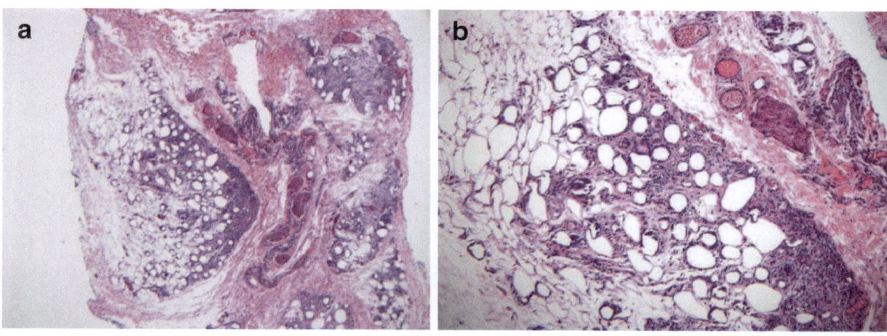

Fig. 9.3 H&E staining of subcutaneous core biopsy. (**a**) Low power consistent with granulomatous, lobular panniculitis composed of lymphohistiocytic infiltrate and giant cells in the subcutaneous fat. (**b**) High power view of adipocytes

Evaluation

Punch biopsies of the upper extremity in areas of lipoatrophy revealed a granulomatous, lobular panniculitis composed of a lymphohistiocytic infiltrate and giant cells in the subcutaneous fat (Fig. 9.3a). Diminution of adipocyte lobule size was also noted on histology (Fig. 9.3b).

Differential Diagnosis

The patient's new onset lipodystrophy was hypothesized to be secondary to her nivolumab therapy given the inflammatory infiltrate seen on biopsy compatible with ICI-related inflammation, temporal relationship with nivolumab therapy, the rarity of generalized lipodystrophy and absence of other triggers or familial predisposition. While another undetermined trigger could be the cause in our patient, it seems unlikely given that the time course was associated with nivolumab administration. After weighing the risk of progressive or recurrent melanoma and the possibility of progression of this irAE, the decision was made to continue nivolumab therapy and manage the adverse effect conservatively.

Treatment

The patient adopted a low calorie diet and restricted carbohydrates and fat. She was initiated on fenofibrate, icosapent ethyl, and metformin for hyperlipidemia and impaired glucose tolerance, respectively.

Although the patient successfully decreased her cholesterol and triglyceride levels and lost weight after diet and medication modifications, there was no reversal of lipodystrophy, which continued to progress slowly on nivolumab therapy. Additionally, her cholesterol and triglycerides, while improved, remained elevated despite medical therapy. She completed 1 year of adjuvant nivolumab therapy, however, no reversal of the process was observed after stopping therapy. Worsening of the lipodystrophy, with new involvement of her facial area, was seen 3 months after completion of nivolumab. She was able to discontinue medical therapy for hyperlipidemia and impaired glucose tolerance a year after discontinuing immunotherapy. She continues to show no evidence of recurrent disease 5 years after diagnosis but subcutaneous adipose redistribution remains stable on physical exam.

Summary

We describe a case of acquired generalized lipodystrophy after nivolumab therapy that was associated with concurrent fatty liver changes, dyslipidemia, hypercholesterolemia and impaired glucose tolerance (Fig. 9.4). She remains without evidence of melanoma 5 years later but adipose redistribution has not resolved.

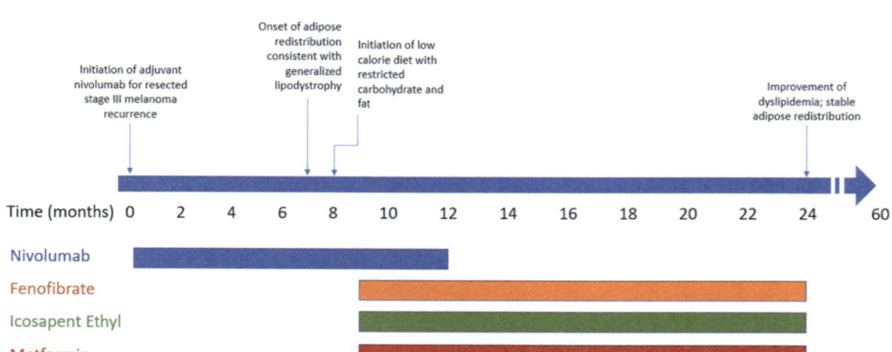

Fig. 9.4 Summary of timeline events (timepoint of 0 is initiation of nivolumab)

Discussion

Immune related adverse events are well described with the use of ICIs involving different organs such as the skin, gastrointestinal tract, and endocrine glands etc. [1–3]. ICI related lipodystrophy is rare and only limited to two case reports. Falcao et al. described the first case of acquired generalized lipodystrophy 2 months after initiation of nivolumab in a 57 year old female with renal cell carcinoma [4]. A similar case was described in a patient receiving pembrolizumab for metastatic melanoma [5].

Lipodystrophy encompasses a large and heterogeneous group of diseases characterized by an abnormal distribution of fat with selective fat loss in some areas and secondary fat accumulation in others. Lipodystrophy can be categorized as congenital or acquired and further subclassified into generalized, partial or localized types [6]. Lipodystrophy is often associated with systemic findings including insulin resistance, diabetes mellitus, dyslipidemia, hypertension, and coronary artery disease, some of which were found in our patient. Histologic findings associated with this disorder can be quite varied, but most often reveals smaller and fewer adipocytes with or without associated inflammation [6, 7]. The most common inflammatory pattern is a panniculitis like pattern [7] which is often observed in acquired generalized forms of lipodystrophy. This inflammatory pattern usually consists of lymphocytes, lipophages, and plasma cells. Granulomatous foci may be present in multiple organ distributions, but uncommon, which is posited to be secondary to an increase in Th17 and its downstream cytokines [8].

The clinical morphology of these granulomatous reactions in the skin vary widely and include granuloma annulare, granulomatous dermatitis, and granulomatous foreign body-like reaction [9–12]. On clinical exam, they can often be mistaken for disease progression or recurrence and can significantly impact patient care. Multiple case reports described various presentations of granulomatous panniculitis from different ICI agents [13–15]. In all the reported cases, the lesions resolved rather rapidly upon discontinuation of the ICI and/or systemic steroids.

Conclusion

A granulomatous panniculitis secondary to immunotherapy presenting as lipodystrophy represents a rare irAE, but one that may result in significant morbidity. Recognition of this novel irAE and appropriate treatment is important for patient care. Traditionally, oral steroids are indicated for irAEs although the theoretic risk of worsening the patient's metabolic syndrome with systemic glucocorticoids makes this treatment option unfavorable. Progression of the lipodystrophy and associated metabolic effects despite conservative management may warrant discontinuation of therapy, especially if such findings are irreversible.

References

1. Wang DY, Salem JE, Cohen JV, et al. Fatal toxic effects associated with immune checkpoint inhibitors: a systematic review and meta-analysis. JAMA. Oncologia. 2018.
2. Mitchell TC, Feld E. Immunotherapy in melanoma. Immunotherapy. 2018 Aug;10(11):987–98.
3. Villadolid J, Amin A. Immune checkpoint inhibitors in clinical practice: update on management of immune-related toxicities. Transl Lung Cancer Res. 2015;4(5):560–75.
4. Falcao CK, Cabral MCS, Mota JM, Arbache ST, Costa-Riquetto AD, Muniz DQB, Cury-Martins J, Almeida MQ, Cukier Kaczemorska P, Nery M, Teles MG. Acquired lipodystrophy associated with nivolumab in a patient with advanced renal cell carcinoma. J Clin Endocrinol Metab. 2019;pii:jc.2018-02221. https://doi.org/10.1210/jc.2018-02221. [Epub ahead of print] PubMed PMID: 30779841.
5. Haddad N, Vidal-Trecan T, Baroudjian B, Zagdanski AM, Arangalage D, Battistella M, Gautier JF, Lebbe C, Delyon J, PATIO group. Acquired generalized lipodystrophy under immune checkpoint inhibition. Br J Dermatol. 2019;182:477–80. https://doi.org/10.1111/bjd.18124. [Epub ahead of print]. PubMed PMID: 31077337.
6. Hussain I, Garg A. Lipodystrophy syndromes. Endocrinol Metab Clin N Am. 2016;45(4):783–97. https://doi.org/10.1016/j.ecl.2016.06.012. Epub 2016 Oct 6. Review. PubMed PMID: 27823605.
7. Peters MS, Winklemann RK. The histopathology of localized lipoatrophy. Br J Dermatol. 1986;114:27–36.
8. Cornejo CM, Haun P, English J 3rd, Rosenbach M. Immune checkpoint inhibitors and the development of granulomatous reactions. J Am Acad Dermatol. 2018;pii: S0190-9622(18):32355–7.
9. Diaz-Perez JA, Beveridge MG, Victor TA, Cibull TL. Granulomatous and lichenoid dermatitis after IgG4 anti-PD-1 monoclonal antibody therapy for advanced cancer. J Cutan Pathol. 2018;45(6):434–8.
10. Martín-Carrasco P, Pérez-Ruiz C, De Zulueta-Dorado T, Conejo-Mir J. Postherpetic granulomatous dermatitis in a man treated with nivolumab. Actas Dermosifiliogr. 2017;108(8):783–4.
11. Birnbaum MR, Ma MW, Fleisig S, et al. Nivolumab-related cutaneous sarcoidosis in a patient with lung adenocarcinoma. JAAD Case Rep. 2017;3(3):208–11.
12. Reule RB, North JP. Cutaneous and pulmonary sarcoidosis-like reaction associated with ipilimumab. J Am Acad Dermatol. 2013;69(5):e272–3.
13. Tetzlaff MT, Jazaeri AA, Torres-Cabala CA, et al. Erythema nodosum-like panniculitis mimicking disease recurrence: a novel toxicity from immune checkpoint blockade therapy-report of 2 patients. J Cutan Pathol. 2017;44(12):1080–6.
14. Jiang B, Patino MM, Gross AJ, Leong SPL, Moretto JC, Kashani-Sabet M, Kim KB. Diffuse granulomatous panniculitis associated with anti PD-1 antibody therapy. JAAD Case Rep. 2017;4(1):13–6. https://doi.org/10.1016/j.jdcr.2017.06.014. eCollection 2018 Jan. PubMed PMID: 29296642; PubMed Central PMCID: PMC5739149.
15. Burillo-Martinez S, Morales-Raya C, Prieto-Barrios M, RodriguezPeralto JL, Ortiz-Romero PL. Pembrolizumab-induced extensive panniculitis and nevus regression: two novel cutaneous manifestations of the post-immunotherapy granulomatous reactions Spectrum. JAMA Dermatol. 2017;153(7):721–2.

Chapter 10
Hypoglycemia Secondary to Anti-PD-1 Therapy

Skyler Burke, Evan Ong, Adam Bograd, Laura Bovee, and Kelly G. Paulson

Abbreviations

BG	Blood glucose
BMI	body mass index
CBC	Complete blood count
CMP	Complete metabolic panel
PD-L1	Programmed death ligand 1
SCC	Squamous cell carcinoma
T1DM	Type 1 Diabetes Mellitus

S. Burke
Elson S Floyd College of Medicine, Washington State University, Spokane, WA, USA
e-mail: skyler.burke@wsu.edu

E. Ong · A. Bograd
Departments of Surgery, Thoracic and Medical Oncology Providence-Swedish Cancer Institute, Seattle, WA, USA
e-mail: Evan.Ong@swedish.org; Adam.Bograd@swedish.org

L. Bovee
Division of Endocrinology, University of Washington, Seattle, WA, USA
e-mail: lbodding@uw.edu

K. G. Paulson (✉)
Elson S Floyd College of Medicine, Washington State University, Spokane, WA, USA

Departments of Surgery, Thoracic and Medical Oncology Providence-Swedish Cancer Institute, Seattle, WA, USA
e-mail: kelly.paulson@providence.org

Y. Wang (ed.), *Challenging Cases in Immunotherapy Related Organ Toxicities*,
https://doi.org/10.1007/978-3-031-83533-9_10

Clinical Presentation and Clinical Course

A male patient in his 60 s presented with a p16-positive, PD-L1 positive T2N2 squamous cell carcinoma (SCC) of the base of tongue. He received initial curative intent therapy with cisplatin based chemoradiation. One year after initial therapy he developed asymptomatic enlarging pulmonary nodules which were biopsy proven to represent recurrent/metastatic disease. He underwent stereotactic radiosurgery followed by pembrolizumab therapy.

Patient initiated pembrolizumab at standard dosing. At the time of treatment initiation, non-fasting plasma glucoses were unremarkable. Several days after his first infusion he developed episodic light headedness, dizziness, fatigue, and inability to ride bike up hills. Three weeks into therapy at his second infusion he presented with a non-fasting mid-morning plasma glucose of 57 mg/dL (Fig. 10.1). He was of normal weight (BMI 19 with no significant recent change). He was not on any antihyperglycemic medications and denied potential exposure to insulin or oral antihyperglycemics; he further denied alcohol or drug use. Patient was advised to eat frequent small meals, with which he complied. He continued to have episodes, although observed they improved with juice intake.

9.5 months after pembrolizumab initiation episodes had worsened in frequency, intensity and character. Patient presented for consideration treatment and underwent afternoon labs after having eaten a lunch meal. Plasma glucose (BG) returned critically low at 38 mg/dL (corroborated with backup blood tube on second clinical instrument) and patient was shaky and with mild confusion. Pembrolizumab was held. He was given an oral glucose load and IV dextrose with improvement in systolic blood pressure (BP) to 113 and improvement in symptoms fulfilling Whipple's triad [1]. The case was discussed with endocrinology. Add-on blood tests were obtained to the original specimen including a normal cortisol (10.3 µg/dL), an

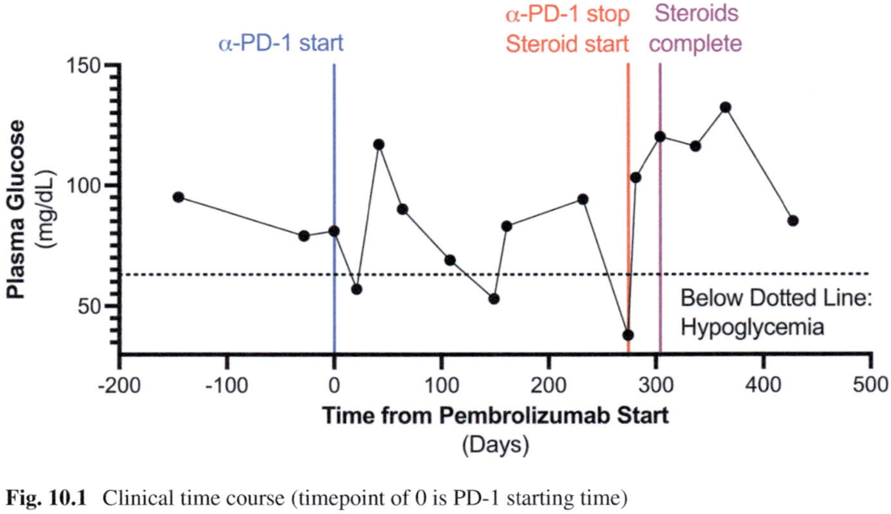

Fig. 10.1 Clinical time course (timepoint of 0 is PD-1 starting time)

insulin level above that expected for hypoglycemia (12.9 μIU/mL; expected findings for BG 38 < 3 μIU/mL), a high C-peptide (4.6 ng/mL, reference range 1.1–4.4 ng/mL), and a negative sulfonylurea hypoglycemics and toxicology panel (ruling out inadvertent medication or toxin ingestion). Islet-cell antibody (IA-2) and insulin antibody were checked and negative. Other routine labs including CBC and CMP were unremarkable. Patient was given a home glucose monitor and noted very low morning glucoses in the 40s and 50s. Urgent MRI of abdomen pancreatic protocol was unremarkable. Oncologic surgery and tumor board recommended treatment of potential autoimmune hypoglycemia before surgical exploration for possible clinically occult insulinoma.

Patient was started on a prednisone taper at 0.5 mg/kg and tapered over a six-week period. With this he noted immediate improvement in energy and resolution of episodes. Morning fasting glucoses on home glucometer were all improved to normal range and non-fasting glucoses in clinic observed to be appropriate for non-fasting range ranging from 84–132 mg/dL. Glucoses have remained normal since taper off of steroids. At last imaging 1 year from therapy start and 3 months from last pembrolizumab patient remained with no evidence of residual cancer.

Clinical Outcome

The hypoglycemia suspected secondary to pembrolizumab resolved with cessation of therapy and prednisone with taper. Patient achieved symptomatic remission.

Summary of the Case

Described here is a case with recurrent squamous cell carcinoma of the head and neck who developed significant persistent unexplained symptomatic episodic hypoglycemia on pembrolizumab monotherapy. A comprehensive workup including endocrinological and autoimmune panel as well as imaging to look for insulinoma were all negative. Withholding pembrolizumab and prednisone treatment achieved normalization of blood glucose and resolution of symptoms.

Discussion

Endocrinopathies are frequently described immune related adverse events to immune checkpoint inhibition including anti-PD-1 therapy including for patients receiving anti-PD-1 for head and neck cancers [2, 3]. Commonly described endocrinopathies include hyper- and hypothyroidism, pituitary dysfunction, adrenal insufficiency, and pancreatic islet beta cell dysfunction (presenting with type 1 type diabetes mellitus:T1DM) [4]. Of all ICI toxicity endocrinopathies, new T1DM is the least common, but is important to be cognizant of due to its potential complication of life threatening diabetic ketoacidosis. Indeed, for this reason T1DM is listed on the FDA label for pembrolizumab as a warning for clinician.

Initial presentation of hypoglycemia as initial indication of ICI mediated pancreatic islet cell inflammation is rare. In at least one other case report, a patient presented with renal cell carcinoma presented with hypoglycemia secondary to ipilimumab and nivolumab [5]. There were no other labs reported at time of hypoglycemia, however the patient subsequently developed T1DM leading the authors to posit the pancreas was inflamed and then 'burned out', similar to a well described recurrent pattern with thyroid endocrinopathies [3].. In our presently reported case the patient had well documented symptomatic hypoglycemia suggesting a possible inflamed (over-producing insulin) phase. The pattern of laboratory workup is consistent with pancreatogenous hypoglycemia without evidence for exogenous insulin or other hypoglycemic agents. There was no evidence for insulinoma, insulin antibodies, adrenal insufficiency or sepsis, and patient had no history of gastric bypass or dumping syndrome. We did not obtain biopsy of pancreas to evaluate for noninsulinoma pancreatogenous hypoglycemia syndrome [6] due to patient's rapid recovery on steroids; of note, patient's laboratory studies are identical for NIPHS [7]. As of writing, patient has not gone on to develop T1DM; it is unclear whether steroids may have stopped an underlying beta cell inflammation/progression to this state.

Conclusion

Hypoglycemia is a rare but clinically significant potential complication of immune checkpoint inhibitor therapy. Laboratory studies in the presently reported patient suggest a mechanism of beta-cell inflammation. Hypoglycemia can in some circumstances be successfully treated with steroids and does not always predict progression to T1DM.

References

1. Whipple AO. The surgical therapy of hyperinsulinism. Int J Surg. 1938:237–76.
2. Harrington KJ, Burtness B, Greil R, et al. Pembrolizumab with or without chemotherapy in recurrent or metastatic head and neck squamous cell carcinoma: updated results of the Phase III KEYNOTE-048 Study. J Clin Oncol. 2023;41(4):790–802. https://doi.org/10.1200/JCO.21.02508.
3. Byun DJ, Wolchok JD, Rosenberg LM, Girotra M. Cancer immunotherapy—immune checkpoint blockade and associated endocrinopathies. Nat Rev Endocrinol. 2017;13(4):195–207. https://doi.org/10.1038/nrendo.2016.205.

4. Schneider BJ, Naidoo J, Santomasso BD, et al. Management of immune-related adverse events in patients treated with immune checkpoint inhibitor therapy: ASCO guideline update. J Clin Oncol. 2021;39(36):4073–126. https://doi.org/10.1200/JCO.21.01440.
5. Kamal RS, Dean A, Dutt H, Rajeh A, Fernandes R. Hypoglycemia as first presentation of presumed immune checkpoint inhibitor-induced type 1 diabetes. Clin Case Rep. 2023;11(9):e7897. https://doi.org/10.1002/ccr3.7897.
6. Service FJ, Natt N, Thompson GB, et al. Noninsulinoma pancreatogenous hypoglycemia: a novel syndrome of hyperinsulinemic hypoglycemia in adults independent of mutations in Kir6.2 and SUR1 genes. J Clin Endocrinol Metab. 1999;84(5):1582–9. https://doi.org/10.1210/jcem.84.5.5645.
7. Dieterle MP, Husari A, Prozmann SN, et al. Diffuse, adult-onset Nesidioblastosis/Non-Insulinoma Pancreatogenous Hypoglycemia Syndrome (NIPHS): review of the literature of a rare cause of hyperinsulinemic hypoglycemia. Biomedicines. 2023;11(6) https://doi.org/10.3390/biomedicines11061732.

Chapter 11
Transient Diabetes Insipidus Related to Immune Checkpoint Inhibitor Therapy

Anna Olsson-Brown

Abbreviations

DI	Diabetes insipidus.
HbA1c	Hemoglobin A1c.
ICI	Immune checkpoint inhibitor.
PD-1	Programmed cell death protein-1.
PS	Performance status.
SACT	Systemic anticancer treatment.
TSH	Thyroid stimulating hormone.
T4	Thyroxine Test.

Clinical Presentation

This is a Caucasian gentleman in his 60's with a history of cutaneous melanoma which had been treated with a wide local excision and a sentinel lymph node biopsy. He was referred for consideration of adjuvant immune checkpoint inhibitor immunotherapy (ICI) with an anti-PD-1 agent, nivolumab, given every 4 weeks. He was of good performance status (PS 0) with no significant past medical history and no regular medication. He was fit and active with a BMI of 30.

Following cycle three he started experiencing excessive thirst and fluid intake (polydipsia) throughout day and night and had an increased urinary frequency

A. Olsson-Brown (✉)
Cancer Division, Sussex Cancer Centre, University Hospitals Sussex NHS Foundation Trust, Worthing Hospital, Worthing, West Sussex, UK

Department of Pharmacology and Theraputics, University of Liverpool, Liverpool, UK
e-mail: a.olsson-brown@nhs.net

Y. Wang (ed.), *Challenging Cases in Immunotherapy Related Organ Toxicities*,
https://doi.org/10.1007/978-3-031-83533-9_11

(polyuria) up to 20 times daily. He had spontaneously tried to restrict his fluid intake which did not reduce his urinary frequency but did lead to increased thirst. He was also reporting significant fatigue, in part potentially related to the interruption in his sleep pattern. In addition to his urinary symptoms he had also developed an increasing headache over the course of 3 weeks.

Evaluations

Initial urinalysis was negative for protein, blood, glucose and leucocytes. His measured urinary volume was 4.5 L/24 h. His random blood glucose was 4.7 mmol/L and HbA1c normal.

His baseline blood work at presentation can be found in Table 11.1. His anterior pituitary hormones and cortisol levels were within the normal range. Due to his hypernatraemia his paired osmolarities were done and illustrated a urine osmolarity of 131 mOsm/kg and a plasma osmolarity of 450 mOsm/kg resulting in a urine/plasma osmolality of 0.29 (Table 11.2).

A Brain MRI with contrast done at the time of presentation showed no evidence of any abnormality. There was no evidence of metastatic disease. Renal ultrasound showed normal renal and urological anatomy.

He underwent a water deprivation test which illustrated an inadequate rise in urinary osmolarity (<600 mOsm/kg) with water deprivation after 2 and 8 h (Fig. 11.1). He then received desmopressin and a significant rise to >600 mOsm/kg was observed.

Table 11.1 Blood results

Parameter	Baseline	Presentation
Sodium (135-145 mmol/L)	136 mmol/L	156 mmol/L
Potassium (3.5–4.5 mmol/L)	4.2 mmol/L	3.0 mmol/L
Urea (2.5–7.8 mmol/L)	4.3 mmol/L	9.0 mmol/L
Creatinine (59–104 μmol/L)	65 μmol/L	170 μmol/L
Corrected calcium (2.2–2.6 mmol/L)	2.26 mmol/L	2.37 mmol/L
Free T4 (10–24 pmol/L)	17.7 pmol/L	19.6 pmol/L
TSH (0.4–4.5 mU/L)	0.66 mU/L	0.80 mU/L
Cortisol (170–690 nmol/L)	592 nmol/L	341 nmol/L

Table 11.2 Biochemical parameters in the differential diagnosis in polydipsia

Parameters	Polydipsia	Cranial diabetes insipidus	Nephrogenic diabetes insipidus
Serum osmolality mOsm/kg (reference range 275–295 mOsm/kg)	<295	>300	>300
Urine osmolality mOsm/kg (reference range 50–1200 mOsm/kg depending on hydration status)	>600	<300 (often <200)	<300
Post desmopressin urinary osmolality mOsm/kg	No or mild response	>600	No response

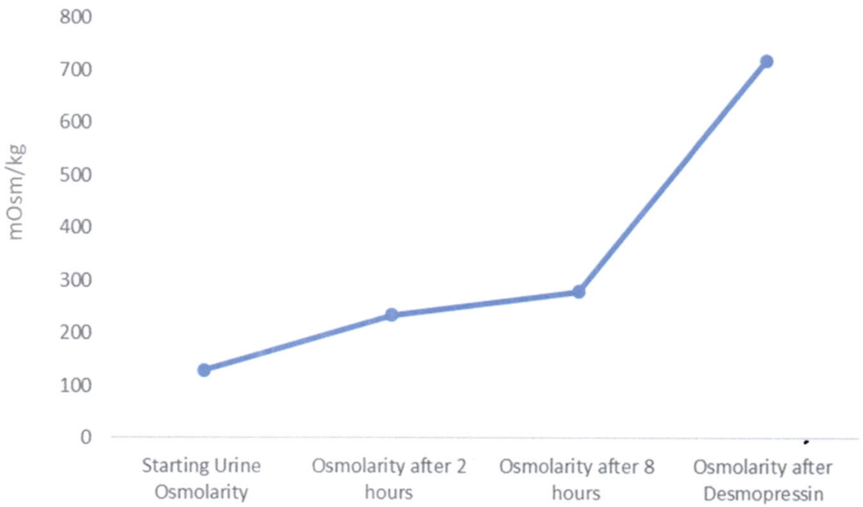

Fig. 11.1 Water deprivation test

Differential Diagnosis

Polydipsia can be caused by diabetes mellitus, psychogenic polydipsia and both cranial and nephrogenic diabetes insipidus (DI). Therefore it is important to establish the patient's glucose management status with both a random blood glucose and a recent HbA1c. This patient had normal work up for diabetes mellitus based on blood work. Psychogenic polydipsia is generally detected in the patient's history but can be borne out by biochemical testing. To differentiate between cranial and nephrogenic diabetes insipidus desmopressin administration is required for diagnosis and may provide therapeutic benefit.

Diabetes insipidus is either a lack of anti-diuretic hormone (cranial DI) or an insensitivity to it (nephrogenic DI). In this case, given the response to desmopressin, although no overt inflammation was seen on MRI imaging, it is likely that subtle inflammation of the posterior pituitary led to a transient reduction in the production of anti-diuretic hormone which resulted in an inadequate concentration and thus reduced effect of anti-diuretic hormone in the kidney leading to a reduction of free water absorption and an increase in solute-free water diuresis.

Management Options

This gentleman was diagnosed with ICI induced cranial diabetes insipidus with clear sensitivity towards desmopressin. Given his renal impairment he was treated with oral fluids in the first instance with the instruction to drink to thirst. Given that he had been trying to reduce his oral intake to limit his polyuria it was felt that oral fluids alone would correct his renal impairment which was what was subsequently observed. Intravenous fluids contain varying amounts of sodium can lead to under or over correction so if it is possible to treat with oral fluids that is preferable and can provide a buffer towards over-rapid changes.

Given the biochemical picture and clinical symptoms he was commenced on desmopressin. Given that he was clinically stable 100 μg of desmopressin was given orally three times per day with symptomatic benefit and a rise in urine osmolarity. The dose of desmopressin was increased to 400 μg daily in divided doses.

Given that this was thought to be an ICI-induced pathology there was discussion regarding the use of corticosteroids in this case. It is unknown as to whether this changes the course of the pathological process and is near-impossible to study given the rarity of the condition. In this case the patient was also treated with 60 mg prednisolone orally followed by a standard weaning course of 10 mg prednisolone every 3 days with a slower wean at the end of the schedule at 10mg and 5mg doses.

Follow Up and Outcome

He completed the course of prednisolone 7 weeks later. Following completion of steroids and observed biochemical stability the desmopressin was weaned with biochemical and symptomatic monitoring. He was weaned to 50 μg three times a day initially before weaning completely. A repeat water deprivation test illustrated near normal results 6 months after the onset of symptoms with a baseline urine osmolality of 190 mOsm/kg rising to 606 mOsm/kg post deprivation. Further follow up with biochemical monitoring and improvement in osmolarities in the presence of a normal sodium confirmed the resolution of the DI. He received no further ICI treatment but had ongoing surveillance with no recurrence of his melanoma in the 4 year follow up period to date.

Summary

This is a rare case with (cranial) DI associated with ICI therapy. The patient presented with classical symptoms of polydipsia and polyuria and suggestive labs with the biochemical picture of hypernatraemia with a low urinary osmolality and a high serum osmolality. The diabetes insipidus was confirmed with a water deprivation test and the correction of the biochemical abnormalities with desmopressin/corticosteroid confirmed and improved his cranial diabetes insipidus. Following a 6 month follow up period the patient's clinical and biochemical picture normalised and withdrawal of pharmacological treatment did not lead to a clinical recurrence leading to the diagnosis of transient diabetes insipidus secondary to ICI therapy. Summary of the timeline events is shown in Fig. 11.2.

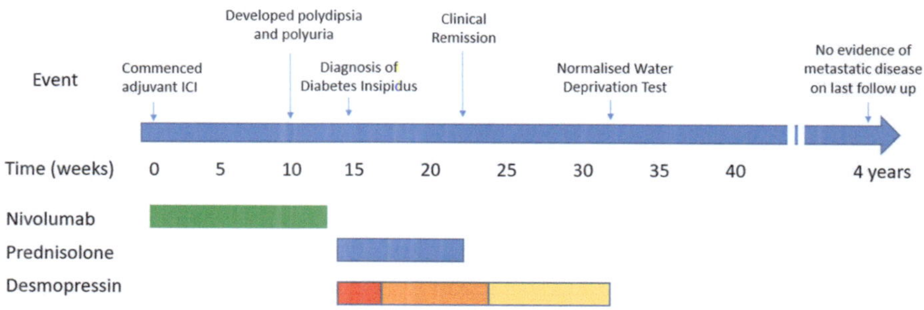

Fig. 11.2 Summary of timeline events: Timepoint of 0 is the commencement of ICI treatment. Desmopressin treatment is illustrated as the time on the starting dose (red, week 13–15), increased dose (orange, week 15–22) and a weaning dose (yellow, week 22–30)

Discussion

DI is a condition whereby there is dysregulation of antidiuretic hormone (ADH) either as a result of reduced production in the posterior pituitary (cranial DI) or by insensitivity to it in the kidney (nephrogenic DI) with a water deprivation test alongside the administration of desmopressin being used to differentiate between the two [1, 2]. Either mechanism results in the excretion of large volumes of hypotonic, dilute urine and patients typically present with polyuria, nocturia and polydipsia [1]. New diabetes mellitus should always be excluded in patients suspected of having DI. In cancer patients, DI can results from structural compression from a malignant mass, occur as a paraneoplastic phenomenon, as a result of prior radiotherapy or as a consequence of systemic anticancer treatment (SACT) including ICIs.

ICI-induced DI is a very rare occurrence, with the WHO global database of individual case safety reports illustrating that it accounts of 0.2% (16/6089) of ICI-related endocrinopathies [3]. Additionally in patients on ICIs DI can co-present with more global hypophysitis so presentation with a headache can occur. Additionally patients may have abnormalities in the other pituitary hormonal axes resulting in a complex biochemical picture. Therefore, it is key in these patients to do a complete workup and evaluation including biochemical investigations and cranial imaging. The ICI-induced cases described in the literature are of cranial DI with response to desmopressin rather than nephrogenic DI. Additionally the majority of cases show a degree of reversibility with patients only requiring desmopressin for a period of weeks which is unusual and out of keeping with the other ICI-induced endocrinopathies which tend to result in permanent hormonal deficit. Interestingly the literature also suggests that the use of corticosteroids in these patients is common, unlike other endocrinopathies [4]. Therefore, if a patient is diagnosed with ICI-induced DI, then weaning of corticosteroids and desmopressin should be considered following clinical stabilisation.

References

1. Baldewag SE, Ball A, Brooke A, et al. Inpatient management of cranial diabetes insipidus; Society for Endocrinology Clinical Guidance. Endocr Connect. 2018;7(7):G8–G11.
2. Wass J. How to do a water deprivation test: interpretation of results. Endocr Abstr. 2008;15:S61.
3. Bai X, Chen X, Wu X, Huang Y, Zhuang Y, Chen Y, et al. Immune checkpoint inhibitor-associated pituitary adverse events: an observational, retrospective, disproportionality study. J Endocrinol Invest. 2020;43:1473–83.
4. Barnabei A, Strigari L, Corsello A, Paragliola RM, Falzone L, Salvatori R, Corsello SM, Torino F. Immune checkpoint inhibitor-induced central diabetes insipidus: looking for the needle in the haystack or a very rare side-effect to promptly diagnose? Front Oncol. 2022;12:798517.

Part IV
Gastroenterology

Chapter 12
Appendicitis Post Immune Checkpoint Inhibitor Therapy

Antony Mathew, Yang Lu, Malek Shatila, Nizar M. Tannir, Bilal Siddiqui, and Yinghong Wang

Abbreviations

CECT	Contrast Enhanced CT
CT	Computed Tomography
ICI	Immune checkpoint inhibitor

Case Presentation

A 50-year-old man with a history of metastatic prostate cancer presented to the emergency room with a 10-day history of abdominal pain, decreased oral intake and nausea. He had previously undergone radical prostatectomy and was subsequently

A. Mathew
Department of Internal Medicine, The University of Texas Health Science Center, Houston, TX, USA
e-mail: AntonyMathew@mhd.com

Y. Lu
Department of Nuclear Medicine, The University of Texas MD Anderson Cancer Center, Houston, TX, USA
e-mail: YLu10@mdanderson.org

M. Shatila · Y. Wang (✉)
Department of Gastroenterology, Hepatology & Nutrition, The University of Texas MD Anderson Cancer Center, Houston, TX, USA
e-mail: ywang59@mdanderson.org

N. M. Tannir · B. Siddiqui
Department of Genitourinary Medical Oncology, The University of Texas MD Anderson Cancer Center, Houston, TX, USA
e-mail: ntannir@mdanderson.org; BASiddiqui@mdanderson.org

Y. Wang (ed.), *Challenging Cases in Immunotherapy Related Organ Toxicities*,
https://doi.org/10.1007/978-3-031-83533-9_12

treated with androgen deprivation therapy. He most recently received ipilimumab for 3 doses approximately 4 months prior to presentation on a clinical trial. He reported bilateral lower quadrant abdominal pain that had been progressively worsening despite the use of tramadol at home. Initially his symptoms were associated with constipation, however, this changed to loose stools after taking Milk of Magnesia. He also reported intermittent fevers and chills with maximal temperature of 102.7 °F at home. Otherwise, the review of systems is negative. Past medical history included hypertension, Hashimoto thyroiditis, acid reflux, and asthma. His home medications included levothyroxine 75 µg daily, lisinopril 10 mg daily, pantoprazole 40 mg daily, albuterol 90 µg Q4 hours as needed. Family history and social history were unremarkable.

On the day of presentation, he was afebrile, normotensive, heart rate 94 beats per minute, saturating 100% on room air. On physical exam he was noted to have mild tenderness to palpation of the right lower quadrant of the abdomen, with no rebound tenderness or guarding. Laboratory results on admission were summarized in Table 12.1, and radiological images at different timepoints were demonstrated in Figs. 12.1 and 12.2.

Table 12.1 Lab Variables

WBC	7.6 × 10^9/L
Hemoglobin	**8.6 g/dL (L)**
Platelets	300 × 10^9/L
Sodium	**133 mEq/L (L)**
Potassium	4.7 mEq/L
Chloride	98 mEq/L
Bicarbonate	30 mEq/L
BUN	9 mg/dL
Creatinine	0.89 mg/dL
Glucose	92 mg/dL
Calcium	8.5 mg/dL
Magnesium	**2.9 mg/dL (H)**
Phosphate	4.5 mg/dL
Albumin	3.4 g/dL
Clostrioides difficile DNA	Negative
Lactoferrin	Negative
Blood cultures	Negative
Urine cultures	Negative

Lab reference range: Hemoglobin—13.3–17.4 g/dL; sodium—136–145 mEq/L; magnesium—1.6–2.6 mg/dL

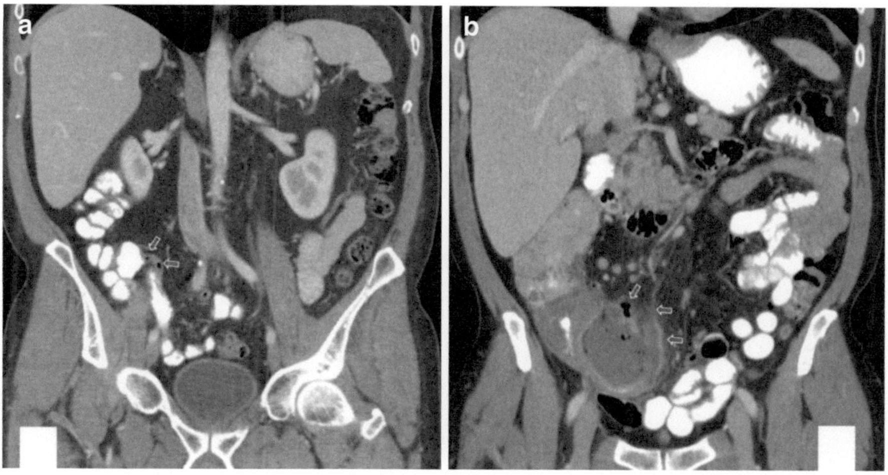

Fig. 12.1 Radiological features of appendicitis and complication: (**a**) Baseline: patent and normal appearing appendix (arrows: coronal view of contrast enhanced CT); (**b**) Event onset: the appendix perforated with large rim-enhancing partially walled off collection containing multiple small pockets of air adjacent to the cecum suggesting a formed abscess, with associated mesentery fat stranding (arrows: coronal view of contrast enhanced CT) [3]

Differential Diagnoses

Both infectious and non-infectious etiologies should be considered in the differential diagnosis. A few differentials include but are not limited to bacterial or viral enteritis/colitis, COVID-19, diverticulitis, immune mediated diarrhea and colitis (IMDC), and appendicitis etc. Given the onset of diarrhea was after laxative use and the lack of evidence supporting infectious etiologies and IMDC with negative lactoferrin, these became less likely. Lastly, with CT imaging showing appendicitis and lack of colitis, this mostly excluded other etiologies.

Follow Up and Outcome

Surgery was promptly consulted based on CT findings. Since the patient was clinically stable with no signs of peritonitis on abdominal exam, it was suspected that the perforation had occurred days prior to presentation. As such, surgical intervention was deferred. He was admitted to the hospital for conservative management with fasting, intravenous fluids and intravenous antibiotics of vancomycin, cefepime and metronidazole. Interventional radiology assessed the feasibility of abscess drain placement but deemed him as high risk given proximity of adjacent small bowel. Subsequently, the patient's condition improved with conservative management. A follow up CT scan 5 days later showed improvement in inflammatory changes when

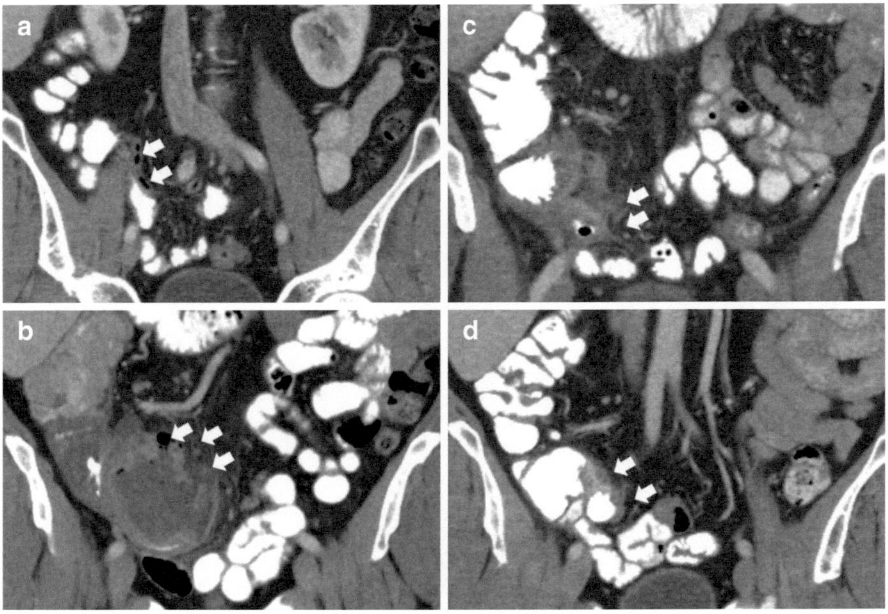

Fig. 12.2 Series of Interval Contrast Enhanced CT (CECT) scans: (**a**) Patent and normal appearing appendix (arrows in a: coronal view of contrast enhanced CT); (**b**) 21 days later, the appendix perforated with large rim-enhancing partially walled off collection containing multiple small pockets of air adjacent to the cecum, with associated mesentery fat stranding (arrows in b: coronal view of CECT). The image features are suggesting perforated appendix with formed abscess; (**c**) Follow up CECT images showed the perforation and local inflammation have improved 1 month later (arrows in c: coronal CECT); (**d**) Resolved at 10 weeks follow up CECT (arrows in **d**: coronal CECT)

compared to initial CT. He was then discharged home with a total 6-week regimen of intravenous ertapenem, oral linezolid and fluconazole. Despite completely recovering from immune checkpoint inhibitor appendicitis the patient had continued progression of his malignancy. He was unable to receive any further cancer treatment after this episode. He passed away while on hospice care 3 months later.

Case Summary

We presented a male patient in his 50s with metastatic prostate cancer on treatment with ipilimumab who presented with 10 days of abdominal pain and was found to have perforated appendicitis with abscess. Given clinical stability, reassuring physical exam and laboratory workup, the patient was managed conservatively with antibiotics and without surgery or abscess drainage. Interval CT imaging on antibiotic treatment showed improvement in intrabdominal findings. Timeline of events are summarized in Fig. 12.3.

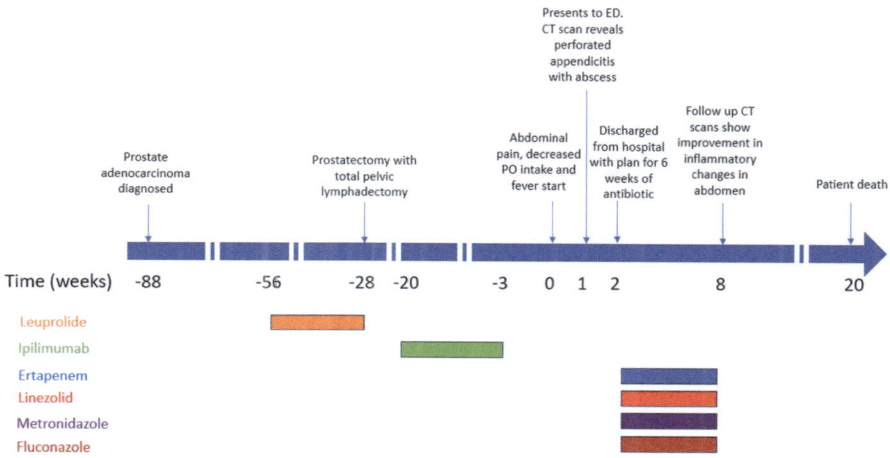

Fig. 12.3 Summary of events on timeline (Timepoint of 0 is the day of appendicitis event)

Discussion

Appendicitis as a possible new irAE is infrequently reported in the literature. Mangas et al. [1] and Papageorgiou et al. [2] initially published case reports about immune checkpoint inhibitor appendicitis and a case series by Wang et al. [3] have further brought this entity to light. These studies suggest that immune checkpoint inhibitor appendicitis is a unique clinical entity. Conventional appendicitis and immune checkpoint inhibitor appendicitis have similar presenting symptoms, radiographic findings, and complication rates but age of onset is higher for immune checkpoint inhibitor appendicitis [4, 5]. Standard management of conventional appendicitis i.e., appendectomy may not be a feasible option for select cancer patients due to medical complexity from the underlying cancer and other comorbid conditions [6]. Non-surgical management with antibiotics or drainage via interventional radiology is common. Broad spectrum antibiotics are the mainstay of treatment, but ideal agent and duration is unknown. Final antibiotic regimen should consider underlying comorbidities, and variance in severity of presenting illness.

References

1. Mangas C, Leoni-Parvex S, Spataro V. Silent acute appendicitis revealed by PET-CT during treatment with ipilimumab and nivolumab: a new immune-related adverse event. Cancer Immunol Immunother. 2020;69(11):2409–10. (In eng). https://doi.org/10.1007/s00262-020-02724-3.
2. Papageorgiou GI, Fergadis E, Skouteris N, et al. Perforated appendicitis induced by pembrolizumab: a case report and review of the literature. Anticancer Drug. 2021. (In eng). https://doi.org/10.1097/cad.0000000000001247.

3. Mathew A, Shatila M, Lai Z, Tan D, Oliva IC, Wang J, Alhalabi O, Zhang HC, Thomas A, Wang Y. Characteristics of appendicitis after immune checkpoint inhibitor therapy among cancer patients. J Cancer Res Clin Oncol. 2022;149:4591–9. https://doi.org/10.1007/s00432-022-04367-6.
4. Körner H, Söndenaa K, Söreide JA, et al. Incidence of acute nonperforated and perforated appendicitis: age-specific and sex-specific analysis. World J Surg. 1997;21(3):313–7. (In eng). https://doi.org/10.1007/s002689900235.
5. Addiss DG, Shaffer N, Fowler BS, et al. The epidemiology of appendicitis and appendectomy in the United States. Am J Epidemiol. 1990;132(5):910–25. (In eng). https://doi.org/10.1093/oxfordjournals.aje.a115734.
6. Carr NJ. The pathology of acute appendicitis. Ann Diagn Pathol. 2000;4(1):46–58. (In eng). https://doi.org/10.1016/s1092-9134(00)90011-x.

Chapter 13
Cholecystitis Related to Immune Checkpoint Inhibitor Therapy

Malek Shatila, Krishnavathana Varatharajalu, Gottumukkala Subba Raju, Anusha S. Thomas, and Yinghong Wang

Abbreviations

BMI	body mass index
CCI	Charlson Comorbidity Index
CT	computed tomography
ECOG	Eastern Cooperative Oncology Group performance status
irAEs	immune-related adverse events
IV	intravenous

Case One

Our first patient is a Hispanic woman in her 50 s (body mass index [BMI] of 26, Charlson Comorbidity Index [CCI] of 7, Eastern Cooperative Oncology Group performance status [ECOG] of 3, and a history of gallstones and chronic diarrhea) who first presented in 2013 with epigastric pain radiating to the back, jaundice, and elevated bilirubin and liver function tests. Imaging at the time showed a mass at the head of the pancreas with suspicious lesions in the liver, and biopsies confirmed metastatic pancreatic cancer. She received multiple treatment regimens over the years but continued to have progressive disease. Most recently, she was enrolled in a clinical trial and started on immune-checkpoint inhibitors with a combination of pembrolizumab and acalabrutinib. One month after starting treatment, the patient was found to have elevated liver enzymes and bilirubin (see Table 13.1). She was started on 60 mg oral prednisone daily on suspicion of treatment-related

M. Shatila · K. Varatharajalu · G. S. Raju · A. S. Thomas · Y. Wang (✉)
Department of Gastroenterology, Hepatology & Nutrition, The University of Texas MD Anderson Cancer Center, Houston, TX, USA
e-mail: MShatila@mdanderson.org; KVaratharajalu@mdanderson.org; GSRaju@mdanderson.org; ASThomas1@mdanderson.org; ywang59@mdanderson.org

Y. Wang (ed.), *Challenging Cases in Immunotherapy Related Organ Toxicities*,
https://doi.org/10.1007/978-3-031-83533-9_13

Table 13.1 Laboratory values at different timepoints in disease course

	Two weeks prior to presentation	One week prior to presentation	Day of presentation	One week after presentation	At discharge
White blood cells (1000 cells/uL) Normal: 4.0–11.0 K/uL	3	–	**12.3 (H)**	5.3	5.1
AST (U/L) Normal: ≤32 U/L	67	**130 (H)**	65	23	24
ALT (U/L) Normal: ≤33 U/L	84	**146 (H)**	**183 (H)**	52	42
Alkaline phosphatase (U/L) Normal: 35–104 U/L	–	–	**263 (H)**	–	**302 (H)**
Total bilirubin (mg/dL) Normal: ≤1.2 mg/dL	0.8	**1.5 (H)**	**1.5 (H)**	1.1	0.8
Direct bilirubin (mg/dL) Normal: ≤0.3 mg/dL	–	**1.1 (H)**	**0.8 (H)**	–	0.6

Abbreviations: *AST* aspartate transaminase, *ALT* alanine transaminase, *H* high value

autoimmune hepatitis. Aside from some intermittent nausea and vomiting, the patient was doing well clinically and hemodynamically stable.

A week after starting steroids, the patient arrived at the emergency department febrile (38.4 °C) with sharp and stabbing abdominal pain that started as severe right upper quadrant pain but quickly generalized to affect the rest of the abdomen. This pain was not associated with food or fluid intake. She was started on intravenous (IV) antibiotics (tazobactam/piperacillin 4.5 g daily) and fluids and was admitted to the hospital for further work-up.

A computed tomography (CT) scan of the abdomen and pelvis on admission showed the stable pancreatic mass, as well as infiltrating/inflammatory changes extending from the head of the pancreas to the pancreaticoduodenal groove, the second portion of the duodenum, the hepatic flexure, and the gallbladder, with wall thickening of the gallbladder. No gallstones were visualized (Fig. 13.1).

She was not considered a good surgical candidate given her acute symptoms, leukocytosis, and severe malnutrition. Percutaneous cholecystostomy was therefore performed with a plan to re-evaluate for surgical intervention in a month after her symptoms and nutrition status improved. She was started on total parenteral nutrition, and blood and bile cultures were obtained. The cultures resulted positive for

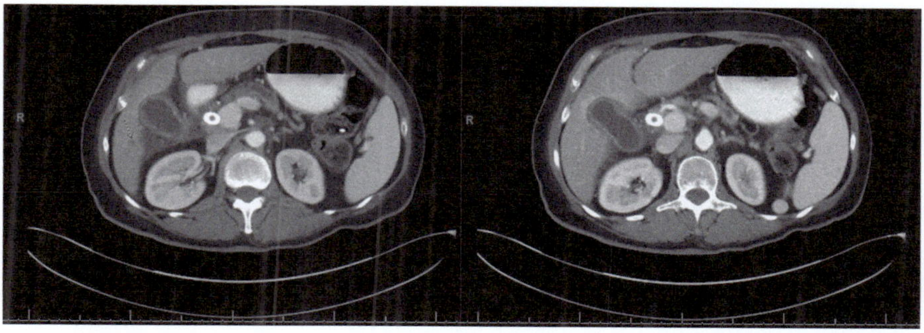

Fig. 13.1 CT abdomen showing signs of gallbladder inflammation

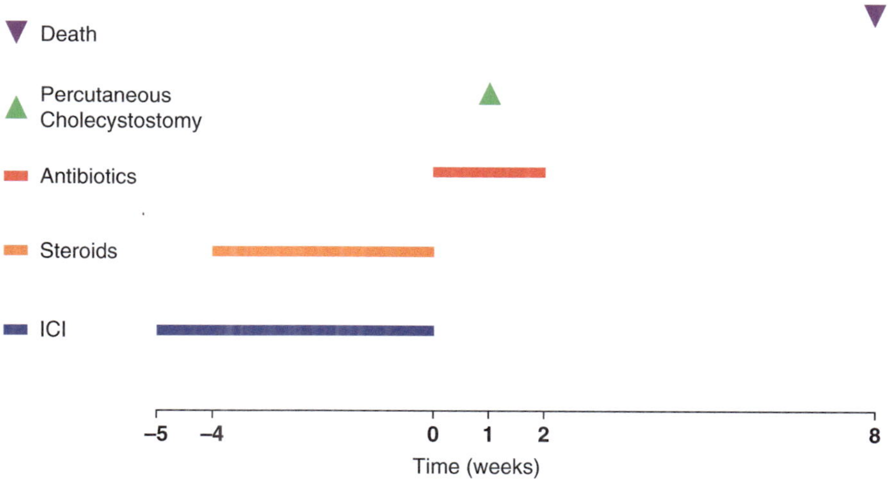

Fig. 13.2 Timeline of Patient #1's disease course with timepoint of 0 referring to symptom onset

Enterococcus faecalis and Stenotrophomonas, for which, the patient was switched to minocycline and ampicillin/sulbactam for the remainder of her hospital stay. Subsequently, she was discharged on oral amoxicillin/clavulanate and minocycline with continued improvement.

She was scheduled to have a follow-up appointment with the surgical oncology team to discuss an elective cholecystectomy, but unfortunately missed her appointment as she was admitted to hospice care and succumb to her malignancy 2 months after discharge. The timeline of her disease course can be found in Fig. 13.2 above.

Case Two

Our second patient is a white man in his 60s (BMI of 23.5, CCI of 8, ECOG of 3, no history of gallstones, and no pertinent comorbidities) who first presented in 2015 with difficulty swallowing that resulted in inadequate food intake and significant weight loss. An esophagogastroduodenoscopy at the time unveiled an esophageal adenocarcinoma at the gastroesophageal junction. The patient was treated with chemotherapy and an esophagectomy but was later found to have metastasis to the appendix. He developed peritoneal carcinomatosis that lead to a chronic, malignant small bowel obstruction that required total parenteral nutrition and the placement of a jejunostomy tube. He was known to have malignant pleural effusions and ascites. Most recently, he was treated with a combination of FOLFIRI (folinic acid, fluorouracil, and irinotecan) and nivolumab, with some signs of improvement.

One month after his eighth dose of nivolumab, the patient presented to the emergency department with fever (39.4 °C), hypotension, vomiting, and altered mental status. He was minimally communicative but expressed neck pain and severe pain upon palpation of the right upper quadrant of the abdomen on physical exam. His blood pressure improved slightly with IV hydration, but there was a significant concern for sepsis, and he was started on IV vancomycin and piperacillin/tazobactam then was switched to cefepime, vancomycin, and ampicillin out of concern for meningitis given the patient's neck pain. His laboratory evaluations can be found (Table 13.2).

Table 13.2 Laboratory values at different timepoints in disease course

	Ten days prior to presentation	Day of presentation	One week after presentation	At discharge
White blood cells (1000 cells/uL) Normal: 4.0–11.0 K/uL	5.4	**13.0 (H)**	6.1	5.7
AST (U/L) Normal: ≤32 U/L	20	34	24	24
ALT (U/L) Normal: ≤33 U/L	29	35	32	25
Alkaline phosphatase (U/L) Normal: 35–104 U/L	116	**192 (H)**	**207 (H)**	**210 (H)**
Total bilirubin (mg/dL) Normal: ≤1.2 mg/dL	0.4	0.7	0.4	0.6
Direct bilirubin (mg/dL) Normal: ≤0.3 mg/dL	**0.4 (H)**	**0.6 (H)**	0.2	0.3

Abbreviations: *AST* aspartate transaminase, *ALT* alanine transaminase, *H* High value

Workup for sepsis was carried out including a lumbar puncture and meningitis panel, urinalysis and culture, respiratory panel, and blood cultures. All of these turned out negative and on the second day of admission a gallbladder ultrasound was ordered (Fig. 13.2) which detected biliary sludge, gallbladder dilation, wall thickening, and pericholecystic fluid, with a suspected perforation as well as a hepatic abscess. This was confirmed with CT imaging showing gallbladder perforation and a hepatic abscess communicating freely with the distended gallbladder (redemonstrated on ultrasound imaging as seen in Fig. 13.3). His antibiotics were switched back to IV piperacillin/tazobactam in light of this.

The patient was deemed not a good candidate for surgical intervention. Instead, an urgent percutaneous cholecystostomy was performed, with cultures drawn from the liver abscess. The patient's fever abated with antibiotics and his blood pressure stabilized, yet his abdominal symptoms persisted. Abscess cultures grow E. coli, and the patient was switched to IV ceftriaxone with total treatment duration of 4 weeks.

Around a week after guided antibiotic treatment, a follow-up CT scan of the abdomen showed worsening malignant pleural effusions and ascites. The decision was made to proceed with drainage of both, and resume chemotherapy while inpatient. He received his first inpatient cycle of chemotherapy around a month after his initial admission given resolution of his fever and leukocytosis and significant improvement of his abdominal symptoms. Despite the fluctuation of abdominal pain and vomiting while receiving chemo, these symptoms resolved with supportive management, and a follow-up ultrasound showed improvement of the hepatic abscess and decompression of the gallbladder. He proceeded to receive a second round of chemotherapy before hospital discharge. He was unable to remove his cholecystostomy tube as it continued to drain until he passed away 4 months later due to his malignancy. A summary of this patient's disease course can be found in Fig. 13.4.

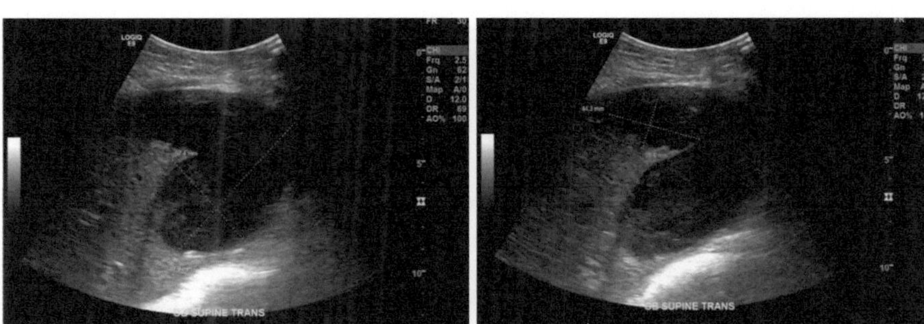

Fig. 13.3 Gallbladder ultrasound suggesting perforation and neighboring hepatic abscess

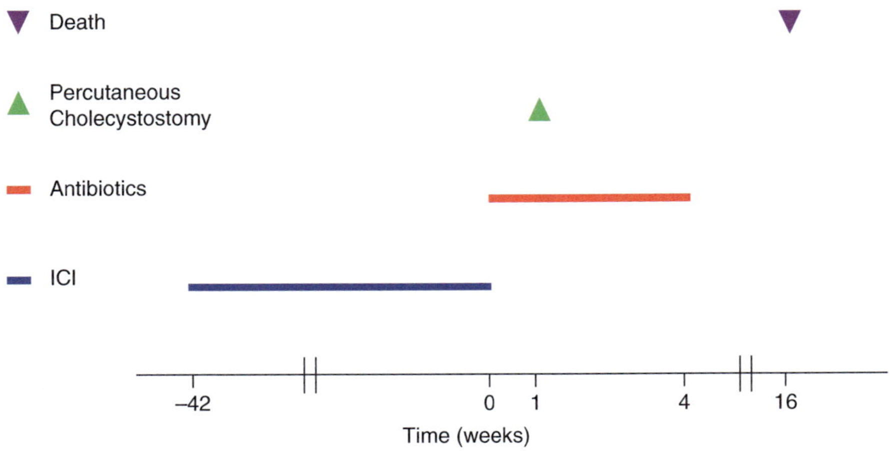

Fig. 13.4 Timeline of Patient #2's disease course with timepoint of 0 referring to symptom onset. Two parallel lines reflect a break in the x-axis

Discussion

Immune-mediated cholecystitis is a rare disease entity that will become more frequently encountered in the clinical setting given the increasing popularity of immune checkpoint inhibitors. The two cases presented here serve to emphasize important clinical themes while also highlighting the need to expand on existing guidelines to accommodate for this relatively novel disease.

The overall clinical picture of immune-mediated cholecystitis is more or less similar to its classical counterpart. The presenting symptoms are similar, and it appears that the standard management for classical cholecystitis is equally effective in the immune-mediated form. However, there are a few themes we can extrapolate from the two cases presented that bear mentioning:

1. Immune-mediated cholecystitis is one of many manifestations of immunotherapy toxicity, and may present in tandem with various other immune-related adverse events (irAEs). The presence of these other AEs complicates the management of these cases. For example, while antibiotics are a staple in the treatment of cholecystitis, there is evidence that they may worsen outcomes in immune-mediated colitis [1]. Moreover, a mild clinical presentation of cholecystitis with liver enzymes reflecting a hepatocellular pattern of injury may be mistaken for immune-mediated hepatitis, and appropriate evaluation and treatment may be delayed. The presence of other irAEs may affect the patient's eligibility for surgical management as well.
2. The role of gallstones or biliary sludge in the pathogenesis of immune-mediated cholecystitis is uncertain. Our first case had a history of gallstones, but they were not a causative factor in her disease. Our second case had no history of gallstones, nor were any detected upon his initial evaluation. For this reason, it may

be safe to consider immune-mediated cholecystitis a form of acalculous cholecystitis. However, there may be a role for gallstones or biliary sludge in precipitating the onset of this irAE.

3. There are a few unique aspects to management of immune-mediated cholecystitis. The role of surgery remains to be elucidated. Conceivably, patients who improve on antibiotics alone with no plan to resume immunotherapy may not have a recurrence of their disease. On the other hand, in patients with cholecystitis severe enough to necessitate discontinuation of their immunotherapy, surgery may not only be curative but also preclude any possibility of disease recurrence, allowing for safe resumption of immunotherapy. Given the complexity of oncological cases however, surgery may not always be a viable option for treatment. In the acute setting, patients may not be stable enough to undergo cholecystectomy. In the longer term, these patients might deteriorate rapidly, as evidenced by our first case who was initially planned to undergo elective cholecystectomy, but rapidly deteriorated after hospital discharge, was admitted to hospice care, and passed away shortly after. It therefore seems that percutaneous cholecystostomy may play a more important role in managing these cases.
4. The role of steroids, which are the mainstay of treatment for most irAEs, is still unclear in immune-mediated cholecystitis.

Conclusion

Immune-mediated cholecystitis is a rare and novel disease entity that is relatively understudied. It shares features in common with classical cholecystitis but also has its idiosyncrasies that make it different enough to warrant special consideration. These differences arise primarily from the unique population—patients with cancer—that is likely to struggle with this affliction as well as the pathophysiology of this disease (immune-mediated rather than mechanical). The cases presented in this chapter encourage a tailored approach to management that accommodates the complexity of oncology patients. They also make salient the potential avenues for research into (1) appropriate treatment options for immune-mediated cholecystitis and (2) the reconciliation of current guidelines for classical cholecystitis with this novel entity and complex demographic.

Reference

1. Abu-Sbeih H, et al. Impact of antibiotic therapy on the development and response to treatment of immune checkpoint inhibitor-mediated diarrhea and colitis. J Immunother Cancer. 2019;7(1):242.

Chapter 14
Colitis Following Immune Checkpoint Inhibitor Therapy

Malek Shatila, Krishnavathana Varatharajalu, Herbert Dupont, Robert Jenq, Franck Carbonnel, Stephen Hanauer, Anusha S. Thomas, and Yinghong Wang

Abbreviations

CT	computed tomography
CTCAE	Common Terminology Criteria for Adverse Events
CTLA-4	cytotoxic T-lymphocyte antigen 4
IBD	inflammatory bowel disease
ICI	immune checkpoint inhibitor
PD—L1	programmed death ligand-1

M. Shatila · K. Varatharajalu · A. S. Thomas · Y. Wang (✉)
Department of Gastroenterology, Hepatology & Nutrition, The University of Texas MD Anderson Cancer Center, Houston, TX, USA
e-mail: MShatila@mdanderson.org; KVaratharajalu@mdanderson.org; ASThomas1@mdanderson.org; ywang59@mdanderson.org

H. Dupont
Department of Infectious Disease, The University of Texas School of Public Health, Houston, TX, USA
e-mail: Herbert.L.Dupont@uth.tmc.edu

R. Jenq
Department of Genomic Medicine, The University of Texas MD Anderson Cancer Center, Houston, TX, USA
e-mail: RRJenq@mdanderson.org

F. Carbonnel
Department of Gastroenterology, Université Paris Saclay 11, Le Kremlin-Bicêtre, France
e-mail: franck.carbonnel@aphp.fr

S. Hanauer
Department of Medicine, Division of Gastroenterology and Hepatology, Northwestern University, Chicago, IL, USA
e-mail: shanauer@northwestern.edu

Y. Wang (ed.), *Challenging Cases in Immunotherapy Related Organ Toxicities*,
https://doi.org/10.1007/978-3-031-83533-9_14

PPI	Proton Pump Inhibitor
SIT	selective immunosuppressive therapy
UCEIS	Ulcerative Colitis Endoscopic Index of Severity

Case Presentation

Our patient was an otherwise healthy female in her 70s diagnosed with small cell lung cancer that initially responded well to treatment with a carboplatin/etoposide combination followed by the PARP inhibitor veliparib. This response was short-lived however, and follow-up imaging showed disease progression with adrenal metastasis. She was started on programmed death ligand-1 (PD-L1) inhibitor atezolizumab interspersed with radiotherapy to the adrenal glands, and she slowly began to improve.

Six months after her initial infusion, she presented to the emergency department complaining of a one-month history of watery diarrhea that started a few days after her last atezolizumab dose and gradually worsened over the month. This was accompanied by epigastric pain, nausea, and vomiting. Laboratory values can be found in Table 14.1 and were unremarkable aside from elevated fecal lactoferrin and calprotectin suggestive of inflammatory bowel disease. Imaging showed mild dilation of the bile duct secondary to an irregular mass at the pancreatic head suspicious for pancreatitis, otherwise the rest of the gastrointestinal tract appeared unremarkable. She was treated for acute pancreatitis with intravenous hydration, pain control, and anti-emetics, and was discharged symptom-free within a week of admission. It was deemed a case of pancreatitis with an unknown cause (endoscopic biopsy of the mass was negative for malignancy and autoimmune pancreatitis was considered unlikely given negative IgG4).

The patient continued her atezolizumab infusions for several months after this incident and was doing well albeit a mild, intermittent diarrhea. This lasted until her 16th ICI cycle, after which she had a sudden worsening of her ailment with 8–12 bowel movements per day (grade 3 diarrhea as per Common Terminology Criteria

Table 14.1 Laboratory evaluations pertaining to immune-mediated colitis at different timepoints in the disease course

Laboratory tests	At presentation	3 months after	6 months after	1.5 years after	3 years after	Final values
Gastrointestinal multiplex panel	Negative	–	Negative	–	Negative	–
C. diff DNA test	Negative	–	Negative	–	Negative	–
Fecal lactoferrin	**Positive**	**Positive**	**Positive**	**Positive**	**Positive**	Negative
Fecal calprotectin (mcg/gm)	**157 (H)**	**170 (H)**	**227 (H)**	**68.6 (H)**	**296 (H)**	<50.0 (N)

Interpretation: (H)—high; (N)—normal; a positive fecal lactoferrin test suggests the presence of inflammation in the colon. Fecal calprotectin (mcg/gm) normal: <50.0 mcg/gm

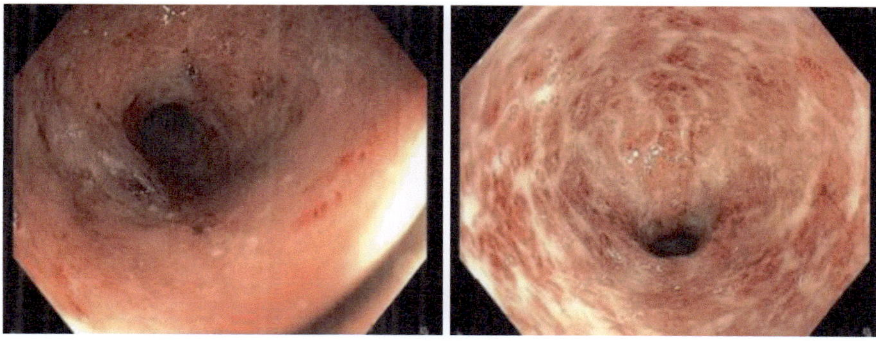

Fig. 14.1 Colonoscopy finding. Mayo grade 3 colitis with erosions, friability, loss of vascularity, and shallow ulceration throughout the colon

for Adverse Events [CTCAE] grading) and hematochezia (grade 2 colitis), warranting a hospital admission and discontinuation of ICI. Upon further conversation with the patient, it was discovered that she had a history of chronic diarrhea that was suspicious for a potential underlying inflammatory bowel disease (IBD) that was not diagnosed. Given negative stool infectious work-up and positive stool inflammatory biomarkers (Table 14.1), she was thus started on high dose steroids and infliximab. Colonoscopy revealed mucosal congestion and ulceration extending from the sigmoid colon to the hepatic flexure, and pathology revealed severe active inflammation suggestive of checkpoint inhibitor associated injury as seen in Fig. 14.1. The scope was not advanced past the hepatic flexure to avoid the risk of perforation.

The patient had an initial improvement on the combination of steroids and infliximab and was discharged with a plan to continue infliximab for two additional doses. However, this failed to adequately control her symptoms and within a few months, she returned to the hospital with new-onset severe hematochezia and abdominal pain. At this point, she underwent another colonoscopy which showed persistent inflammation, and the decision was made to switch the patient to vedolizumab.

Vedolizumab proved to be an effective treatment for her condition. Her symptoms resolved, and a follow-up scope after her second dose showed only mild patchy inflammation in the ascending colon (Fig. 14.2)—a significant improvement from her previous findings. Unfortunately, the patient developed arthralgias as well as symptoms of an upper respiratory tract infection like sinus congestion, coughing, and fever (100.6 °F) soon after her second dose, which were thought to be a reaction to the vedolizumab. Her symptoms quickly improved after treatment with prednisone and diphenhydramine. The primary oncology team resumed ICI promptly given cancer progression on restaging, considering the patient's previous good response to it. The patient was symptom-free at this point in time, but there was a significant concern for recurrence of her diarrhea upon resumption of atezolizumab. She had originally been planned to resume atezolizumab with concurrent

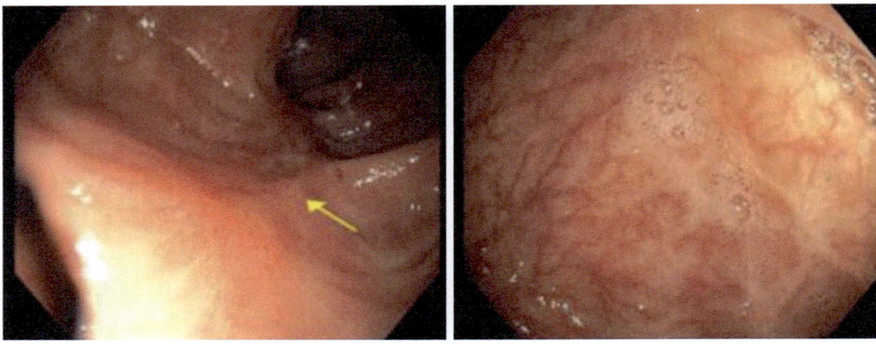

Fig. 14.2 Endoscopy slide showing improvement in previous inflammation with mild patchy inflammation in the ascending colon and a healing ulcer in the transverse colon (yellow arrow)

vedolizumab therapy to ensure sustained control of her diarrhea, but because of her previous adverse reaction to the drug, she was started on ustekinumab instead. Atezolizumab was successfully resumed and she continued to improve from an oncology standpoint, with a laparoscopic adrenalectomy performed to eliminate the last vestiges of her disease.

As ideal as it would be for her to case to end here, it is unfortunately only the beginning. One month after her surgery, she developed upper respiratory tract symptoms similar to what she experienced before—a suspected adverse reaction to ustekinumab this time—with a recurrence of her diarrhea and hematochezia not long after her ustekinumab infusions were discontinued. The decision was then made to proceed with fecal microbiota transplantation. Her symptoms resolved within 1 week of her procedure, and she was able to safely resume maintenance atezolizumab for another 9 months. She had a brief period of mild diarrhea which resolved with loperamide, and her calprotectin at this time was the lowest it had been at 68.6 mcg/gm (Table 14.1).

At around 3 years after first starting ICI, our patient had her third major episode of diarrheal illness with up to 13 bowel movements per day (CTCAE grade 3). Stool infectious work-up was negative, and fecal calprotectin had risen to 296 mcg/gm (Table 14.1). Prednisone was prescribed while the patient was frantically scheduled for a second FMT, and atezolizumab was held. Despite the success of her first procedure, the second FMT did not achieve the complete resolution of her GI symptom. Her diarrhea improved to grade 1 within a few days of the procedure. She also had persistent inflammation with no change in histology on follow-up colonoscopy 2 months later. Though not a full remission, the patient was satisfied with this improvement, and the oncology team had no immediate plans to resume ICI.

Almost a year after this second FMT, it was discovered that her primary cancer had metastasized to the brain and there was suddenly an urgent need to restart her previous ICI; the only obstacle in the way was her mild but persistent loose stool. For this reason, our patient underwent a third FMT which effectively cured her

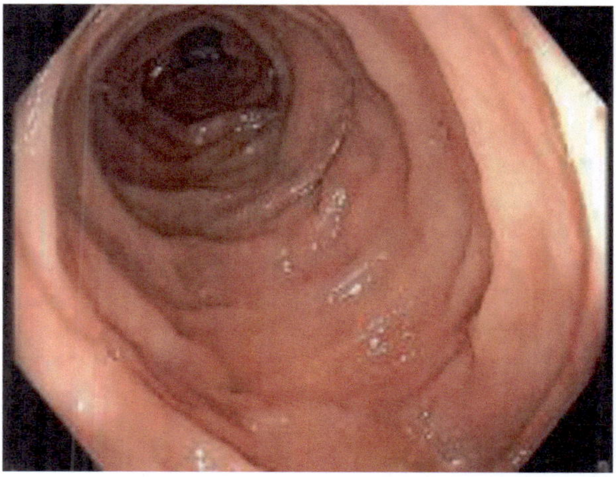

Fig. 14.3 Image of final endoscopic findings with entire colon normal except for some edema

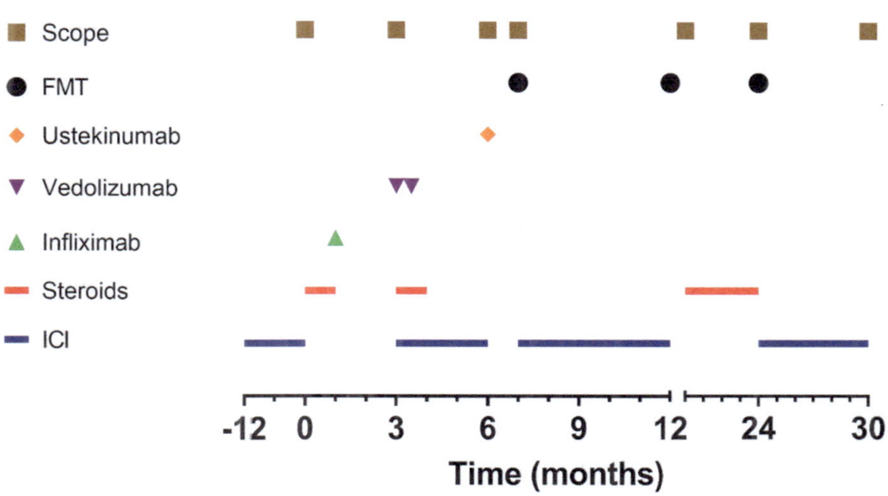

Fig. 14.4 Timeline of the patient's IMC disease course with timepoint of 0 reflecting symptom onset

colitis. Within 2 weeks, she had a complete and sustained resolution of her diarrhea, and the inflammation in her colon improved significantly on follow-up scope a few months later, with a macroscopically normal examination and only mild inflammation on histology (Fig. 14.3). After a long and arduous colitis course with multiple lines of treatment, her symptoms had finally resolved. She was able to resume atezolizumab following the third FMT and underwent Gamma Knife surgery and remained in great condition until today. A summary of her disease course can be found in Fig. 14.4.

Case Summary

Our case was that of an elderly woman with small cell lung cancer who presented with grade 3 diarrhea and grade 2 colitis after 1 year of immune checkpoint inhibition with atezolizumab that was refractory to treatment with steroids and infliximab. Her symptoms improved after administration of vedolizumab and ustekinumab, but she was unable to take these medications due to a severe allergic reaction (sinusitis and arthralgias). Her condition stabilized after fecal microbiota transplant which enabled her to resume atezolizumab long term with favorable cancer outcome, however, had recurrent colitis symptom after 1 year, which benefited from repeat fecal transplant treatment.

Discussion

Immune mediated colitis is the most common form of gastrointestinal toxicity to ICI therapy and can affect anywhere from 9–37% of patients [1]. It is typically more severe among patients receiving anti-CTLA-4 inhibition [2, 3] and its presentation and pathophysiology are highly reminiscent of IBD. Because of this, most treatment strategies have been adapted from IBD guidelines.

Symptom severity of IMC is measured by the Common Terminology Criteria for Adverse Events and has been shown to correlate poorly with endoscopic or histologic inflammation [4]. Endoscopic evaluation is therefore an essential aspect of management as early scoping has been associated with shorter symptom and steroid treatment durations, and certain high risk features such as deep or large ulcers, or extensive inflammation predicted the need for selective immunosuppressive therapy and longer and more frequent hospitalizations [5]. To date, no endoscopic scoring system has been validated specifically for use in IMC, but many such as the UCEIS and the Mayo score have been adopted from IBD practice and shown to have prognostic value [6]. Biopsies are equally important to identify the underlying pathology and histological findings may predict the risk for recurrent symptoms [5].

Stool inflammatory biomarkers such as fecal lactoferrin and calprotectin can be used to stratify patient need for endoscopic evaluation. Lactoferrin was found to have a sensitivity of 90% and 70% in detecting histological and endoscopic inflammation respectively [5], and serial fecal calprotectin levels may be an effective means of monitoring disease activity and predicting remission [7]. Other forms of evaluation such as C-reactive protein levels and CT imaging have been shown to have a limited role in the work-up of IMC [4, 8, 9].

Though most instances of IMC are not as complex as the one presented here, several themes emerge that can be generalized to the management of other cases:

1. Various risk factors have been identified and linked to worse disease course in IMC including previous PPI use [10], specific intestinal microbiome signals [11], and concurrent gastrointestinal infections [12]. Previous inflammatory

bowel disease as suspected in this patient has been associated with an earlier time to onset and more severe clinical grade of colitis as well as a potentially higher incidence of IMC [13, 14]. This may in part explain our patient's difficult disease course. The long term outcomes of IMC have yet to be elucidated, but patients with this condition may be at a higher risk of developing colon adenomas [15]

2. While milder forms of IMC do not necessitate the discontinuation of ICI, more severe cases do. This creates a dynamic struggle between the need to restart ICI in order to combat the patient's primary disease, and the need to control the patient's colitis. A common question that arises is whether it is safe to restart immunotherapy following the development of immune mediated diarrhea and colitis. Up to 36% of cases recur following ICI resumption [16], but this risk can be significantly mitigated by introducing concurrent SIT alongside immunotherapy infusions [17], as seen with our patient. Unfortunately, our patient was unable to continue maintenance therapy given her adverse reactions to the medication—in these cases, FMT has proven to be a valuable treatment option that has great success at achieving clinical remission [18].
3. Selective immunosuppressive therapy (SIT) with infliximab or vedolizumab is the mainstay of treating steroid-refractory IMC. They have been shown to be equally effective at achieving clinical remission though infliximab is associated with a shorter time to clinical improvement at the cost of more frequent hospitalizations and recurrence [19]. Ustekinumab is an IL-12/23 inhibitor that is receiving increasing attention as a viable treatment for refractory disease [20]. Regardless of the type of SIT used, early treatment introduction was associated with fewer hospitalizations and steroid tapering attempts and a shorter steroid treatment course and symptom duration. Patients receiving three or more doses of SIT were more likely to achieve endoscopic and histological remission [21]. While our patient was able to complete three doses of infliximab, she had to prematurely discontinue both vedolizumab infusions and ustekinumab injections due to the adverse reaction she experienced. For this reason, it is hard to say whether SIT alone would have been enough to control her disease. Previous research suggests that vedolizumab can help achieve clinical remission in up to two thirds of patients who have previously failed infliximab [22]. Our patient showed significant improvement after treatment with vedolizumab, but it is unknown whether this response would have been sustained.
4. FMT has been shown to be effective as both a first-line and salvage treatment for IMC, achieving clinical remission in up to 71.4% and 85.1% of patients respectively [18, 23]. There are a few clinical trials in this field that are actively enrolling patients for FMT treatment (NCT04038619; NCT03819296). However, multiple FMTs may be needed to ensure symptom resolution as evidenced by this case. Our patient received different donor stool at each FMT she received, with manifestly variable results. This is in large part due to the different microbiome compositions of each donor sample and highlights the need for in depth research into specific intestinal microbiome patterns that are associated with better and worse outcomes. In our own clinical practice, we have noticed that there

are certain "superdonors" whose samples are particularly effective at improving symptoms across patients while other donor stools may not be as effective in all patients. Further research into this phenomenon could help enhance the efficacy of FMT.

References

1. Michot JM, et al. Immune-related adverse events with immune checkpoint blockade: a comprehensive review. Eur J Cancer. 2016;54:139–48.
2. Tran AN, et al. Immune checkpoint inhibitor-associated diarrhea and colitis: a systematic review and meta-analysis of observational studies. J Immunother. 2021;44(8):325–34.
3. Nielsen DL, et al. Immune checkpoint inhibitor-induced diarrhea and colitis: incidence and management. A systematic review and meta-analysis. Cancer Treat Rev. 2022;109:102440.
4. Wang Y, et al. Endoscopic and histologic features of immune checkpoint inhibitor-related colitis. Inflamm Bowel Dis. 2018;24(8):1695–705.
5. Abu-Sbeih H, et al. Importance of endoscopic and histological evaluation in the management of immune checkpoint inhibitor-induced colitis. J Immunother Cancer. 2018;6(1):95.
6. Cheung VTF, et al. Immune checkpoint inhibitor-related colitis assessment and prognosis: can IBD scoring point the way? Br J Cancer. 2020;123(2):207–15.
7. Zou F, et al. Fecal calprotectin concentration to assess endoscopic and histologic remission in patients with cancer with immune-mediated diarrhea and colitis. J Immunother Cancer. 2021;9(1)
8. Liu C, et al. Role of C-reactive protein in predicting the severity and response of immune-mediated diarrhea and colitis in patients with cancer. J Cancer. 2023;14(10):1913–9.
9. Ibarra Rovira J, et al. Role of abdominal and pelvic CT scans in diagnosis of patients with immunotherapy-induced colitis. J Immunother Precis Oncol. 2022;5(2):32–6.
10. Yin J, et al. Chronic use of proton pump inhibitors is associated with an increased risk of immune checkpoint inhibitor colitis in renal cell carcinoma. Clin Genitourin Cancer. 2022;20(3):260–9.
11. Dubin K, et al. Intestinal microbiome analyses identify melanoma patients at risk for checkpoint-blockade-induced colitis. Nat Commun. 2016;7:10391.
12. Ma W, et al. Outcomes of immune checkpoint inhibitor-related Diarrhea or colitis in cancer patients with superimposed gastrointestinal infections. Am J Clin Oncol. 2021;44(8):402–8.
13. Sleiman J, et al. Incidence of immune checkpoint inhibitor-mediated diarrhea and colitis (imDC) in patients with cancer and preexisting inflammatory bowel disease: a propensity score-matched retrospective study. J Immunother Cancer. 2021;9(6)
14. Abu-Sbeih H, et al. Immune checkpoint inhibitor therapy in patients with Preexisting inflammatory bowel disease. J Clin Oncol. 2020;38(6):576–83.
15. Machado AP, Shatila M, De Toni EN, Török HP, Philpott J, Zhao D, Zhou Y, Varatharajalu K, Shafi MA, Zhang HC, Thomas AS, Wang Y. Colon adenoma after diagnosis of immune checkpoint inhibitor–mediated colitis. J Cancer. 2023;14(14):2686–93.
16. Abu-Sbeih H, et al. Resumption of immune checkpoint inhibitor therapy after immune-mediated colitis. J Clin Oncol. 2019;37(30):2738–45.
17. Abu-Sbeih H, Zou F, Dutra B, Altan M, McQuade JL, Thompson JA, Thomas A, Wang Y. Maintenance immunosuppressive therapy with resumption of immune checkpoint inhibitor treatment to reduce recurrence of immune-mediated colitis. J Clin Oncol. 2021;39(15):2642.
18. Wang Y, Varatharajalu K, Shatila M, Shen SE, Herrera M, Gonzalez E, Wang XS, Thomas A, Jiang ZD, DuPont H. Effect of fecal transplantation on patients' reported outcome after immune checkpoint inhibitor colitis. J Clin Oncol. 2023;41(16):2645.

19. Zou F, et al. Efficacy and safety of vedolizumab and infliximab treatment for immune-mediated diarrhea and colitis in patients with cancer: a two-center observational study. J Immunother Cancer. 2021;9(11)
20. Shirwaikar Thomas A, et al. IL12/23 blockade for refractory immune-mediated colitis: 2-center experience. Am J Gastroenterol. 2023;118:1679–83.
21. Abu-Sbeih H, et al. Early introduction of selective immunosuppressive therapy associated with favorable clinical outcomes in patients with immune checkpoint inhibitor-induced colitis. J Immunother Cancer. 2019;7(1):93.
22. Abu-Sbeih H, et al. Outcomes of vedolizumab therapy in patients with immune checkpoint inhibitor-induced colitis: a multi-center study. J Immunother Cancer. 2018;6(1):142.
23. Wang Y, Varatharajalu K, Shatila M, Campbell MT, Msaouel P, Kovitz CA. First-line treatment of fecal microbiota transplantation for immune-mediated colitis. J Clin Oncol. 2023;41(16):2510.

Chapter 15
CMV Colitis with Perforation Post Immune Checkpoint Inhibitor Therapy with Multi-Organ Failure

Nitish Mittal, Christine Catinis, Yang Lu, Swaminathan Padmanabhan Iyer, Pablo C. Okhuysen, and Yinghong Wang

Abbreviations

ABVD	Doxorubicin, bleomycin, vinblastine, dacarbazine
BAL	Broncho-alveolar lavage
CT	Computed Tomography
CMV	Cytomegalovirus
DLCO	Diffuse capacity of the lungs for carbon monoxide
GI	Gastro-intestinal
ICI	Immune checkpoint inhibitor

N. Mittal · C. Catinis
Department of Internal Medicine, The University of Texas Health Science Center, Houston, TX, USA
e-mail: nitish.mittal@uth.tmc.edu; Christine.catinis@uth.tmc.edu

Y. Lu
Department of Nuclear Medicine, The University of Texas MD Anderson Cancer, Houston, TX, USA
e-mail: YLu10@mdanderson.org

S. P. Iyer
Department of Lymphoma and Myeloma, The University of Texas MD Anderson Cancer, Houston, TX, USA
e-mail: SPIyer@mdanderson.org

P. C. Okhuysen
Department of Infectious Diseases, Infection Control, and Employee Health, The University of Texas MD Anderson Cancer, Houston, TX, USA
e-mail: PCOkhuysen@mdanderson.org

Y. Wang (✉)
Department of Gastroenterology, Hepatology & Nutrition, The University of Texas MD Anderson Cancer Center, Houston, TX, USA
e-mail: ywang59@mdanderson.org

Y. Wang (ed.), *Challenging Cases in Immunotherapy Related Organ Toxicities*,
https://doi.org/10.1007/978-3-031-83533-9_15

IMDC	Immune-mediated diarrhea and colitis
irAEs	Immune-related adverse events

Case Presentation

This is a female in 70s with a history of atrial fibrillation s/p ablation, Hodgkin Lymphoma (received doxorubicin, bleomycin, vinblastine, dacarbazine (ABVD) about 20 years ago, four cycles of doxorubicin, radiation), metastatic urothelial carcinoma of the right renal pelvis 10 years ago who initially received gemcitabine and cisplatin with cancer progression based on 4 month follow up imaging, subsequently, switched to nivolumab and ipilimumab 5 months later. She developed significant diarrhea after first infusion of immune-checkpoint inhibitor (ICI) leading to hospitalization and received 4 days of methylprednisolone 1 mg/kg due to concern for immune-mediated diarrhea before being tested positive for Clostridioides difficile toxin and steroid was discontinued. Patient responded to oral vancomycin for 14 days. Patient received second cycle of ICI. Within 2 weeks, she was admitted to hospital for creamy loose stools with concern of ICI related gastro-intestinal (GI) toxicity. At this time, the Infectious work up (stool culture, stool ova and parasites, clostridioides difficile toxin) came back negative, however, lactoferrin was positive. Colonoscopy/histology was performed that showed no inflammation but only two adenoma polyps. The steroids were not initiated this time as no inflammation was noted. She received loperamide with symptomatic improvement, and patient got discharged on loperamide on as needed basis. She received another 3 cycles of ICI, then reported slight worsening shortness of breath above the baseline. Chest X-ray was ordered that showed atelectasis bilaterally at lower bases. The patient was started on inhaler and incentive spirometry. In the light of this, the ICI therapy was switched to just nivolumab monotherapy. Within 2 weeks, patient complained again about persistent shortness of breath which raised the concern of lung toxicity. Therefore, ICI therapy was halted.

Video bronchoscopy showed hemosiderin-laden macrophages suggestive of alveolar hemorrhage and decreased CD4:CD8 which was suggestive of pneumonitis related to ICI. Pulmonary function test showed improvement in diffuse capacity of the lungs for carbon monoxide (DLCO) from 40 to 60% after discontinuing ICI therapy. She was started on methylprednisolone 1 mg/kg for 7 days followed by oral prednisone 160 mg a day and tapered down to 80 mg daily in 4 weeks. She got admitted again with shortness of breath and diarrhea, CT (Computed tomography) of the chest showed new innumerable small sub-centimeter nodules measuring 1–2 mm with predominance in the bilateral upper lobes. No evidence of cavitation or consolidation was noted. Bronchoscopy was performed with broncho-alveolar lavage (BAL) that tested positive for cytomegalovirus (CMV). In the setting of elevated CMV titers, she was diagnosed with CMV pneumonitis and received ganciclovir. For diarrhea and hematochezia with severe abdominal pain, she underwent emergent sigmoidoscopy with biopsy revealing CMV inclusion body with ulceration. Her abdominal pain kept worsening and within 5 days of this acute presentation, the CT Abdomen and Pelvis confirmed sigmoid colon perforation (Fig. 15.1).

Laboratory testing is summarized in the Table 15.1 with remarkable abnormalities on the last hospital admission:

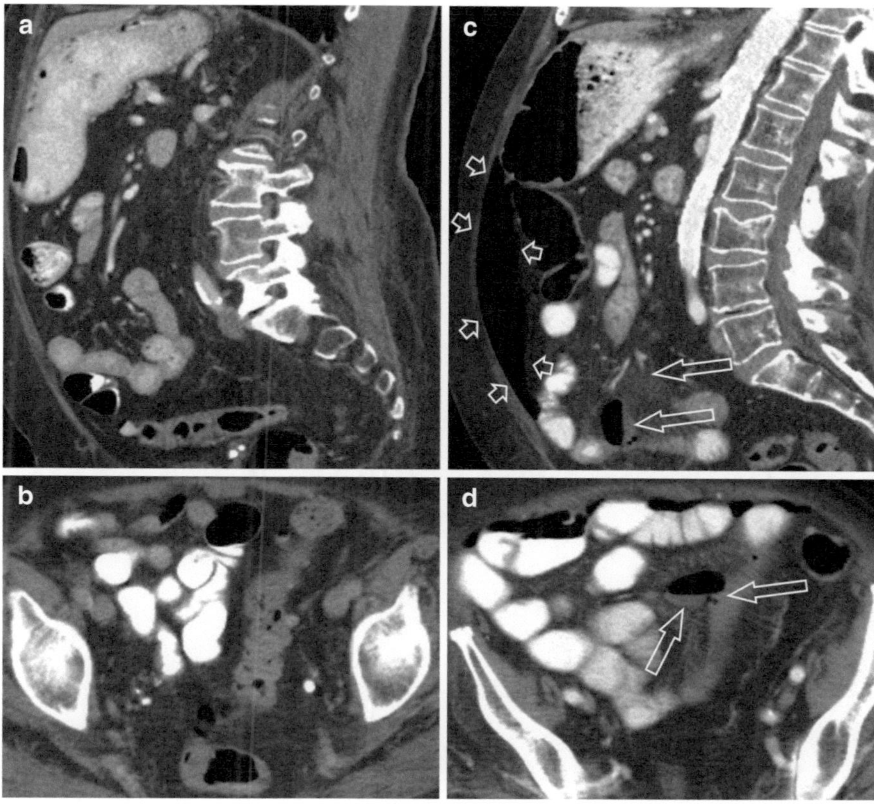

Fig. 15.1 CECT on initial presentation: (**a**) CECT sagittal view, (**b**) triangulated coronal view, showed no perforation of sigmoid colon; CECT 5 weeks later, (**c**) CECT sagittal view, (**d**) triangulated coronal view, showed perforation of sigmoid colon with local air fluid level and adjacent fat stranding (long arrows), and large peritoneal air collections (short arrows in **c**)

Table 15.1 Lab variables

WBC (4.0–11.0 K/μL)	3.9 K/μL
Hemoglobin (14.0–18.0 g/dL)	7.4 g/dL (low)
Platelets (140–440 K/μL)	40 K/μL (low)
Sodium (136–145 mEq/L)	131 mEq/L (low)
Potassium (3.5–5.1 mEq/L)	4.3 mEq/L
Chloride (98–107 mEq/L)	105 mEq/L
Bicarbonate (22–29 mEq/L)	27 mEq/L
BUN (6–23 mg/dL)	85 mg/dL (high)
Creatinine (0.67–1.17 mg/dL)	1.5 mg/dL (high)
Glucose (70–99 mg/dL)	233 mg/dL (high)
Magnesium (1.6–2.6 mg/dL)	1.6 mg/dL (low)
Calcium (8.4–10.2 mg/dL)	7.9 mg/dL
Phosphorus (2.5–4.5 mg/dL)	2.8 mg/dL
Albumin (3.5–5.2 g/dL)	2.2 g/dL (low)

Differential Diagnosis

The patient's presentation can have a list of differential diagnosis given the complexity of the cancer, cancer treatment, and surgical history. Given the multiple episodes of diarrhea after the start of ICI therapy, immune-mediated colitis, and/or concurrent infectious colitis (bacterial or viral colitis) were highest on differential. CT imaging confirmed perforated colitis likely secondary to cytomegalovirus colitis with background of immunotherapy colitis which was diagnosed with biopsy of sigmoid colon (Fig. 15.2).

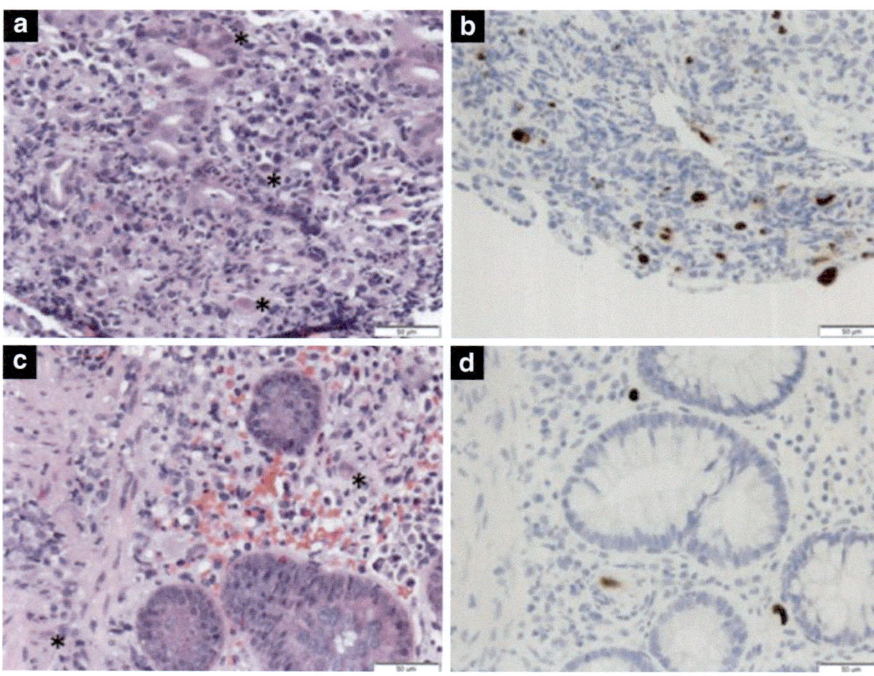

Fig. 15.2 (**a**) and (**c**) are hematoxylin and eosin stain with typical "owl's eyes" or basophilic intranuclear inclusion bodies; (**b**) and (**d**) are immunohistochemical stain (magnification, 20×). (Ref. [2])

Follow Up and Outcome

Surgery was promptly consulted based on CT findings. The surgery team performed sigmoid colectomy with end colostomy and abdominal washout. Unfortunately, despite surgery, due to severity of medical condition with co-morbidities, the patient continued to deteriorate with multi-organ failure. She was transitioned to hospice and passed away 20 days after surgery.

Case Summary

We present a case with metastatic urothelial carcinoma on ICI treatment, then developed multi-organ toxicities with complicated disease course of CMV pneumonitis and colitis, and bowel perforation post immunosuppressive therapy. The patient eventually passed away from multi-organ failure despite CMV treatment, and prompt surgery for perforation. Summary of the events is shown in Fig. 15.3.

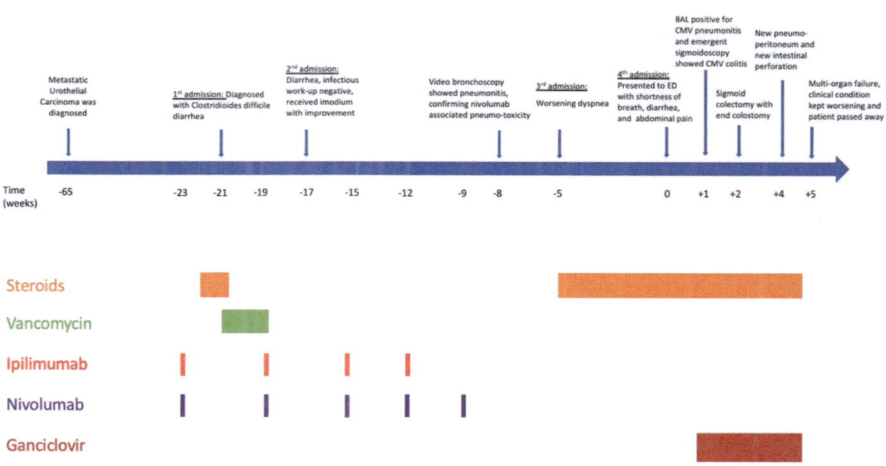

Fig. 15.3 Summary of events on timeline (Timepoint of 0 is the day of shortness of breath, diarrhea, and abdominal pain admission)

Discussion

Gastrointestinal side effects such as diarrhea and colitis are quite common related to cancer immunotherapy that are frequently associated with complicated disease course. Vasavada et al. showed that Clostridioides difficile infection can also be encountered in cancer patients treated with ICI, with overlapping symptoms, especially in the setting of immune-mediated diarrhea and colitis requiring immunosuppressants [1]. Moreover, evidence also reported that CMV and common GI bacterial and viral infections in cancer patients treated with ICI could increase the severity of the GI symptoms and even lead to perforation [2–5]. Interestingly, the anti-microbial treatments have not been found to be associated with better survival which raised the notion that these infections could be bystanders complicating the pre-existing inflammatory damage to the organs involved.

On the other hand, there have been data on intestinal perforation in patient receiving ICI treatment without infections. There are case series indicating a low incidence of bowel perforation after ICI treatment (0.6%), and about 40% of patients also had co-existing bowel inflammation as a potential contributing factor [6, 7]. Thus, early recognition and prompt intervention is critical to improve the patient outcomes. Clinicians should advise the patient about these side effects and closely monitor for early signs to ensure prompt treatments. The role of anti-microbial treatment in these vulnerable cases remains to be investigated in the context of standard ICI related organ toxicity management.

References

1. Vasavada S, Panneerselvam K, Amin R, Varatharajalu K, Okhuysen PC, Oliva IC, Wang J, Grivas P, Thomas AS, Wang Y. Clostridioides difficile infection in cancer patients receiving immune checkpoint inhibitors. Ann Gastroenterol. 2022;35(4):393.
2. Panneerselvam K, Szafron D, Amin RN, Wei D, Tan D, Altan M, Okhuysen PC, Shatila M, Raju GS, Thomas AS, Wang Y. Cytomegalovirus infection among patients with cancer receiving immune checkpoint inhibitors. Ann Gastroenterol. 2022;35(5):522.
3. Ma W, Gong Z, Abu-Sbeih H, Peng Y, Peng F, Zou F, Charabaty A, Okhuysen PC, McQuade JL, Altan M, Zhang HC. Outcomes of immune checkpoint inhibitor–related diarrhea or colitis in cancer patients with superimposed gastrointestinal infections. Am J Clin Oncol. 2021;44(8):402–8.
4. Cho HJ, Kim WR, Kim JH, Kim DH, Kim DJ, Kang H. Colonic perforation after treatment with nivolumab in esophageal cancer: a case report. Ann Coloproctol. 2021;37(Suppl 1):S39.
5. Barling DR, Tucker S, Varia H, Isaacs P. Large bowel perforation secondary to CMV colitis: an unusual primary presentation of HIV infection. BMJ Case Rep. 2016;2016:bcr2016217221.
6. Pizuorno Machado A, Shatila M, Liu C, Lu Y, Altan M, Glitza Oliva IC, Zhao D, Zhang HC, Thomas A, Wang Y. Characteristics, treatment, and outcome of patients with bowel perforation after immune checkpoint inhibitor exposure. J Cancer Res Clin Oncol. 2023;8:1.
7. Yasuda K, Tanaka T, Ishihara S, Otani K, Nishikawa T, Kiyomatsu T, Kawai K, Hata K, Nozawa H, Masui Y, Shintani Y. Intestinal perforation after nivolumab immunotherapy for a malignant melanoma: a case report. Surg Case Rep. 2017;3:1–4.

Chapter 16
Diverticulitis Post Immune Checkpoint Inhibitor Therapy

Austin R. Thomas, Yang Lu, Karen Amelia Nahmod, Dongfeng Tan, Mehmet Altan, Mehnaz A. Shafi, and Yinghong Wang

Abbreviations

CT	Computed tomography
GI	Gastrointestinal
ICI	Immune checkpoint inhibitor
SCAD	Segmental colitis associated with diverticulosis

A. R. Thomas
Department of General Internal Medicine, The University of Texas Health Science Center, Houston, TX, USA
e-mail: Austin.R.Thomas@uth.tmc.edu

Y. Lu
Department of Nuclear Medicine, The University of Texas MD Anderson Cancer Center, Houston, TX, USA
e-mail: YLu10@mdanderson.org

K. A. Nahmod · D. Tan
Division of Pathology/Laboratory Medicine, The University of Texas MD Anderson Cancer Center, Houston, TX, USA
e-mail: KANahmod@mdanderson.org; dtan@mdanderson.org

M. Altan
Department of Thoracic/Head and Neck Medical Oncology, The University of Texas MD Anderson Cancer Center, Houston, TX, USA
e-mail: MAltan@mdanderson.org

M. A. Shafi · Y. Wang (✉)
Department of Gastroenterology, Hepatology & Nutrition, The University of Texas MD Anderson Cancer Center, Houston, TX, USA
e-mail: mashafi@mdanderson.org; ywang59@mdanderson.org

Y. Wang (ed.), *Challenging Cases in Immunotherapy Related Organ Toxicities*,
https://doi.org/10.1007/978-3-031-83533-9_16

Clinical Presentation

A woman in her 70s presented with severe explosive diarrhea for 2 days after receiving chemotherapy. She had a history of locoregional early-stage squamous cell cancer of the tongue diagnosed at age of 56 which was treated with surgical resection. She also had a history of diverticulosis, hypothyroidism, tobacco use, cholelithiasis, and hyperlipidemia. Seventeen years after her initial cancer diagnosis the patient presented with a second primary oral cavity cancer that was metastatic at the time of diagnosis. She was started on first line palliative systemic therapy with pembrolizumab, carboplatin, and docetaxel combination therapy followed by pembrolizumab maintenance monotherapy. She developed weekly severe explosive diarrhea and occasional fecal incontinence that began a couple of days after her second dose of pembrolizumab, which was approximately 40 days after her initial dose. Computed tomography (CT) of the abdomen and pelvis (AP) obtained shortly after her second pembrolizumab dose did not reveal infectious or inflammatory changes. The patient continued to have weekly explosive diarrhea with baseline 1–2 loose bowel movements per day in between the diarrheal episodes. She used loperamide as needed. Cancer restaging imaging about 6 months later revealed CT scan findings suggestive of a colovaginal fistula with acute inflammatory changes (Fig. 16.1).

Thirteen months after her initial dose of pembrolizumab (after receiving a total of 17 doses, with the most recent dose administered 1 month prior) she presented to the gastroenterology clinic with complaints of increasing frequency of diarrhea of 1–2 episodes per day. She denied vaginal symptoms at this time. Stool testing revealed fecal calprotectin >1000 μg/g and positive fecal lactoferrin (Table 16.1). Colonoscopy was attempted but the scope could not be advanced beyond the sigmoid colon due to tortuosity. Visualized areas of the rectum and sigmoid colon revealed moderate congestion and a localized area of granular mucosa in the distal rectum (Fig. 16.2). Random rectal and distal colon biopsies did not reveal active inflammation or infection. The diarrhea gradually resolved without the need for anti-diarrheal medications. Two months later she reported vaginal stool leakage. Three months after the onset of vaginal stool leakage, she had diarrhea recurrence and a fecal calprotectin level of 787 μg/g after restarting pembrolizumab for newly

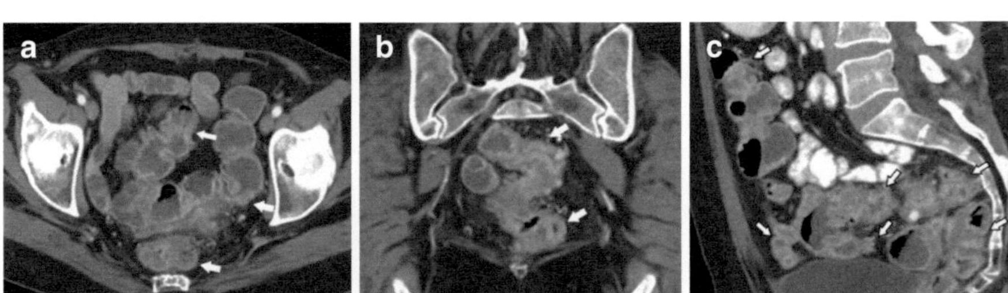

Fig. 16.1 Contrast enhanced CT images (**a**: axial, **b**: coronal, **c**: sagittal) shows diffusely enhanced wall thickening in the sigmoid colon and descending colon (arrows in **a–c**), suggestive of colitis and rectovaginal fistula. (Photo credit: Yang Lu, MD, PhD; Department of Nuclear Medicine)

Table 16.1 Lab values

Test	Value at onset of diarrhea	Value after complete resolution of diarrhea
Fecal calprotectin	**>1000 μg/g (ref: 0–50 μg/g)**	113 μg/g
Fecal lactoferrin	**Positive (ref: negative)**	Negative
Urine culture	**>100 k CFU/mL ESBL *Escherichia coli***	**>100 k CFU/mL ESBL *Escherichia coli***
Fecal ova and parasite	Negative	Negative
Enteric pathogen panel	No results available	Negative
White blood cell	5.9 K/μL	6.2 K/μL
Hemoglobin	**10.3 g/dL (ref: 14–18 g/dL)**	**11.3 g/dL (ref: 14–18 g/dL)**
Platelet	254 K/μL	245 K/μL
Clostridioides difficile DNA	No results available	Negative

μg microgram, *g* gram, *ref* normal reference range, *CFU* colony forming unit, *mL* milliliter, *K* thousand, *μL* microliter, *dL* deciliter, *ESBL* extended spectrum beta-lactamase, *DNA* deoxyribonucleic acid
Abnormal values are bolded in the table

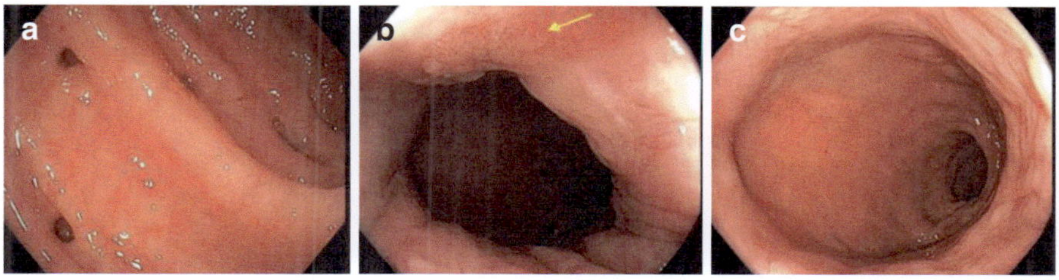

Fig. 16.2 Colonoscopy 1 month after initial presentation. (**a**) Sigmoid diverticula; (**b**) Granular mucosa of anus (yellow arrow); (**c**) Edematous mucosa of rectum

diagnosed brain metastases. The pembrolizumab was discontinued after three doses. She was subsequently started on vedolizumab for suspected immune mediated diarrhea and colitis. A repeat CT scan showed chronic diverticulitis, a small chronic diverticular abscess, and a stable colovaginal fistula. Gastrointestinal (GI) enteric pathogen panel was negative for infectious etiologies. She did not respond adequately to 2 doses of vedolizumab and was switched to ustekinumab. A second attempt at colonoscopy was successful and showed mild colitis vs. segmental colitis associated with diverticulosis (SCAD) in the rectosigmoid colon without any obvious fistula tract visualized (Fig. 16.3). Biopsies of this area revealed collagenous colitis (Fig. 16.4). Her diarrhea slowly resolved after receiving 1 dose of ustekinumab. Fecal calprotectin decreased to 113 μg/g and fecal lactoferrin was negative. No further doses of ustekinumab were given due to the nearly complete resolution of her GI symptoms and termination of the immune checkpoint inhibitor (ICI) therapy. A follow up CT scan still did not show any active inflammatory changes but did show a persistent colovaginal fistula.

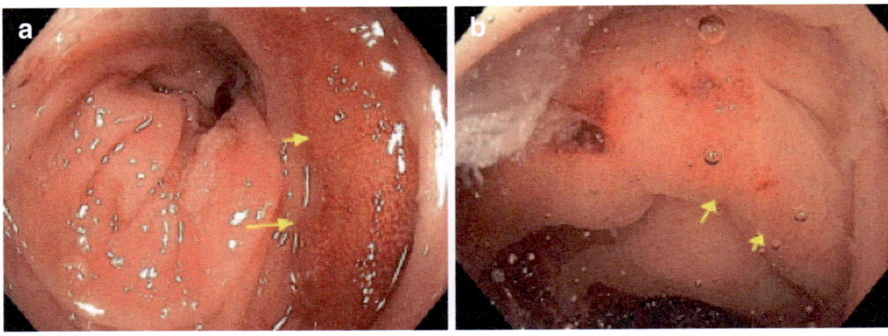

Fig. 16.3 Colonoscopy 10 months after initial presentation. (**a**) Rectosigmoid junction with patchy erythema (yellow arrows). Unable to identify presence of fistula tract due to sharp angulation. (**b**) Rectosigmoid junction with patchy erythema (yellow arrows)

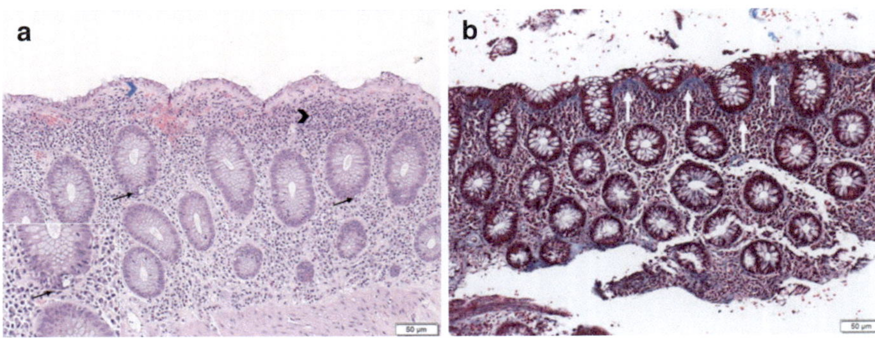

Fig. 16.4 Pathology. (**a**) Histological sections show colonic mucosa with expanded lamina propria by a lymphoplasmacytic infiltrate (black arrowhead), increased crypt apoptosis (black arrows) and thickened subepithelial collagen layer (blue arrowhead) (Hematoxylin and eosin stain ×200). (**b**) Trichrome stain highlights subepithelial collagen deposition (white arrows) (Trichrome stain ×200)

Clinical Outcome

The patient's diarrhea did not recur after receiving ustekinumab and discontinuing the pembrolizumab. CT imaging after resolution of diarrhea showed a persistent colovaginal fistula. She continued to decline secondary to cancer progression and decided to transition to home hospice where she later passed away about 7 months later.

Summary of the Case

This is a female in her 70s with a medical history of diverticulosis and squamous cell carcinoma of the tongue who underwent treatment with pembrolizumab, carboplatin, and docetaxel who subsequently developed diarrhea and vaginal stool leakage. She was later diagnosed with diverticulitis complicated by diverticular abscess and a colovaginal fistula, in addition to collagenous colitis. Pembrolizumab was discontinued and her colitis was initially treated with vedolizumab but then changed to ustekinumab due to lack of response. Ustekinumab resulted in complete resolution of colitis and she had no further complications from her diverticulitis. Unfortunately, the patient continued to decline due to cancer progression and died 7 months following resolution of diarrhea. Timeline events are summarized in Fig. 16.5.

Discussion

Little is known about diverticulitis related to ICI therapy or the optimum management strategies. Current management of post-ICI diverticulitis without colitis is similar to that of traditional diverticulitis. This consists of symptomatic support, antibiotics, and less commonly, surgical intervention for complicated cases (e.g., abscesses, colonic perforation, bowel obstruction). If there is concomitant ICI-mediated colitis then treatment could include glucocorticoids, biologics (e.g.,

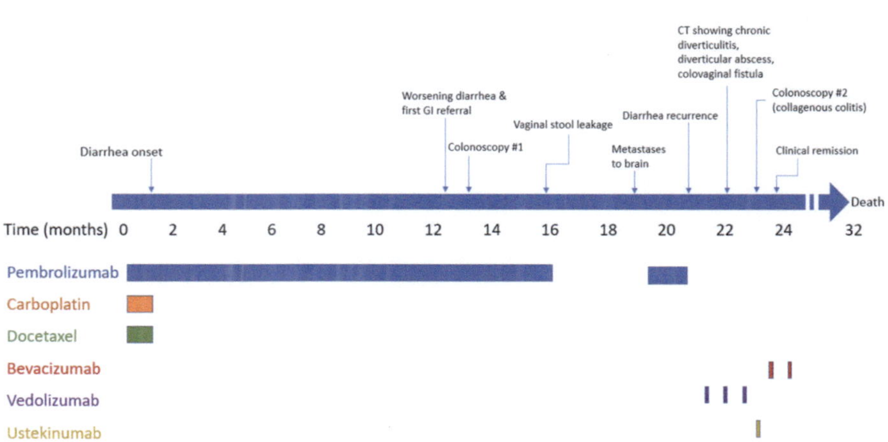

Fig. 16.5 Clinical course and timeline of the events. (Timepoint 0 is the initiation of ICI)

vedolizumab, ustekinumab, infliximab), and fecal microbiota transplant [1, 2]. Another entity that might complicate the clinical picture is SCAD. Treatment of SCAD is similar to that of other colitides which includes antibiotics, mesalamine, glucocorticoids, and occasionally immunomodulators (e.g., infliximab, azathioprine) [3]. Prior studies have suggested higher complication rates requiring surgical or interventional radiology procedures in patients with post-ICI diverticulitis [4]. Those patients with complications also had an increased need for hospitalization and lower overall survival. Similar to traditional diverticulitis [5], GI luminal cancer appears to be more common in those who develop complicated diverticulitis after ICI exposure. Recurrence rate of post-ICI diverticulitis appears to be comparable to that of traditional diverticulitis.

Conclusion

Post-ICI diverticulitis appears to have a similar clinical presentation, evaluation, and management as traditional diverticulitis, but it is associated with a more severe index event and higher rates of complications, which may require surgical intervention and decreased overall survival. The role of glucocorticoids in the management of post-ICI diverticulitis remains unclear unless it is given for concurrent ICI-mediated colitis or SCAD. Recurrence of diverticulitis seems to occur at comparable rates to that of traditional diverticulitis.

References

1. Abu-Sbeih H, Ali FS, Alsaadi D, Jennings J, Luo W, Gong Z, et al. Outcomes of vedolizumab therapy in patients with immune checkpoint inhibitor-induced colitis: a multi-center study. J Immunother Cancer. 2018;6(1):142. https://doi.org/10.1186/s40425-018-0461-4.
2. Brahmer JR, Lacchetti C, Schneider BJ, Atkins MB, Brassil KJ, Caterino JM, et al. Management of immune-related adverse events in patients treated with immune checkpoint inhibitor therapy: American Society of Clinical Oncology Clinical Practice Guideline. J Clin Oncol. 2018;36(17):1714–68. https://doi.org/10.1200/JCO.2017.77.6385.
3. Kucejko RJ, Poggio JL. Considerations and changes in the evaluation, management, and outcomes in the management of diverticular disease: the diagnosis, pathology, and treatment of diverticular colitis. Clin Colon Rectal Surg. 2018;31(4):221–5. https://doi.org/10.1055/s-0037-1607467.
4. Thomas AR, Eyada M, Kono M, Varatharajalu K, Lu Y, Xu G, et al. Characteristics, treatment, and outcome of diverticulitis after immune checkpoint inhibitor treatment in patients with malignancies. J Cancer Res Clin Oncol. 2023;149:4805–16. https://doi.org/10.1007/s00432-022-04405-3.
5. Rottier SJ, van Dijk ST, van Geloven AAW, Schreurs WH, Draaisma WA, van Enst WA, et al. Meta-analysis of the role of colonoscopy after an episode of left-sided acute diverticulitis. Br J Surg. 2019;106(8):988–97. https://doi.org/10.1002/bjs.11191.

Chapter 17
Enteritis and Venous Thromboembolism Related to Immune Checkpoint Inhibitor Therapy

Sidra Naz, Yang Lu, Anusha S. Thomas, and Yinghong Wang

Abbreviations

CT Computed tomography
DVT Deep venous thrombosis
ICI Immune checkpoint inhibitor
irAEs Immune related adverse events
PE Pulmonary embolism
VTE Venous thromboembolism

Clinical Presentation

This is a female patient in her 60s with lung cancer on treatment with pembrolizumab and past medical history of venous thromboembolism (VTE) on apixaban. She presented with acute onset of severe abdominal pain, constipation, and significant weight loss after 6 doses of pembrolizumab. Notably, there were no bloody stools or signs of sepsis.

S. Naz · A. S. Thomas · Y. Wang (✉)
Department of Gastroenterology, Hepatology & Nutrition, The University of Texas MD Anderson Cancer Center, Houston, TX, USA
e-mail: SNaz@mdanderson.org; ASThomas1@mdanderson.org; ywang59@mdanderson.org

Y. Lu
Department of Nuclear Medicine, The University of Texas MD Anderson Cancer Center, Houston, TX, USA
e-mail: YLu10@mdanderson.org

Y. Wang (ed.), *Challenging Cases in Immunotherapy Related Organ Toxicities*,
https://doi.org/10.1007/978-3-031-83533-9_17

Evaluations

Lab investigations revealed fecal calprotectin 1084 μg/g and positive lactoferrin, indicating underlying GI tract inflammation (Table 17.1). Celiac serology and lactic acid were within normal range (Table 17.1). Imaging identified an isolated segment of small bowel wall thickening, without visible thrombus or superior mesenteric artery (SMA) blockage (Fig. 17.1).

Table 17.1 Lab values

Test	Value at onset of GI symptoms	Value after complete resolution of GI symptoms post treatment	Normal range
Lactic acid	1.4 mmol/L	1.2 mmol/L	0.5–1.6 mmol/L
Fecal lactoferrin	Positive	Negative	0–6.4 μg/mL
Fecal calprotectin	1084 μg/g	380 μg/g	50–120 μg/g
White blood cell	5.2 K/μL	5.4 K/μL	4–11 K/μL
Hemoglobin	8.9 g/dL	9.9 g/dL	12–16 g/dL
Platelet	548 K/μL	689 K/μL	140–440 K/μL

μg microgram, *g* gram, *mL* milliliter, *K* thousand, *μL* microliter, *dL* deciliter

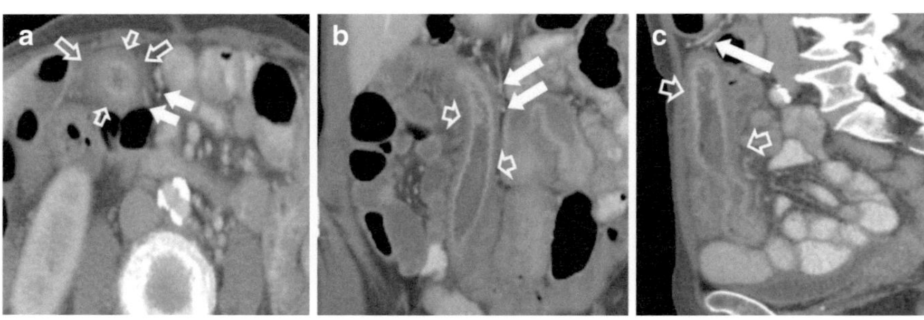

Fig. 17.1 CECT (**a**: axial; **b**: coronal; **c**: sagittal images) showed segmental wall thickening of small bowel loop (short arrows), with associated adjacent fat stranding (long hollow arrows in **a**), suggestive of enteritis. Meanwhile, the supplying branches of a superior mesenteric artery are patent with contrast filling (long solid arrows in **a**–**c**). (Photo credit: Yang Lu MD, PhD Department of Nuclear Medicine)

Differential Diagnosis

This case highlights the challenges in diagnosing and managing ICI related GI complications, particularly in the context of concurrent history of VTE and cancer. Prior reports suggest that ICI treatment is associated with a fourfold increased risk of VTE [2]. Our patient on anticoagulation presented with an isolated segmental small bowel wall thickening in absence of VTE on imaging or signs of enterocolitis clinically. An elevated fecal calprotectin favored the diagnosis of ICI related enteritis.

Treatment and Disease Course

She initially received budesonide 9 mg/day for 1 month, along with dietary modifications for presumed ICI enteritis, but experienced no improvement and consequently, after multi-disciplinary discussion, a trial of vedolizumab was initiated. She achieved a favorable clinical response after 3 doses and resumed cancer therapy with pembrolizumab. On follow up, the calprotectin levels improved to 380 μg/g. Despite resuming pembrolizumab treatment, her cancer course was complicated by obstructive jaundice due to pancreatic metastasis, requiring endoscopic decompression. Additionally, she underwent portal vein stent placement for new-onset portal vein hypertension and recurrent ascites. However, the procedure was complicated by bloody peritoneal fluid and spontaneous bacterial infection and eventual demise of the patient. Disease course is shown in Fig. 17.2.

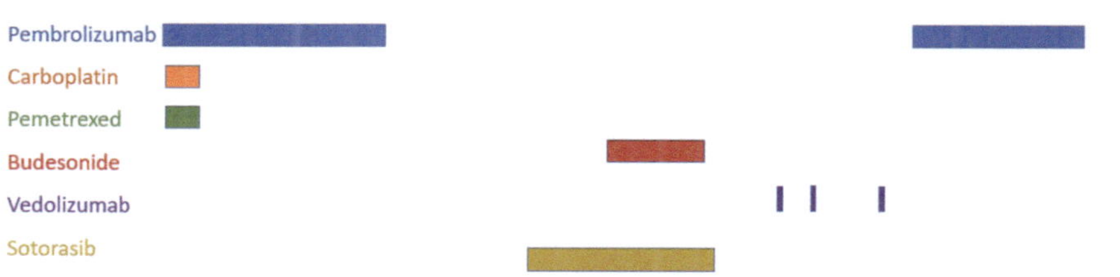

Fig. 17.2 Summary of disease course with timeline (timepoint of 0 is ICI initiation)

Summary

This is a case with metastatic lung cancer, and a history of venous thrombosis on apixaban developed abdominal pain and constipation after 6 doses of pembrolizumab. CT scan indicated isolated segment of small bowel inflammation without mesenteric artery blockage. A diagnosis of ICI-induced enteritis was made despite atypical clinical presentation after excluding the thromboembolic event based on labs and imaging, that eventually responded to vedolizumab. Despite resuming pembrolizumab, she died due to cancer progression and its related complications.

Discussion

Isolated enteritis associated with the use of ICIs is an uncommon but potentially severe irAE [1]. It can manifest with common symptoms such as diarrhea, abdominal pain, and, in severe cases, bowel perforation, but may also present with atypical symptom of constipation. Venous thrombosis, including DVT and pulmonary embolism (PE) is a common complication in cancer patients, and anticoagulation is the standard treatment. The coexistence of venous thrombosis and cancer is a well-established risk factor for recurrent thrombotic events [2]. The interplay between venous thrombosis history and ICI-induced gastrointestinal inflammation raises several important considerations: (1) ICIs can lead to an enhanced immune response, which theoretically could exacerbate inflammation in thrombosed vessels [3, 4] which may raise concerns about the potential risk of thrombosis recurrence in patients with a history of venous thrombosis; (2) managing patients with a history of venous thrombosis and cancer who require ICIs necessitates a coordinated approach between oncologists and hematologists. Balancing anticoagulation for thrombosis prevention and the potential for irAEs is challenging but critical [5]; (3) patient-specific risk assessment should be conducted before initiating ICIs in individuals with a history of venous thrombosis. The potential benefits of ICI therapy in cancer management must be weighed against the risks of both recurrent thrombosis and irAEs.

Conclusion

The real world clinical practice recognizes the increasing complexity of ICI related gastrointestinal toxicities. Thorough evaluation, early recognition and appropriate management for accurate diagnosis are crucial to optimize patient outcomes in this challenging clinical scenario.

References

1. Abu-Sbeih H, Ali FS, Alsaadi D, Jennings J, Luo W, Gong Z, et al. Outcomes of vedolizumab therapy in patients with immune checkpoint inhibitor-induced colitis: a multi-center study. J Immunother Cancer. 2018;6(1):142. https://doi.org/10.1186/s40425-018-0461-4.
2. Wang DY, et al. Immune checkpoint inhibitor cancer therapy: a new risk factor for thromboembolism? J Immunother Cancer. 2019;7(1):71.
3. Chen JH, et al. Immune-related gastrointestinal adverse events during immune checkpoint inhibitor treatment: mechanisms and management. Therap Adv Gastroenterol. 2019;12:1756284819870917.
4. Khorana AA, et al. Thromboembolism is a leading cause of death in cancer patients receiving outpatient chemotherapy. J Thromb Haemost. 2007;5(3):632–4.
5. Abu-Sbeih H, et al. Immune checkpoint inhibitor-induced gastrointestinal and hepatic injury: pathologists' perspective. J Clin Pathol. 2020;73(3):135–47.

Chapter 18
Stomach Perforation Post Immune Checkpoint Inhibitors Treatment

Antonio Pizuorno Machado, Yang Lu, and Yinghong Wang

Abbreviations

ICI Immune checkpoint inhibitors
GI Gastrointestinal

Clinical Presentation

This is a male in 60s with a past medical history of renal cell carcinoma with metastasis to the lungs, pleura, intrathoracic lymph nodes and bones diagnosed a few years ago. He has been on multiple lines of treatments including pazopanib, axitinib, cabozantinib, then transitioned to everolimus and nivolumab. However, cancer continued to progress which lead to termination of this regimen. Three weeks after, he started developing epigastric pain, nausea and vomiting. The abdominal pain was

A. P. Machado
Department of Internal Medicine, The University of Texas Health Science Center, Houston, TX, USA
e-mail: antonio.pizuornomachado@utsouthwestern.edu

Y. Lu
Department of Nuclear Medicine, The University of Texas MD Anderson Cancer Center, Houston, TX, USA
e-mail: YLu10@mdanderson.org

Y. Wang (✉)
Department of Gastroenterology, Hepatology & Nutrition, The University of Texas MD Anderson Cancer Center, Houston, TX, USA
e-mail: ywang59@mdanderson.org

Y. Wang (ed.), *Challenging Cases in Immunotherapy Related Organ Toxicities*, https://doi.org/10.1007/978-3-031-83533-9_18

progressive, 8 out of 10 in a scale of intensity, aching, sharp and shooting type, with no response to home analgesia which lead to emergency room evaluation.

Upon arrival to the emergency department, patient was found to be tachycardic, hypothermic, with physical exam remarkable for generalized tenderness in the abdominal area with guarding and rebound along with decreased intensity of his bowel movements. The laboratory tests (Table 18.1) were entirely normal comparable to the ones done 4 weeks ago before the last dose of nivolumab. An X-ray of the abdomen showed paucity of bowel gas with a possible bowel obstruction for which a CT was obtained (Fig. 18.1) that revealed large peritoneal free air in the anterior abdomen with numerous small pockets of peritoneal air. There was wall thickening of the stomach and a defect along the greater curvature of the stomach measuring 1.7 cm. In addition, it also revealed large amount of ascites, as well as numerous hepatic metastasis and upper abdomen retroperitoneal lymphadenopathy.

Table 18.1 Laboratory characteristics

Test	Value at last dose of ICI 3 weeks prior	Value at the onset of stomach perforation
White blood cell counts K/μL	3.8	**2.8 ↓**
Hemoglobin g/dL	12.5	16.0
Platelets K/μL	221	443
Sodium level mEq/L	139	138
Potassium level mEq/L	4.3	**5.5 ↑**
Chloride level mEq/L	101	98
Bicarbonate level mEq/L	30	23
Creatinine level mg/dL	1.00	**1.36 ↑**
Glucose level mg/dL	103	139
Calcium level mEq/L	8.1	8.9
Magnesium level mEq/L	2.0	2.0
Phosphorous level mEq/L	3.2	**5.4 ↑**
Albumin level g/dL	3.2	3.3
Bilirubin total mg/dL	0.5	**1.2 ↑**
Bilirubin direct mg/dL	0.5	0.6
AST level U/L	81	**110 ↑**
ALT level U/L	64	**140 ↑**
Amylase level U/L	<26	<26
Lipase level U/L	51	<25
Lactic acid level mmol/L	1.2	**4.3 ↑**

ALT alanine aminotransferase, *AST* aspartate aminotransferase
Laboratory reference: White blood cell counts 4–11 K/μL. Potassium level 3.5–5.0 mEq/L. Creatinine level 0.7–1.3 mg/dL. Phosphorous level 2.5–4.5 mEq/L. Bilirubin total 0.2–1.1 mg/dL. AST level 15–46 U/L. ALT level 7–56 U/L. Lactic acid level 0.7–2.1 mmol/L

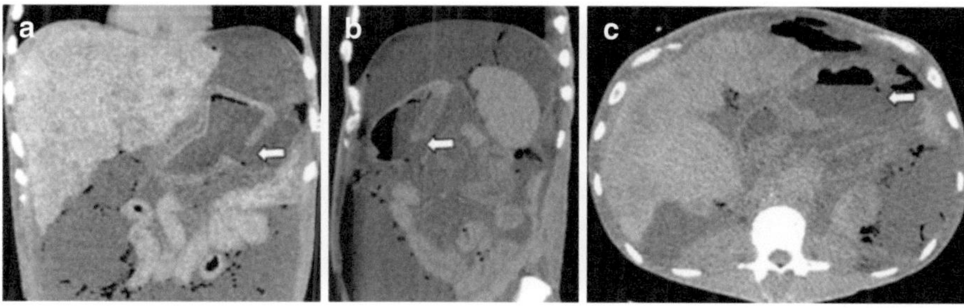

Fig. 18.1 Computed tomography (CT) of the abdomen demonstrating large defect or perforation along the stomach great curvature (arrow in panel **a**, coronal; arrow in panel **b**, sagittal; arrow in panel **c**, axial) [2]

In the lieu of the laboratory tests and imaging, the consensus was reached among inpatient oncology team, surgical team and interventional radiology that he would not be a surgical candidate given the advanced stage of cancer and his overall condition. The working diagnosis for the stomach perforation was due to immune checkpoint inhibitor (ICI) related toxicity given the absence of metastatic disease in the stomach and upper gastrointestinal tract based on previous and current imaging without other identifiable risk factors.

Clinical Outcome

Supportive treatment with broad spectrum antibiotics and antifungals was started with caspofungin, linezolid, metronidazole and piperacillin-tazobactam. However, his lactic acidosis continued to worsen without response to fluids or antibiotics with subsequent multi-organ failure, he was transitioned to comfort measures and passed away during the same hospital admission.

Case Summary

Case was comprised by a 60's year old male patient with a previous diagnosis of metastatic renal cell carcinoma whom failed multiple lines of therapy and transitioned to nivolumab and everolimus. The later was further discontinued due to cancer progression, however, was followed by acute stomach perforation that was deemed to be caused by the immunotherapy. Given the patient was not a surgical candidate, therefore, supportive and then comfort measures were established with further passing of the patient. Summary of events is depicted in Fig. 18.2.

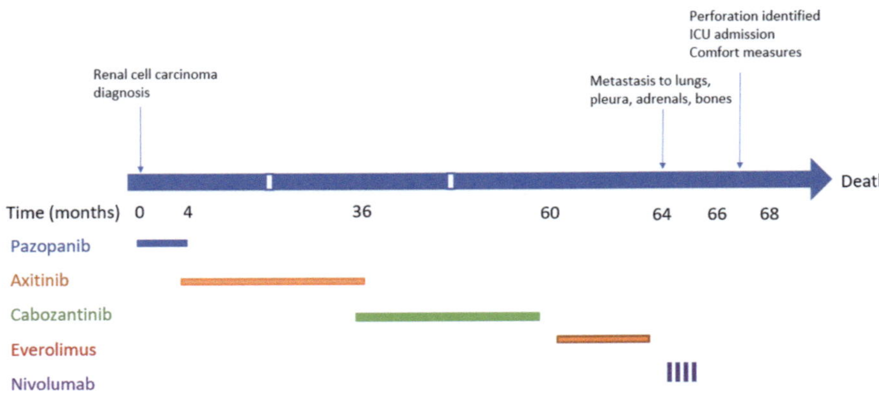

Fig. 18.2 Clinical course and timeline (timepoint of 0 is the diagnosis of renal cell carcinoma)

Discussion

Bowel perforation is a serious medical emergency and is characterized by high mortality specially in patients with cancer [1]. This complication is typically seen in patients with either trauma, metastasis or other diseases such as colitis which is a common complication of ICI. It has overlapping clinical presentations with many other differentials in cancer patients. The incidence of ICI related bowel perforation is rare, described to be 0.6% [2] even without having a previous GI pathology. No known underlying mechanism has been proposed or found so far in the correlation between ICI and bowel perforation. The management of this complication is depending on a multidisciplinary team approach from surgeons and oncologists to assess the overall health state that the patient has, to offer surgical approach or conservative strategy e.g. aggressive antibiotic treatment with potential drainage by interventional radiology etc. The standardization of the diagnosis and management of this condition is still to be established.

References

1. Banaszkiewicz Z, Woda Ł, Tojek K, Jarmocik P, Jawień A. Colorectal cancer with intestinal perforation—a retrospective analysis of treatment outcomes. Contemp Oncol. 2014;18(6):414–8.
2. Pizuorno Machado A, Shatila M, Liu C, et al. Characteristics, treatment, and outcome of patients with bowel perforation after immune checkpoint inhibitor exposure. J Cancer Res Clin Oncol. 2023;149(9):5989–98.

Chapter 19
Sclerosing Mesenteritis After Immune Checkpoint Inhibitor Therapy

Andrew G. Kuang, Yang Lu, Dongfeng Tan, Malek Shatila, John A. Thompson, and Yinghong Wang

Abbreviations

CT Computed tomography
SM Sclerosing mesenteritis

A. G. Kuang
Division of Gastroenterology, Department of Medicine, University of Pennsylvania Health System, Philadelphia, PA, USA
e-mail: andrew.kuang@pennmedicine.upenn.edu

Y. Lu
Department of Nuclear Medicine, The University of Texas MD Anderson Cancer Center, Houston, TX, USA
e-mail: YLu10@mdanderson.org

D. Tan
Division of Pathology/Laboratory Medicine, The University of Texas MD Anderson Cancer Center, Houston, TX, USA
e-mail: dtan@mdanderson.org

M. Shatila · Y. Wang (✉)
Department of Gastroenterology, Hepatology & Nutrition, The University of Texas MD Anderson Cancer Center, Houston, TX, USA
e-mail: MShatila@mdanderson.org; ywang59@mdanderson.org

J. A. Thompson
Department of Medicine, Fred Hutchinson Cancer Center, University of Washington, Seattle, WA, USA
e-mail: jat@uw.edu

Y. Wang (ed.), *Challenging Cases in Immunotherapy Related Organ Toxicities*, https://doi.org/10.1007/978-3-031-83533-9_19

Clinical Presentation

The patient is a woman in her 60s with past medical history of stage IIIB right triple negative invasive ductal breast carcinoma treated with 2 cycles of paclitaxel, carboplatin, and pembrolizumab. She received her most recent cancer therapy cycle 22 days prior to presentation. She presented to the hospital after having 1 day of fever measured at home to be 100.8 F associated with mild shortness of breath. She was found to have stable laboratory testing and computed tomography (CT) imaging of her chest and was discharged from the emergency room with a course of levofloxacin. She returned 2 days later to the hospital with a fever of 102.4 F and reported one episode of non-bloody, loose bowel movement but denied any nausea, vomiting, abdominal pain, dysuria, hematochezia, or melena. Her shortness of breath had resolved but she reported dry cough for the past several weeks. Her past medical history included anemia of chronic disease, hypertension, and pre-diabetes. She had no prior surgical history. Her medications as outpatient included amlodipine 5 mg daily, chlorthalidone 25 mg daily, quinapril 40 mg daily. Her laboratory testing revealed hemoglobin of 10.2 g/dL and platelet count of $85 \times 10^3/\mu L$ which were similar to prior results (Table 19.1). Infectious work-up including blood and urine cultures were negative. Clostridioides difficile stool panel and gastrointestinal stool pathogen panel were negative. Contrast-enhanced CT imaging of the abdomen and pelvis (Fig. 19.1) showed new focal soft tissue stranding within the central midgut mesentery suggestive of sclerosing mesenteritis (SM).

Hospital Course and Management

She was admitted to the hospital and started on empiric antibiotic therapy with vancomycin and piperacillin-tazobactam. Infectious disease was consulted, and vancomycin was later switched to daptomycin. On hospital day 2, she had a temperature of 101.2 ° F and reported mild abdominal tenderness. She also was noted to have two aphthous ulcers on her tongue which were swabbed and negative for HSV and VZV. She continued to have occasional loose stools. The rest of her infectious work-up remained unrevealing. She did not have recurrence of fever. The multidisciplinary consensus for the patient's overall clinical picture was that it was most likely related to sclerosing mesenteritis which was suspected to be related to immune checkpoint inhibitor therapy. She was discharged home to start on a short prednisone taper starting at 60 mg for a total of 8 days.

Table 19.1 Laboratory findings

Laboratory test	Value
White blood count	$4.8 \times 10^3/\mu L$
Hemoglobin	**10.2 g/dL**
Platelet count	**$85 \times 10^3/\mu L$**
Sodium	**135 mmol/L**
Potassium	3.6 mmol/L
Chloride	**96 mmol/L**
Carbon dioxide	23 mmol/L
Blood urea nitrogen	18 mg/dL
Creatinine	0.81 mg/dL
Glucose	115 mg/dL
Calcium	9.1 mg/dL
ALT	27 U/L
AST	44 U/L
Alkaline phosphatase	68 U/L
Total bilirubin	0.4 mg/dL
Total protein	6.7 g/dL
Albumin	3.5 g/dL
International normalization ratio	1.18
Blood culture (2 sets)	Negative
Urine culture	Negative
Clostridioides difficile stool panel	Negative
Gastrointestinal stool PCR panel	Negative
Respiratory PCR panel	Negative

Abbreviations: *AST* aspartate aminotransferase, *ALT* alanine transaminase, *HSV* herpes simplex virus, *NAAT* nucleic acid amplification test, *PCR* polymerase chain reaction
Laboratory reference values: hemoglobin 12.0–16.0 g/dL, platelet count 140–440 K/μL, sodium 136–145 mEq/L, chloride 98–107 mEq/L

Case Outcome

Patient was followed-up by telephone by her primary oncologist 3 days after her discharge. At that time, she had remained afebrile and her other symptoms had improved. She resumed her cancer therapy regimen of pembrolizumab, paclitaxel, and carboplatin after 14 days post-discharge. She did not have later recurrence of these symptoms or complications of SM. She did not receive repeat abdominal imaging to assess for imaging resolution of SM afterwards given resolution of her symptoms.

Summary

This is a case report of a woman with metastatic triple negative breast cancer who had received two cycles of chemotherapy and pembrolizumab who subsequently developed fever with CT findings of central midgut mesenteric soft tissue stranding

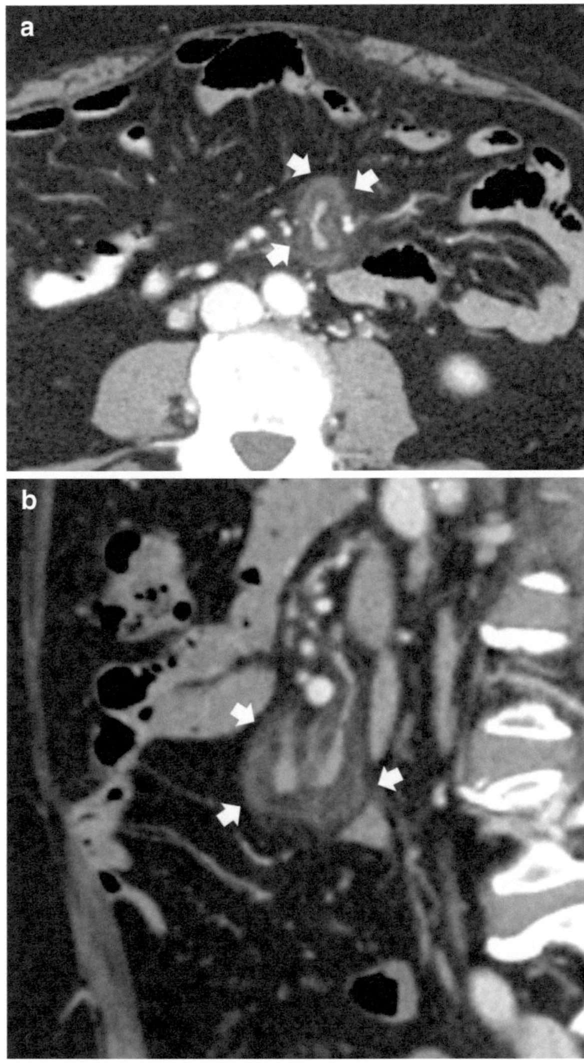

Fig. 19.1 Contrast-enhanced CT images (**a.** axial abdomen; **b.** triangulated sagittal abdomen) show new focal soft tissue stranding within the central midgut mesentery (arrows in **a**, **b**), suggestive of SM. (Taken from Kuang et al. 2023)

concerning for SM. This patient was treated with a short course of corticosteroids and had resolution of her symptoms and no further recurrence of SM. The patient was able to resume her previous cancer therapy including immune checkpoint inhibitor therapy. The summary of the disease course is depicted in Fig. 19.2.

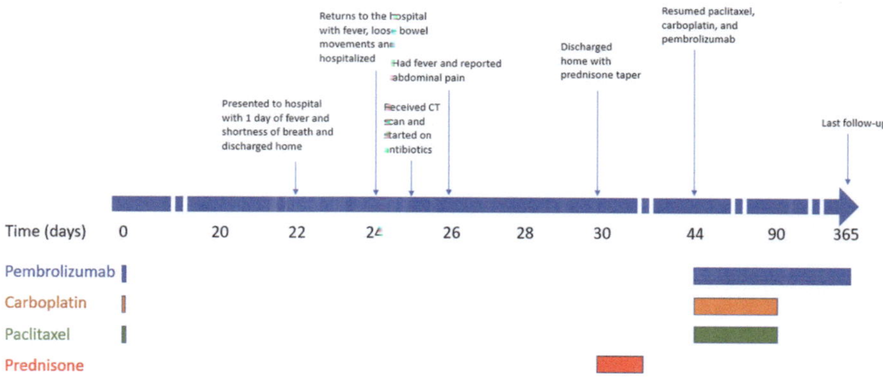

Fig. 19.2 Timeline depicting sequence of events of diagnosis and management of sclerosing mesenteritis. (timepoint of 0 is the initiation of ICI)

Discussion

SM is a rare inflammatory disorder affecting the mesentery, with various potential causes, including immune checkpoint inhibitor toxicity [1–9]. The pathophysiology and natural progression of SM remain inadequately understood, particularly among cancer patients [8, 10–13]. Some have hypothesized that SM may be a paraneoplastic phenomenon, but the correlation between SM remission and cancer outcomes is unclear [8, 9]. While many instances of SM are reported as incidental and asymptomatic, some cases manifest common gastrointestinal complaints like abdominal pain, nausea, and vomiting. Many patients exhibit no physical examination findings [14–16]. The diagnosis is made based on cross-sectional imaging or histological findings. Findings such as hyper-attenuation of adipose tissue, pseudocapsule formation, and mesenteric fatty masses may be seen on computed tomography [2]. Histologic findings include mesenteric fat necrosis, fibrosis of adipose tissue, and lymphocyte infiltration [14] (Fig. 19.3).

The most suitable treatment for SM remains uncertain due to the absence of high-quality, large-scale cohort studies. Generally, therapies like corticosteroids, tamoxifen, and occasionally azathioprine, thalidomide, colchicine, progesterone, and pentoxifylline have been documented [2, 15, 17–19]. The American College of Gastroenterology recommends a combination of corticosteroid taper and long-term tamoxifen for most symptomatic SM patients [2]. Most individuals with SM seem to have favorable outcomes although 20% experience chronic morbidity [7, 14] and death on rare occasion [15].

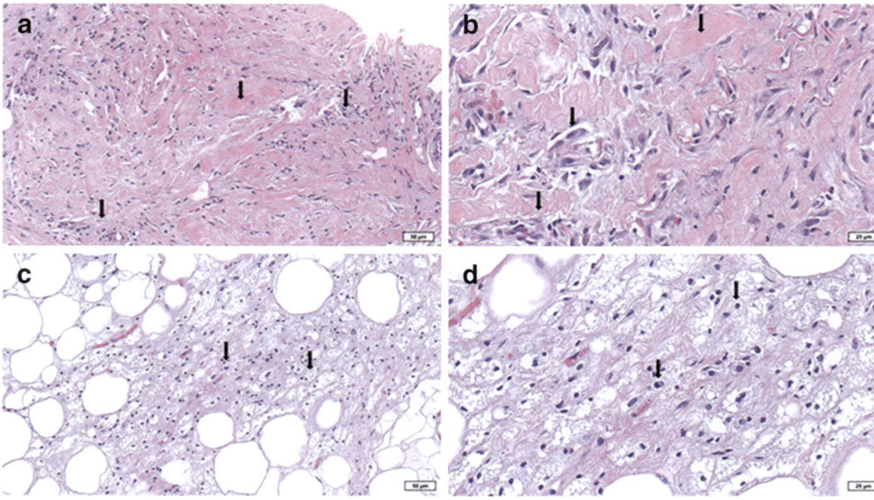

Fig. 19.3 Histopathology of SM. Microscopic photographs of histopathology samples stained with hematoxylin-and-eosin from patients with SM. (**a**) Fibrosis with dense collagen, reactive fibroblasts, and chronic inflammatory cells (arrow; hematoxylin-and-eosin [H&E] 200×). (**b**) High-power view of dense eosinophilic collagen and reactive fibroblasts in a background of lymphocytes, plasma cells, and scattered eosinophils (arrow; H&E 400×). (**c**) Mesenteric fibroadipose tissue with an infiltrate of foamy histiocytes and chronic inflammatory cells (arrow; H&E 200×). (**d**) High-power view of abundant foamy histiocytes in a background of lymphocytes and plasma cells (arrow; H&E 400×). (Taken from Kuang et al. 2023)

References

1. Kuang AG, Sperling G, Liang TZ, Lu Y, Tan D, Bollin K, et al. Sclerosing mesenteritis following immune checkpoint inhibitor therapy. J Cancer Res Clin Oncol. 2023;149(11):9221–7. https://doi.org/10.1007/s00432-023-04802-2.
2. Danford CJ, Lin SC, Wolf JL. Sclerosing mesenteritis. Am J Gastroenterol. 2019;114:867–73. https://doi.org/10.14309/ajg.0000000000000167.
3. Michael P, Gratiot J. Mesenteric panniculitis associated with trauma. Calif Med. 1964;100:285–7.
4. Nomura Y, Naito Y, Eriguchi N, Kume T, Itai N, Sonoda H, Hayashida S, et al. A case of IgG4-related sclerosing mesenteritis. Pathol Res Pract. 2011;207:518–21. https://doi.org/10.1016/j.prp.2011.05.009.
5. Venkataramani A, Behling CA, Lyche KD. Sclerosing mesenteritis (SM): an unusual cause of abdominal pain in an HIV-positive patient. Am J Gastroenterol. 1997;92:1059–60.
6. Artigues Serra F, García-Gasalla M, Campins A, González de Cabo M, Morales R, Peña RR, et al. Sclerosing mesenteritis due to mycobacterium genavense infection: a case report. Medicine (Baltimore). 2022;101:1–4. https://doi.org/10.1097/MD.0000000000030351.
7. Sharma P, Yadav S, Needham CM, Feuerstadt P. Sclerosing mesenteritis (SM): a systematic review of 192 cases. Clin J Gastroenterol. 2017;10:103–11. https://doi.org/10.1007/s12328-017-0716-5.
8. Buchwald P, Diesing L, Dixon L, Wakeman C, Eglinton T, Dobbs B. Cohort study of mesenteric panniculitis and its relationship to malignancy. Br J Surg. 2016;103:1727–30. https://doi.org/10.1002/bjs.10229.

9. Gögebakan Ö, Albrecht T, Osterhoff MA, Reimann A. Is mesenteric panniculitis truly a paraneoplastic phenomenon? A matched pair analysis. Eur J Radiol. 2013;82:1853–9. https://doi.org/10.1016/j.ejrad.2013.06.023.
10. Khasminsky V, Ram E, Atar E, Steinmintz A, Issa N, Bachar GN. Is there an association between mesenteric panniculitis and lymphoma? A case control analysis. Clin Radiol. 2017;72:844–9. https://doi.org/10.1016/j.crad.2017.05.008.
11. Protin-Catteau L, Thiéfin G, Barbe C, Jolly D, Soyer P, Hoeffel C. Mesenteric panniculitis: review of consecutive abdominal MDCT examinations with a matched-pair analysis. Acta Radiol. 2016;57:1438–44. https://doi.org/10.1177/0284185116629829.
12. Smith ZL, Sifuentes H, Deepak P, Ecanow DB, Ehrenpreis ED. Relationship between mesenteric abnormalities on computed tomography and malignancy: clinical findings and outcomes of 359 patients. J Clin Gastroenterol. 2013;47:409–14. https://doi.org/10.1097/MCG.0b013e3182703148.
13. van Putte-Katier N, van Bommel EF, Elgersma OE, Hendriksz TR. Mesenteric panniculitis: prevalence, clinicoradiological presentation and 5-year follow-up. Br J Radiol. 2014;87:1–9. https://doi.org/10.1259/bjr.2014045[illegible].
14. Emory TS, Monihan JM, Carr NJ, Sobin LH. Sclerosing mesenteritis, mesenteric panniculitis and mesenteric lipodystrophy: a single entity? Am J Surg Pathol. 1997;21:392–8. https://doi.org/10.1097/00000478-199704000-00004.
15. Akram S, Pardi DS, Schaffner JA, Smyrk TC. Sclerosing mesenteritis (SM): clinical features, treatment, and outcome in ninety-two patients. Clin Gastroenterol Hepatol. 2007;5:589–94. https://doi.org/10.1016/j.cgh.2007.02.032.
16. Kipfer RE, Moertel CG, Dahlin DC. Mesenteric lipodystrophy. Ann Intern Med. 1974;80:582–8. https://doi.org/10.7326/0003-4819-80-5-582.
17. Généreau T, Bellin MF, Wechsler B, Le TH, Bellanger J, Grellet J, et al. Demonstration of efficacy of combining corticosteroids and colchicine in two patients with idiopathic sclerosing mesenteritis. Dig Dis Sci. 1996;41:684–8. https://doi.org/10.1007/BF02213123.
18. Bala A, Coderre S, Johnson D, et al. Treatment of sclerosing mesenteritis with corticosteroids and azathioprine. Can J Gastroenterol. 2001;15:533–5.
19. Ginsburg PM, Ehrenpreis ED. A pilot study of thalidomide for patients with symptomatic mesenteric panniculitis. Aliment Pharmacol Ther. 2002;16:2115–22. https://doi.org/10.1046/j.1365-2036.2002.01383.x.

Chapter 20
Pneumatosis Intestinalis Following Immune Checkpoint Inhibitor Therapy

Gabriel Sperling, Yang Lu, Malek Shatila, Krishnavathana Varatharajalu, Bryan Schneider, Anam Khan, and Yinghong Wang

Abbreviations

ALT	Alanine transaminase
AST	Aspartate aminotransferase
CT	Computerized tomography
GI	Gastrointestinal
ICI	Immune checkpoint inhibitor
IMDC	Immune mediated diarrhea and colitis
PEG	Percutaneous endoscopic gastrostomy
PI	Pneumatosis intestinalis

G. Sperling
John Sealy School of Medicine, The University of Texas Medical Branch, Galveston, TX, USA
e-mail: gasperli@utmb.edu

Y. Lu
Department of Nuclear Medicine, The University of Texas MD Anderson Cancer Center, Houston, TX, USA
e-mail: YLu10@mdanderson.org

M. Shatila · K. Varatharajalu · A. Khan · Y. Wang (✉)
Department of Gastroenterology, Hepatology & Nutrition, The University of Texas MD Anderson Cancer Center, Houston, TX, USA
e-mail: MShatila@mdanderson.org; KVaratharajalu@mdanderson.org; anam.khan@mdanderson.org; ywang59@mdanderson.org

B. Schneider
Department of Thoracic Medical Oncology, The University of Michigan, Ann Arbor, MI, USA
e-mail: bryansch@med.umich.edu

Y. Wang (ed.), *Challenging Cases in Immunotherapy Related Organ Toxicities*, https://doi.org/10.1007/978-3-031-83533-9_20

Clinical Presentation

This is a Caucasian male in 50s with a medical history that is notable for stage IV anaplastic thyroid cancer status-post thyroidectomy on a pembrolizumab and lenvatinib. He received 2 cycles of pembrolizumab, with the most recent dose administered 1 month prior to presentation. He presented with severe, diffuse abdominal pain for several days associated with multiple episodes of loose stools per day. He denied fever, chills, chest pain, or shortness breath. He had no other past medical history on file, and his only surgical history included a thyroidectomy and planned tracheostomy and percutaneous endoscopic gastrostomy (PEG) tube. His outpatient medications include levothyroxine for post-procedural hypothyroidism, scopolamine for secretions and nausea/vomiting, and tramadol for pain. On admission, he was normotensive and breathing comfortably on room air but tachycardic into the 140 s. Admission labs were notable for leukocytosis with a white cell count of $14.5 \times 10^3/\mu L$, thrombocytosis with platelet count of $464 \times 10^3/\mu L$, mild hyponatremia at 133 mmol/L, and lactic acid of 3.5 mmol/L (normal 0.5–1.6 mmol/L) (Table 20.1). Gastrointestinal multiplex panel, Clostridioides difficile, urine

Table 20.1 Laboratory findings

Laboratory test	Value
White blood count (4.0–11.0 × $10^3/\mu L$)	**14.5 × $10^3/\mu L$**
Hemoglobin (12.0–16.0 g/dL)	15.4 g/dL
Platelet count (140–440 × $10^3/\mu L$)	**464 × $10^3/\mu L$**
Sodium (136–145 mEq/L)	**133 mmol/L**
Potassium (3.5–5.1 mEq/L)	3.9 mmol/L
Chloride (98–107 mEq/L)	94 mmol/L
Carbon dioxide (22–29 mEq/L)	23 mmol/L
Blood urea nitrogen (6–23 mg/dL)	39 mg/dL
Creatinine (0.67–1.17 mg/dL)	1.01 mg/dL
Glucose (70–99 mg/dL)	152 mg/dL
Calcium (8.4–10.2 mg/dL)	9.3 mg/dL
ALT (<41 U/L)	40 U/L
AST (<40 U/L)	44 U/L
Alkaline phosphatase (40–129 U/L)	119 U/L
Total bilirubin (<1.2 mg/dL)	0.4 mg/dL
Total protein (6.4–8.3 g/dL)	6.6 g/dL
Albumin (3.5–5.2 g/dL)	3.4 g/dL
International normalization ratio (0.9–1.10)	1.17
Blood culture	–
Urine culture	Negative
Stool culture	Negative
Clostridioides difficile stool panel	Negative
Gastrointestinal stool PCR panel	Negative
Lactoferrin	**Positive**
Fecal calprotectin (<50 μg/g)	**541 μg/g**

[a]Lab values in bold are abnormal

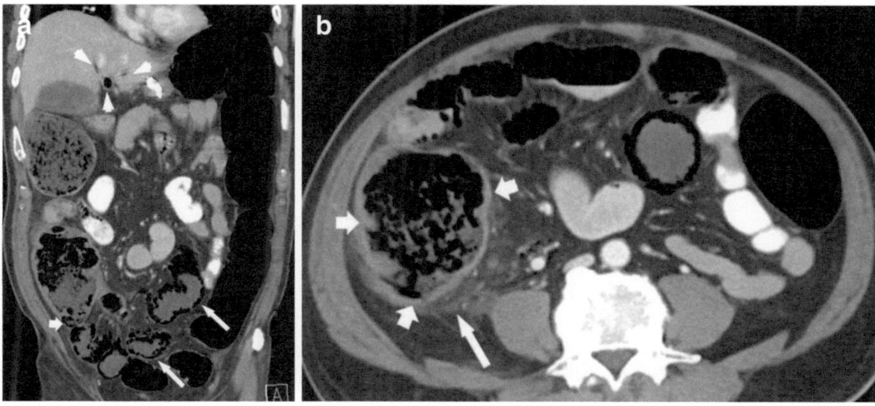

Fig. 20.1 (**a**) Contrast enhanced CT on admission (coronal view) showed dilated loops of distal small bowel (long arrows) and cecum (short arrow) with diffuse pneumatosis; additionally, there is evidence of air tracking into the liver causing pneumobilia (arrowheads). (Sperling et al. 2023 [3]). (**b**) Axial images showed dilated ascending colon with wall thickening (short arrows) and associated adjacent fat stranding (long arrow), suggestive of co-existing colitis

cultures, stool cultures, and vancomycin-resistant enterococci cultures were all negative. However, lactoferrin was positive and fecal calprotectin was elevated at 541 μg/g (normal <50 μg/g). Imaging studies done on admission revealed dilated loops of distal small bowel and colon with diffuse pneumatosis and air trapping, consistent with a diagnosis of pneumatosis intestinalis (PI) of the small and large bowel. Further, there was evidence of colitis present on computerized tomography (CT) scan (Fig. 20.1).

Differential Diagnosis

Pneumatosis is not a primary disease, but rather a clinical sign of an underlying pathology. On initial presentation, the underlying etiology of pneumatosis was unclear. There are many known contributing factors to PI, including chronic obstructive pulmonary disease (COPD), asthma, autoimmune diseases including lupus, polymyositis, dermatomyositis, and drug-induced including corticosteroids. Additional gastrointestinal conditions with associations to PI include inflammatory bowel disease, colitis, Clostridioides difficile infection, and peptic ulcers. Lastly, infectious causes such as human immunodeficiency virus and iatrogenic causes such as blunt trauma, endoscopy, and barium enemas are all associated with PI [1]. However, given that our patient lacked all of these risk factors based on history, close attention was directed towards medications as the possible culprit. Unlike chemotherapy-related diarrhea, immune checkpoint inhibitor (ICI)-mediated diarrhea is typically persistent regardless of administering or holding ICI cycles, as with our patient. Although no colonoscopy with biopsy was conducted to confirm specific histologic changes related with ICI diarrhea/colitis, the patient's calprotectin elevation, rapid symptomatic and radiologic response to high-dose steroids are consistent with this potential etiology. Colitis may precipitate development of PI in general; however, it could also be caused simultaneously by ICI therapy. Finally, there are also limited case reports of lenvatinib associated with PI, which could also contribute to this patient's scenario.

Hospital Course and Management

He was admitted to the intensive care unit and received empiric piperacillin-tazobactam, aggressive hydration, and high flow oxygen for pneumatosis. He was also started on 1 mg/kg of intravenous methylprednisolone for potential immune-mediated diarrhea and colitis. His lenvatinib and pembrolizumab were on hold due to this event. Surgical oncology recommended no surgical intervention given that he would require a total abdominal colectomy and resection of a large amount of small bowel, placing the operative mortality in excess of 50%. The gastroenterology (GI) team believed the risks of endoscopic evaluation outweighed the limited contribution to the medical decision making, and therefore no endoscopy was performed. By hospital day 7, the patient's clinical symptoms resolved and repeat X-ray revealed resolution of PI. Antibiotics were continued, but high flow oxygen was weaned down and the patient was advised to follow-up outpatient with the GI team. A multidisciplinary team suspected that the pneumatosis as well as colitis were related to pembrolizumab and so it was permanently discontinued. This suspicion was based on clinical symptoms, imaging, positive lactoferrin, and elevated fecal calprotectin in the setting of pembrolizumab use and lack of other risk factors. Patient was subsequently consented to restart lenvatinib monotherapy following hospitalization.

Case Outcome

Patient followed up with oncology team 2 days after discharge but failed to follow up with the GI team. Overall, he continued to do well symptomatically but was having occasional loose stool. His cancer disease had been responding to lenvatinib without further progression, so the plan was to continue the treatment. However, 3 weeks after discharge, the patient unexpectedly died after cardiac arrest.

Case Summary

This is a patient with anaplastic thyroid cancer who had received two cycles of lenvatinib and pembrolizumab and subsequently developed acute pneumatosis intestinalis and immune-mediated colitis He was treated with antibiotics, oxygen, and bowel rest with symptomatic remission and resolution on repeat imaging after 7 days. The patient unfortunately expired from cardiac arrest 3 weeks after hospital discharge. Summary of timeline event is shown in Fig. 20.2.

Discussion

Pneumatosis intestinalis is a radiologic finding defined as gas and free air in the extraluminal space of the intestines that is most often secondary to an underlying etiology which may include immune checkpoint inhibitor toxicity. Most patients are asymptomatic; however, symptomatic patients often present with general GI complaints including abdominal pain, diarrhea, and nausea/vomiting. Symptomatic patients may be treated with antibiotics, bowel rest, oxygen, or surgical intervention depending on symptom severity and the affected region of bowel [2]. Most cancer patients with this condition appear to have favorable outcomes with full recovery without the need for surgical intervention. An additional consideration is the use of corticosteroids for concurrent immune-related adverse events including colitis, as steroids may also contribute to the development of PI [3]. Therefore, one must conduct a critical analysis of risks and benefits prior to initiating corticosteroids for patients with PI and simultaneous immune-related adverse events. Importantly, the decision to restart cancer therapy following PI resolution has not been established in literature and this decision should be made on an individual basis with a multidisciplinary team.

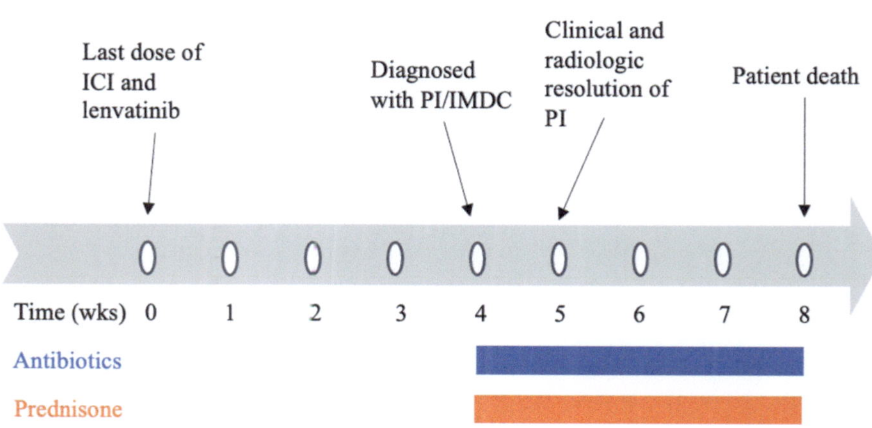

Fig. 20.2 Summary of timeline events

References

1. Zhang T, Cao M, Zhao B, et al. Pneumatosis intestinalis post steroid use in a patient with immune-related adverse events: case report, literature review and FAERS analysis. Front Pharmacol. 2023;14:1133551. Published 2023 Mar 14. https://doi.org/10.3389/fphar.2023.1133551.
2. Im J, Anjum F. Pneumatosis intestinalis. In: StatPearls. Treasure Island, FL: StatPearls; 2022.
3. Sperling G, Shatila M, Varatharajalu K, et al. Pneumatosis intestinalis in cancer patients who received immune checkpoint inhibitors. J Cancer Res Clin Oncol. 2023;149:17597–605. https://doi.org/10.1007/s00432-023-05461-z.

Chapter 21
Pouchitis Post Immune Checkpoint Inhibitor Therapy

Gabriel Sperling, Malek Shatila, Dan Zhao, Yan Zhou, and Yinghong Wang

Abbreviations

ALT	Alanine transaminase
AST	Aspartate aminotransferase
CT	Computerized tomography
CTCAE	Common terminology criteria for adverse events
IBD	Inflammatory bowel disease
ICI	Immune checkpoint inhibitor
IPAA	Ileal pouch anal anastomosis
GI	Gastrointestinal
PCR	Polymerase chain reaction

G. Sperling
John Sealy School of Medicine, The University of Texas Medical Branch,
Galveston, TX, USA
e-mail: gasperli@utmb.edu

M. Shatila · Y. Wang (✉)
Department of Gastroenterology, Hepatology & Nutrition, The University of Texas MD Anderson Cancer Center, Houston, TX, USA
e-mail: MShatila@mdanderson.org; ywang59@mdanderson.org

D. Zhao
Department of Gastrointestinal Medical Oncology, The University of Texas MD Anderson Cancer Center, Houston, TX, USA
e-mail: DZhao3@mdanderson.org

Y. Zhou
Department of Hospital Medicine, The University of Texas MD Anderson Cancer Center,
Houston, TX, USA
e-mail: YZhou@mdanderson.org

Y. Wang (ed.), *Challenging Cases in Immunotherapy Related Organ Toxicities*,
https://doi.org/10.1007/978-3-031-83533-9_21

Patient A

Clinical Presentation, Hospital Course, and Management

The patient is a man in his 70s with past medical history of ulcerative colitis for which he received a colectomy with ileal pouch anal anastomosis (IPAA: J pouch) over 20 years prior. He has stage IVB squamous cell carcinoma of the mid-esophagus treated previously with chemoradiation with FOLFOX and then pembrolizumab every 3 weeks for 8 total doses. Five weeks after his last pembrolizumab dose, the patient presented to the hospital with sudden onset of worsening, grade 3 diarrhea based on common terminology criteria for adverse events (CTCAE). He also had increased frequency, incontinence, and nightly episodes. Admission labs were notable for positive lactoferrin, and stool infectious testing was negative for Clostridioides difficile and gastrointestinal multiplex panel. Subsequent sigmoidoscopy revealed an inflamed pouch with superficial ulceration along the afferent limb of the pouch to the neo-terminal ileum near the anastomosis as seen in Fig. 21.1. Histologic findings showed focal active inflammation with epithelial apoptosis and erosion. The nonspecific findings were deemed to be an immune checkpoint inhibitor (ICI)-induced injury in the context of recent pembrolizumab use given the lack of other risk factors, and therefore ICI therapy was withheld. After 3 days in the hospital, he was discharged on a 60 mg/day oral prednisone taper for 4 weeks with complete symptomatic resolution by his follow-up appointment 2 weeks later.

Six weeks after discharge, the patient was readmitted with new rectal bleeding. Admission labs were notable for anemia with hemoglobin of 10.6 g/dL, leukocytosis at $11.5 \times 10^3/\mu L$, positive lactoferrin, elevated calprotectin at 96.6 μg/g, and a negative infectious stool work-up (Table 21.1). A subsequent pouchoscopy showed multiple oozing ulcers in the pouch and nonbleeding vessels along the dentate line, suspicious for persistent and aggressive pouchitis despite discontinuation of ICI therapy. Pouch biopsies revealed ulcerated mucosa and regenerative changes in the background of chronic inflammation. During this presentation, the patient was already receiving oral prednisone at 100 mg/day with a 6-week taper from a recent hospitalization for ICI-mediated pneumonitis. Despite the resolution of respiratory symptoms, recurrent pouchitis symptoms persisted on steroids. Consequently, the decision was made to escalate care to 300 mg intravenous vedolizumab, which he received 3 total doses at 0, 2, and 6 weeks.

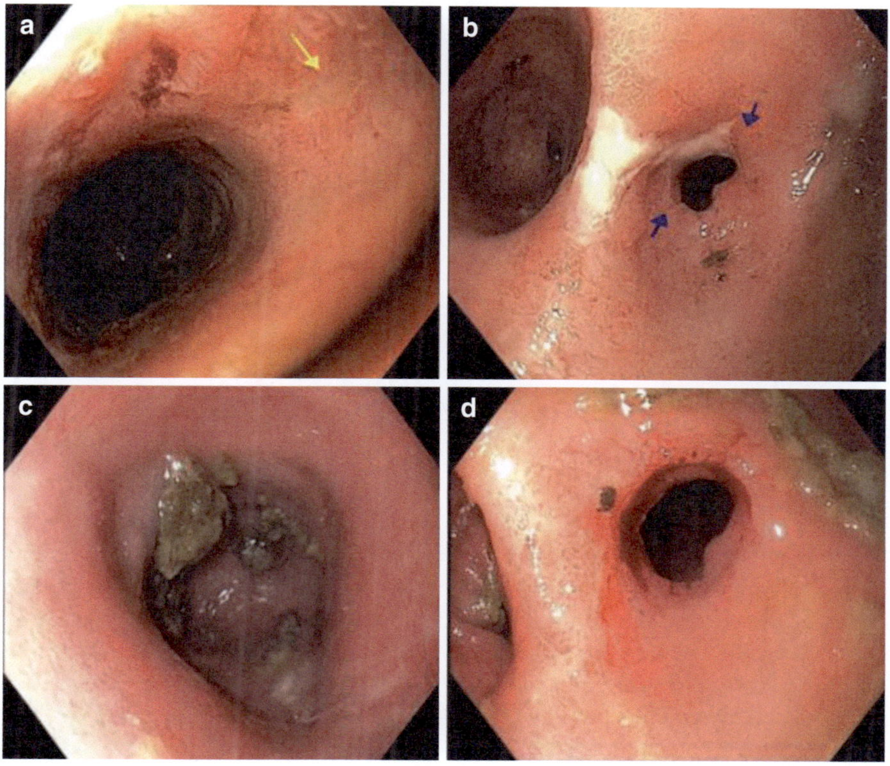

Fig. 21.1 Pouchoscopy images. Superficial ulcers at the afferent limb of the pouch to the neo-terminal ileum, erosions, erythema (**a**, **b**; before treatment); mild erythema with resolution of ulcers (**c**, **d**; after treatment)

Table 21.1 Laboratory findings for Patient A

Laboratory test	Admission #1	Admission #2
White blood count (4.0–11.0 × 10^3/μL)	5.1 × 10^3/μL	**11.5 × 10^3/μL**
Hemoglobin (12.0–16.0 g/dL)	**11.5 g/dL**	**10.6 g/dL**
Platelet count (140–440 × 10^3/μL)	**126 × 10^3/μL**	284 × 10^3/μL
Sodium (136–145 mEq/L)	**127 mmol/L**	**131 mmol/L**
Potassium (3.5–5.1 mEq/L)	4.3 mmol/L	5 mmol/L
Chloride (98–107 mEq/L)	**90 mmol/L**	100 mmol/L
Carbon dioxide (22–29 mEq/L)	23 mmol/L	22 mmol/L
Blood urea nitrogen (6–23 mg/dL)	**26 mg/dL**	**33 mg/dL**
Creatinine (0.67–1.17 mg/dL)	**2.45 mg/dL**	**1.46 mg/dL**
Glucose (70–99 mg/dL)	**108 mg/dL**	**121 mg/dL**
Calcium (8.4–10.2 mg/dL)	8.9 mg/dL	9 mg/dL
ALT (<41 U/L)	13 U/L	13 U/L
AST (<40 U/L)	17 U/L	17 U/L

(continued)

Table 21.1 (continued)

Laboratory test	Admission #1	Admission #2
Alkaline phosphatase (40–129 U/L)	47 U/L	51 U/L
Total bilirubin (<1.2 mg/dL)	0.5 mg/dL	0.3 mg/dL
Total protein (6.4–8.3 g/dL)	**6.2 g/dL**	**5.2 g/dL**
Albumin (3.5–5.2 g/dL)	3.9 g/dL	3.5 g/dL
International normalization ratio (0.9–1.10)	–	1.09
Blood culture (2 sets)	–	Negative
Urine culture	–	–
Clostridioides difficile stool panel	Negative	Negative
Gastrointestinal stool PCR panel	Negative	Negative
Lactoferrin	**Positive**	**Positive**
Fecal calprotectin (<50 μg/g)	20.2 μg/g	**96.6 μg/g**

Case Outcome

The patient did well symptomatically for the following 2 months after hospital discharge, although repeat pouchoscopy showing persistent active inflammation and ulcers of the pouch. Due to these endoscopic findings, the decision was made to continue vedolizumab for an additional 2 doses at weeks 14 and 22. The following pouchoscopy 4 months after the most recent procedure showed an ulcerated anastomotic site but overall much improved from the previous exam, as seen in Fig. 21.1. Biopsies of the pouch confirmed mild chronic inflammation with crypt apoptotic bodies. Repeat stool calprotectin at this time was within normal range at <50 μg/g. The patient's gastrointestinal (GI) symptoms remained at baseline for another 29 months without further pouchitis flares, though the most recent pouchoscopy still showed mild residual pouch inflammation. From a cancer perspective, he has not received any further cancer treatment since discontinuing pembrolizumab; however, his cancer has remained in stable condition with frequent surveillance every 6 months.

Case Summary

This is a patient with stage IVB esophageal squamous cell carcinoma who received eight cycles of pembrolizumab and subsequently developed pouchitis in the J-pouch from IPAA surgery. His prolonged disease course was complicated by diarrhea and rectal bleeding requiring hospitalizations and treatment with both steroids and vedolizumab. He achieved sustained clinical and endoscopic remission after treatment, and his cancer has remained stable off pembrolizumab and any other systemic chemotherapy for 2.5 years of follow-up surveillance. Timeline of events are summarized in Fig. 21.2.

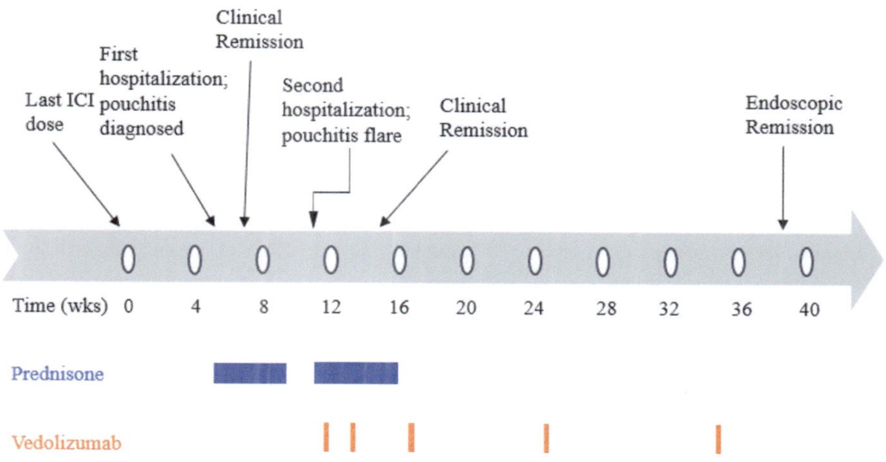

Fig. 21.2 Summary of timeline events for Patient A (timepoint of 0 is the last dose of ICI)

Patient B

Clinical Presentation, Hospital Course, and Management

The patient is a man in his 60s with a past medical history of ulcerative colitis for which he underwent a colectomy with IPAA over 30 years prior. Notably, he had an episode of pouchitis several years prior which resolved. He was diagnosed with stage IIIB hepatocellular carcinoma, for which he had received multiple lines of treatments including lenvatinib, Y90, nivolumab, STAT3 inhibitor, bevacizumab and atezolizumab, radiation, and cabozantinib. Most recently, he was started on durvalumab and tremelimumab. Four weeks after receiving the first dose of this regimen, the patient was admitted to the hospital with progressive right lower quadrant pain and worsening grade 3 diarrhea. He was having about 8–10 watery bowel movements daily, an increase in his baseline frequency of 3–5 solid bowel movements, in addition to fecal incontinence. On admission, he was hypotensive and tachycardic. Labs were notable for a fecal calprotectin >3000 μg/g, positive lactoferrin, ALT of 46 U/L, AST of 51 U/L, and creatinine of 1.71 mg/dL (Table 21.2). Subsequent computerized tomography (CT) scan of the abdomen and pelvis demonstrated thickening of the distal small bowel to the level of the J-pouch, suspicious for enteritis/pouchitis. A pouchoscopy revealed diffuse erythema with inflammatory exudate of the pouch body, as seen in Fig. 21.3, and pathology demonstrated focal active inflammation. He was started on intravenous methylprednisolone 50 mg/day for 8 days without symptomatic improvement. He then received a dose of 300 mg vedolizumab intravenously for steroid-refractory pouchitis, and he was discharged in an overall improved condition. He was discharged on a 4-week, 60 mg/day oral steroid taper and received a second dose of vedolizumab 2 weeks after the first.

Table 21.2 Laboratory findings for Patient B

Laboratory test	Admission #1	Admission #2
White blood count (4.0–11.0 K/μL)	6.4 × 10^3/μL	5.9 × 10^3/μL
Hemoglobin (12.0–16.0 g/dL)	12.4 g/dL	**10.7 g/dL**
Platelet count (140–440 K/μL)	221 × 10^3/μL	143 × 10^3/μL
Sodium (136–145 mEq/L)	**133 mmol/L**	**134 mmol/L**
Potassium (3.5–5.1 mEq/L)	4.3 mmol/L	4.0 mmol/L
Chloride (98–107 mEq/L)	**97 mmol/L**	100 mmol/L
Carbon dioxide (22–29 mEq/L)	**20 mmol/L**	23 mmol/L
Blood urea nitrogen (6–23 mg/dL)	**25 mg/dL**	**27 mg/dL**
Creatinine (0.67–1.17 mg/dL)	**1.71 mg/dL**	**2.10 mg/dL**
Glucose (70–99 mg/dL)	91 mg/dL	96 mg/dL
Calcium (8.4–10.2 mg/dL)	**11.1 mg/dL**	9.5 mg/dL
ALT (<41 U/L)	**46 U/L**	**48 U/L**
AST (<40 U/L)	**51 U/L**	31 U/L
Alkaline phosphatase (40–129 U/L)	**241 U/L**	**298 U/L**
Total bilirubin (<1.2 mg/dL)	0.7 mg/dL	0.6 mg/dL
Total protein (6.4–8.3 g/dL)	**9.3 g/dL**	6.8 g/dL
Albumin (3.5–5.2 g/dL)	4.5 g/dL	3.5 g/dL
International normalization ratio (0.9–1.10)	–	–
Blood culture (2 sets)	–	–
Urine culture	Negative	Negative
Clostridioides difficile stool panel	Negative	Negative
Gastrointestinal stool PCR panel	Negative	Negative
Lactoferrin	**Positive**	**Positive**
Fecal calprotectin (<50 μg/g)	**>3000 μg/g**	**51.7 μg/g**

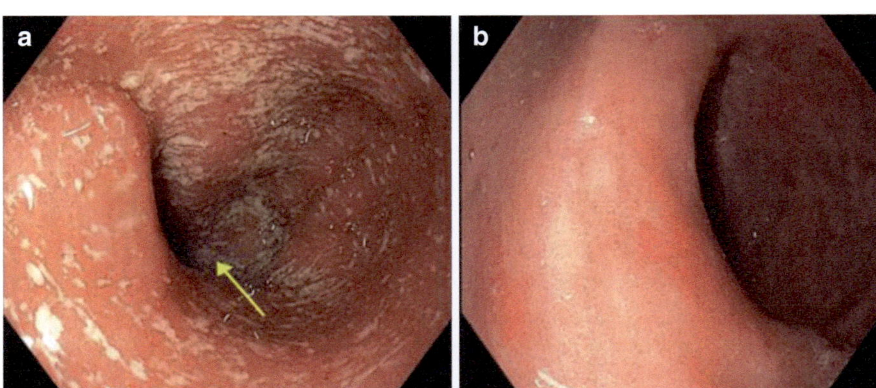

Fig. 21.3 J-pouch with diffuse erythema, inflammatory exudate (**a**; before treatment); mild erythema (**b**; after treatment)

Three weeks after discharge, the patient returned to the emergency department with grade 3 diarrhea again. He noted temporary improvement for several days after each dose of vedolizumab but otherwise he was symptomatically unchanged from the last admission. Admission labs were notable for a hemoglobin of 10.7 g/dL, creatinine of 2.10 mg/dL, ALT of 48 U/L, and positive lactoferrin. CT scan of the abdomen and pelvis revealed persistent inflammation of the pouch. A repeat pouchoscopy demonstrated mucosal ulceration and erythema, and pathology was consistent with acute enteritis/ileitis. Given the elevated liver enzymes likely related to an ICI-mediated adverse event, 260 mg of intravenous ustekinumab was started before discharge from the hospital.

Case Outcome

His GI symptoms were at his baseline condition at 1 and 2 months follow-up and he received a second dose of ustekinumab 8 weeks after the first. Calprotectin at this time returned to 88.0 μg/g. A subsequent pouchoscopy 2 weeks later revealed minimally erythematous mucosa in the pouch, as seen in Fig. 21.2, but greatly improved from his prior procedure. Given that he was in clinical and endoscopic remission at this point, pouchitis treatment was discontinued and he will continue to receive a yearly surveillance pouchoscopy. He proceeded to receive transarterial chemoembolization (TACE) followed by sorafenib therapy for his cancer. At his most recent follow-up to date, his cancer is overall stable.

Case Summary

This is a unique case of a patient with hepatocellular carcinoma who developed pouchitis after one dose of durvalumab and tremelimumab. He had a prolonged disease course with severe diarrhea leading to two hospitalizations. He required high-dose steroids, vedolizumab, and ustekinumab over the course of 5 months before ultimately achieving clinical and endoscopic remission for pouchitis. Given his notable history of pouchitis 3 years prior, this was most likely a pouchitis flare after receiving ICI therapy. Fortunately, he has done well without further flares for 5 months. He recently was able to resume chemotherapy and his cancer is overall stable and monitored with regular follow-up appointments. Timeline of events are summarized in Fig. 21.4.

Pouchitis is a complex disease characterized by inflammation of the pouch. It is a common complication found in patients who have had a proctocolectomy with ileal pouch anal anastomosis for ulcerative colitis, familial adenomatous polyposis, or another GI pathology [1]. Presentations vary widely but may include increased stool frequency, urgency, pelvic pain, incontinence, or abdominal cramping and pain. Many underlying risk factors have been identified including metabolic factors,

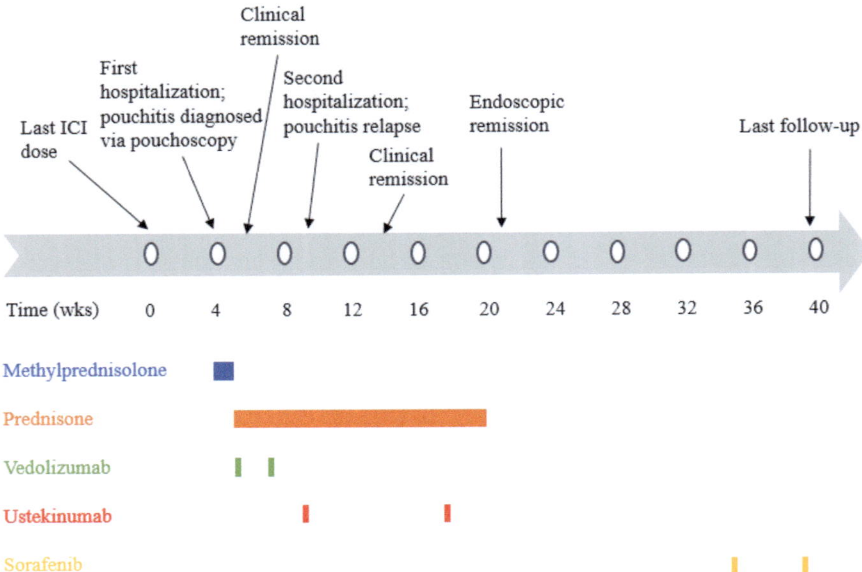

Fig. 21.4 Summary of timeline events (timepoint of 0 is the last ICI dose)

lifestyle factors, and medication use [2, 3]; however, to our knowledge, there have only been two cases reported in literature of ICI-induced pouchitis from our group which are included here [4]. For this reason, its standard treatment is unclear. Treatment of lower GI toxicities from ICI therapy have been well-established, though, and include steroids followed by immunosuppressants such as vedolizumab or infliximab in cases of steroid-refractory disease [5]. Raising awareness about this uncommon pathology is crucial, especially as an increasing number of patients with a history of inflammatory bowel disease (IBD) are undergoing ICI treatments, a standard approach in modern cancer care. This can potentially worsen their underlying inflammatory condition, highlighting the need for understanding and vigilance [4]. Hypothetically, this risk certainly applies to IBD patients with IPAA surgery with J-pouch even though the pouch condition could have remained quiescent for years. Future studies are still required to further clarify the optimal treatment options for this unique population.

References

1. Stocchi L, Pemberton JH. Pouch and pouchitis. Gastroenterol Clin North Am. 2001;30:223–41. [PMID: 11394032]. https://doi.org/10.1016/s0889-8553(05)70175-8.
2. Shen B. Acute and chronic pouchitis—pathogenesis, diagnosis and treatment. Nat Rev Gastroenterol Hepatol. 2012;9:323–33. [PMID: 22508158]. https://doi.org/10.1038/nrgastro.2012.58.

3. Shen B, Kochhar GS, Rubin DT, et al. Treatment of pouchitis, Crohn's disease, cuffitis, and other inflammatory disorders of the pouch: consensus guidelines from the International Ileal Pouch Consortium. Lancet Gastroenterol Hepatol. 2022;7:69–95. [PMID: 34774224]. https://doi.org/10.1016/S2468-1253(21)00214-4.
4. Sperling G, Wang Y. Pouchitis after immune checkpoint inhibitors. AIM Clin Cases. 2023;2:e230414. https://doi.org/10.7326/aimcc.2023.0414.
5. Rajha E, Chaftari P, Kamal M, et al. Gastrointestinal adverse events associated with immune checkpoint inhibitor therapy. Gastroenterol Rep (Oxf). 2019;8:25–30. [PMID: 32104583]. https://doi.org/10.1093/gastro/goz065.

Chapter 22
Rectal Ulcer and Perianal Fistula in a Cancer Patient on Immune Checkpoint Inhibitor Therapy

Christine Catinis, Nitish Mittal, Maya Sarihan, Abdullah Aleem, Jianbo Wang, Matthew T. Campbell, and Yinghong Wang

Abbreviations

CT	Computed tomography
GI	Gastrointestinal
ICI	Immune checkpoint inhibitors
MRI	Magnetic resonance imaging

Clinical Presentation and Clinical Course

This is a male in his 60s with renal cell carcinoma with metastases to the bilateral lungs and brain who presented to the emergency department with progressively worsening diarrhea, abdominal bloating, and decreased appetite. He was receiving treatment with nivolumab/ipilimumab and cabozantinib and completed cycle 3 of

C. Catinis · N. Mittal · M. Sarihan · A. Aleem
Department of Internal Medicine, The University of Texas Health Science Center, Houston, TX, USA
e-mail: christine.catinis@uth.tmc.edu; nitish.mittal@uth.tmc.edu; maya.c.sarihan@uth.tmc.edu; abdullah.aleem@uth.tmc.edu

J. Wang · M. T. Campbell
Department of Genitourinary Medical Oncology, The University of Texas MD Anderson Cancer Center, Houston, TX, USA
e-mail: JWang38@mdanderson.org; MCampbell3@mdanderson.org

Y. Wang (✉)
Department of Gastroenterology, Hepatology & Nutrition, The University of Texas MD Anderson Cancer Center, Houston, TX, USA
e-mail: ywang59@mdanderson.org

Y. Wang (ed.), *Challenging Cases in Immunotherapy Related Organ Toxicities*,
https://doi.org/10.1007/978-3-031-83533-9_22

nivolumab/ipilimumab three weeks prior. Otherwise, he has a past medical history of atrial fibrillation and hyperlipidemia.

One month prior to this presentation, he was hospitalized with neutropenic fever and *E. Coli* bacteremia secondary to sigmoid diverticulitis. He was treated with cefepime, vancomycin, and metronidazole, and was ultimately transitioned to oral ciprofloxacin and metronidazole to complete a 14-day antibiotic course. Cabozantinib was held at that time, as it was thought to have contributed to his agranulocytosis. Given resolution of symptoms, however, it was re-started a few weeks later.

A few days prior to his presentation to the emergency department, he started to experience intractable diarrhea. Cabozantinib was held once again, but his symptoms continued to worsen to the point where he was having as many as 14 to 16 diarrheal episodes daily. He denied any fevers, nausea, vomiting, or blood in the stool, but endorsed associated increased urgency, decreased appetite, and abdominal cramping.

Evaluations

Initial testing revealed a negative enteric stool pathogen panel, negative C. difficile PCR/antigen, positive lactoferrin, and calprotectin of 955 μg/g (reference range <50 μg/g) (Table 22.1). Colonoscopy revealed a single 15 mm rectal ulcer distorting the anal canal and distal rectum alongside a fistula opening (Fig. 22.1). Biopsies were obtained and showed a nonspecific ulcer base with inflamed granulation tissue and inflammatory exudate. Pathology of the remaining colon was normal.

Table 22.1 Lab values

Test	Value at onset of GI symptoms	Value after complete resolution of GI symptoms (2 months later)
Fecal calprotectin (Normal <50.0 μg/g)	**955 μg/g (H)**	<50 μg/g
Fecal lactoferrin	**Positive**	Negative
Fecal ova and parasite	Negative	Negative
Enteric pathogen panel	Negative	Negative
White blood cell (Normal 4.0–11.0 K/μL)	4.8 K/μL	6.2 K/μL
Hemoglobin (Normal 14.0–18.0 g/dL)	14.2 g/dL	**10.8 g/dL (L)**
Platelet (Normal 140–440 K/μL)	358 K/μL	207 K/μL
Clostridioides difficile DNA, antigen	Negative	Negative

μg microgram, *g* gram, *CFU* colony forming unit, *mL* milliliter, *K* thousand, *μL* microliter, *dL* deciliter, *ESBL* extended spectrum beta-lactamase, *DNA* deoxyribonucleic acid
Abnormal lab values are in bold

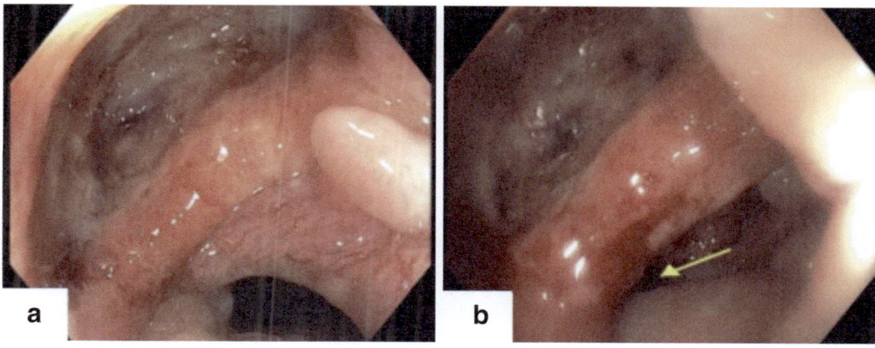

Fig. 22.1 Colonoscopy during initial presentation. (**a**) shows a single 15 mm ulcer found in the rectum. (**b**) shows a rectal fistula opening (yellow arrow)

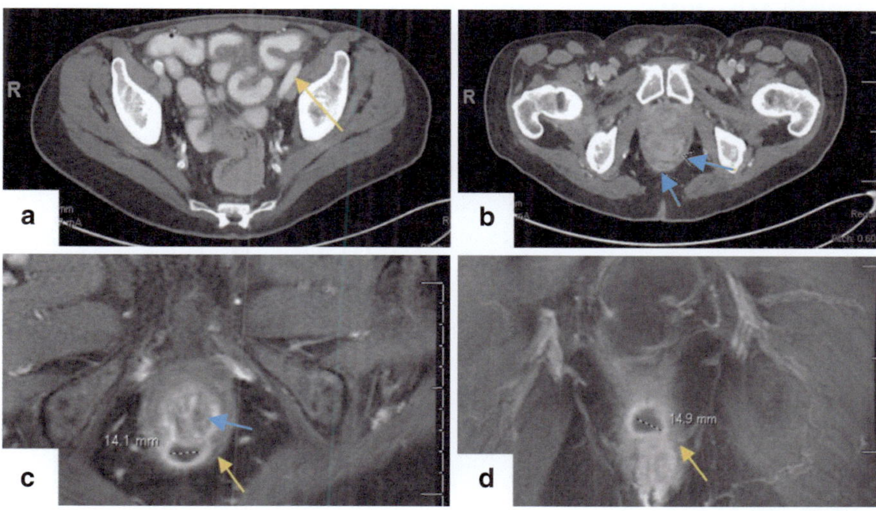

Fig. 22.2 Contrast enhanced CT images (coronal) showing (**a**) thickened wall of the small bowel with peri-enteric stranding (yellow arrow), suggestive of immunotherapy related enteritis, and (**b**) thin perianal enhancing tracts (blue arrows). Contrast enhanced MRI images (coronal) showing (**c**) a perianal fistulous tract (blue arrow) associated with a 0.9 cm fluid collection (yellow arrow) and (**d**) a 1.4 cm fluid collection (yellow arrow)

Esophagogastroduodenoscopy (EGD) was also performed, which showed diffuse inflammation in the stomach and multiple 2–5 mm flat polyps in the second portion of the duodenum. Biopsies revealed chronic gastritis, chronic duodenitis, and fragments of tubular adenoma. Computed tomography (CT) of abdomen and pelvis (AP) showed interval development of immune-mediated enteritis and possible thin perianal enhancing tracts. Further evaluation with contrast-enhanced magnetic resonance imaging (MRI) of the pelvis confirmed the presence of two perianal fistulous tracts with associated small fluid collections (Fig. 22.2). Interventional radiology and surgical oncology were consulted for possible drainage or aspiration of the fluid collections, but they were deemed to be too small for surgical intervention.

Treatment

The patient was thus started on empiric ampicillin/sulbactam, which was ultimately transitioned to oral amoxicillin/clavulanic acid to complete a 14-day antibiotic course. Given the patient's persistent diarrhea secondary to presumed immune-mediated enteritis, he was started on budesonide and vedolizumab.

Clinical Outcome

Our patient noted significant improvement in his symptoms after starting budesonide and vedolizumab. After his second dose of vedolizumab 2 weeks later, his diarrheal symptoms completely resolved. A repeat CT AP 3 weeks later revealed resolution of the enteritis and rectal fistula. In addition, a repeat calprotectin level 4 months later was <50 μg/g, therefore, treatment with budesonide was discontinued. The patient received a total of three doses of vedolizumab. Cabozantinib was re-started at a lower dose, together with nivolumab monotherapy. Two months later, he started having diarrheal symptoms again with repeat calprotectin level of 298 μg/g with negative infectious workup. Because of the evidence of recurrent bowel inflammation, he will plan to receive 3 additional maintenance vedolizumab treatments every eight weeks and repeat sigmoidoscopy in three months.

Summary of the Case

This is a male with metastatic renal cell carcinoma on nivolumab/ipilimumab and cabozantinib who presented with progressively worsening diarrhea and was found to have duodenitis, rectal ulcer, and perianal fistula/fluid collection. He was treated with antibiotics, budesonide, and 3 doses of vedolizumab with significant symptom response and resolution of fistula on follow up imaging 3 weeks later. He was successfully resumed on cabozantinib and remained on nivolumab during the entire GI event. Summary of the events is depicted in Fig. 22.3.

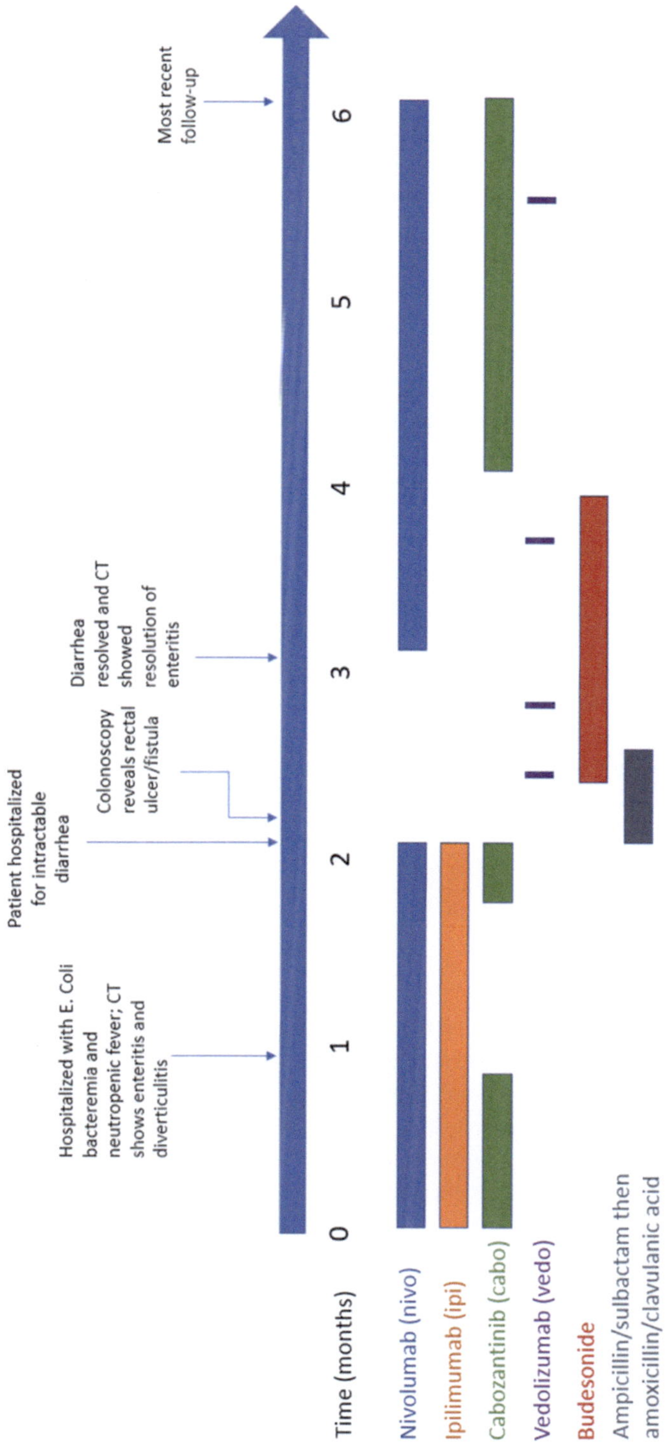

Fig. 22.3 Clinical course and timeline of the events. (Timepoint of 0 is the initiation of ICI)

Discussion

Gastrointestinal symptoms including diarrhea and colitis [1–4] are commonly reported after ICI treatment, though there have been few reports associating ICI therapy with the development of diverticulitis and subsequent luminal GI tract fistula/abscess formation [5, 6]. Perianal abscesses and fistulas as the predominant presentations of GI toxicity post ICI exposure were rarely seen [1, 7]. Given the rarity of its presentation and the fact that it is always reported in conjunction with findings of enterocolitis, it appears as though abscess and fistula formation occur as sequelae of ICI related enterocolitis rather than as isolated GI toxicities. Therefore, prompt diagnosis and management of colitis is paramount.

Historically, initiation of corticosteroid therapy has been implemented in the treatment of ICI related colitis, though some patients have inadequate response to steroid therapy despite optimized dosing and multiple attempts at tapering. Additional immunosuppressive therapy with infliximab and vedolizumab have been used in the treatment of severe, steroid-refractory ICI related colitis with high efficacy [8, 9].

The successful treatment outcome from a combination regimen of antibiotics, budesonide, and vedolizumab in this particularly challenging case provides a great reference for our future clinical practice. In such patients, medical therapy may be sufficient in the treatment of ICI related ulcers and fistulas. However, similar to the management of fistula formation in IBD, further surgical management with fistulectomy and fistulotomy or even colectomy may be indicated if medical management is insufficient. Importantly, restarting immunotherapy after successful treatment and resolution of ICI related GI toxicity poses a high risk of relapse [10] and should be considered on a case-by-case basis.

Conclusion

In summary, perianal abscesses and fistulas could be a rare presentation of GI toxicity that may or may not be associated with enterocolitis post-ICI exposure. Its management is primarily based on anecdotal evidence. The successful treatment outcome from a combination regimen of antibiotics, budesonide, and vedolizumab in this particularly challenging case illustrated the importance of early diagnosis and initiation of the appropriate therapy. Failure to initiate prompt therapy may lead to disease progression which ultimately will require operative management.

References

1. Rocha M, et al. Management of Gastrointestinal Toxicity from Immune Checkpoint Inhibitor. 2019; 268-274.; Wei W, Luo Z. Risk of gastrointestinal toxicities with PD-1 inhibitors in cancer patients: a meta-analysis of randomized clinical trials. Medicine (Baltimore). 2017;96(48):e8931.
2. Mearns ES, Bell JA, Galaznik A, Puglielli SM, Cichewicz AB, Boulanger T, Garcia-Ribas I. Gastrointestinal adverse events with combination of checkpoint inhibitors in advanced melanoma: a systematic review. Melanoma Manag. 2018;5(1):MMT01.
3. Pereira ROL, Patel PR, Guru PK, Sanghavi DK. Tumour-bowel fistula as a possible complication of pazopanib therapy in retroperitoneal leiomyosarcoma. BMJ Case Rep. 2019;12(11):e230727.
4. Thomas AR, Wang Y. Complicated diverticulitis after immune checkpoint inhibitor therapy. Am J Gastroenterol. 2021;116:S831.
5. Tursi A. Immune checkpoint inhibitors-induced acute diverticulitis. Eur J Gastroenterol Hepatol. 2020;32:893–5.
6. Marthey L, Mateus C, Mussini C, Nachury M, Nancey S, Grange F, et al. Cancer immunotherapy with antiCTLA-4 monoclonal antibodies induces an inflammatory bowel disease. J Crohns Colitis. 2016;10(4):395–401.
7. Abu-Sbeih H, Ali FS, Luo W, et al. Importance of endoscopic and histological evaluation in the management of immune checkpoint inhibitor-induced colitis. J Immunother Cancer. 2018;6:95.
8. Johnson D, Zobniw C, Trinh V, Ma J, Bassett R, Anderson J, Davis J, Joseph J, Ali N, Abu-Sbeih H, Davies M, Wong M, Hwu W-J, Hwu P, Wang Y, Diab A. Infliximab associated with faster symptom resolution compared with corticosteroids alone for the management of immune-related enterocolitis. J Immunother Cancer. 2018;6(1):103.
9. Zou F, Faleck D, Thomas A, Harris J, Satish D, Wang X, Charabaty A, Ernstoff MS, Glitza Oliva IC, Hanauer S, McQuade J, Obeid M, Shah A, Richards DM, Sharon E, Wolchok J, Thompson J, Wang Y. Efficacy and safety of vedolizumab and infliximab treatment for immune-mediated diarrhea and colitis in patients with cancer: a two-center observational study. J Immunother Cancer. 2021;9(11):e003277. https://doi.org/10.1136/jitc-2021-003277.
10. Abu-Sbeih H, Ali FS, Naqash AR, Owen DH, Patel S, Otterson GA, Kendra K, Ricciuti B, Chiari R, De Giglio A, Sleiman J, Funchain P, Wills B, Zhang J, Naidoo J, Philpott J, Gao J, Subudhi SK, Wang Y. Immune–mediated colitis after resumption of immune checkpoint inhibitor therapy. J Clin Oncol. 2019;37(30):2738–45.

Chapter 23
Recurrent Clostridioides Difficile Infection and Colitis Post Immune Checkpoint Inhibitor Therapy

Elliot Baerman, Kristin Junek, Rey Cerbas Lavilla, Xin Shelley Wang, and Yinghong Wang

Abbreviations

CT Computed tomography
DNA Deoxyribonucleic acid
FMT Fecal microbiota transplantation
ICI Immune checkpoint inhibitor
rCDI Recurrent Clostridioides difficile colitis

Case Presentation

Our patient is a female in her 70s with history of low-grade B-cell lymphoma, who underwent multiple lines of chemotherapy including rituximab, bendamustine, and copanalisib and then 9 cycles of atezolizumab over 6 months with the last cycle 3 months prior, and presented with watery diarrhea, fever and chills. Otherwise, she had past medical history of chronic obstructive pulmonary disease, peripheral arterial disease, hypothyroidism, hypertension, and Nissen fundoplication.

E. Baerman
Department of Internal Medicine, Baylor College of Medicine, Houston, TX, USA
e-mail: Elliot.Baerman@bcm.edu

K. Junek · R. C. Lavilla · Y. Wang (✉)
Department of Gastroenterology, Hepatology & Nutrition, The University of Texas MD Anderson Cancer Center, Houston, TX, USA
e-mail: KNJunek@mdanderson.org; RCLavilla@mdanderson.org; YWang59@mdanderson.org

X. S. Wang
Department of Symptom Research, The University of Texas MD Anderson Cancer Center, Houston, TX, USA
e-mail: xswang@mdanderson.org

Y. Wang (ed.), *Challenging Cases in Immunotherapy Related Organ Toxicities*,
https://doi.org/10.1007/978-3-031-83533-9_23

In the preceding 6 months, she was exposed to multiple courses of antibiotics for urinary tract infections including nitrofurantoin, trimethoprim/sulfamethoxazole, and cefpodoxime. She had several previous episodes of Clostridioides difficile infection (CDI) including a hospitalization 1 month prior to presentation for which she received vancomycin and intravenous hydration with resolution of diarrhea. 15 days before arrival, she had been admitted for worsening diarrhea and was found to have congested mucosa in the rectum, recto-sigmoid, sigmoid colon, and descending colon along with ulcers in the same areas on flexible sigmoidoscopy. Biopsies demonstrated colonic mucosa with focal erosions, ulceration, and acute colitis with changes confirming the presence of pseudomembranous colitis. Given negative C. diff deoxyribonucleic acid and toxin during that hospitalization, she was diagnosed with immune checkpoint inhibitor colitis (Table 23.1). She received intravenous methylprednisolone with rapid improvement in diarrhea and was discharged on oral prednisone with taper alongside prophylactic trimethoprim/sulfamethoxazole. However, 10 days later, she developed watery stools again with 5 to 6 episodes per day along with intermittent lower abdominal pain. She also endorsed increased fatigue, chills, and fevers with no melena or hematochezia. Repeat C. diff testing was negative. Other medications include amlodipine 5 mg daily, clopidogrel 75 mg daily, albuterol 2 puffs every 6 h PRN, gabapentin 100 mg, vitamin D 500,000 U q weekly, levothyroxine 25 μg daily, pantoprazole 40 mg daily, prochlorperazine

Table 23.1 Lab variables on the presentation

WBC (4–11 × 10^9/L)	11.3 × 10^9/L
Hemoglobin (12–16 g/dL)	**11.4 g/dL (L)**
Platelets (140–440 × 10^9/L)	283 × 10^9/L
Neutrophil Abs (1.7–7.3 × 10^9/L)	9.08 × 10^9/L
Sodium (135–145 mEq/L)	136 mEq/L
Potassium (3.5–5.1 mEq/L)	**3 mEq/L (L)**
Chloride (98–107 mEq/L)	98 mEq/L
Bicarbonate (22–29 mg/dL)	24 mEq/L
BUN (6–23 mg/dL)	14 mg/dL
Creatinine (0.51–0.95 mg/dL)	0.69 mg/dL
Glucose (70–99 mg/dL)	118 mg/dL
Calcium (8.4–10.2 mg/dL)	8.5 mg/dL
Magnesium (1.6–2.6 mg/dL)	2.1 mg/dL
Phosphate (2.5–4.5 mg/dL)	2.9 mg/dL
Albumin (3.5–5.2 mg/dL)	3.9 mg/dL
ALT (≤33 mg/dL)	29 mg/dL
AST (≤32 mg/dL)	34 mg/dL
Alkaline phosphatase (35–104 mg/dL)	68 mg/dL
Total bilirubin (≤1.2 mg/dL)	0.2 mg/dL
Clostridioides difficile toxin	**Positive**
Clostridioides difficile DNA	**Positive**
Blood cultures	Negative
Urine culture	Negative

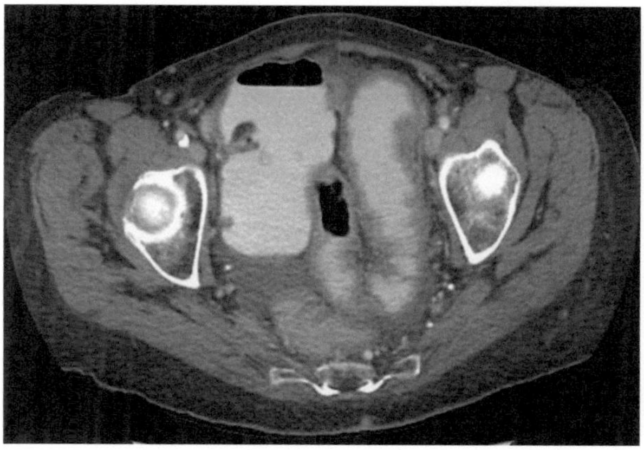

Fig. 23.1 CT abdomen and pelvis with contrast on the current admission

5 mg every 6 h as needed, spironolactone 50 mg daily, trimethoprim/sulfamethoxazole 3 times per week, and valacyclovir 500 mg daily.

On day of presentation, she was tachycardic to 106 beats/min and hemodynamically stable with a fever to 101.8 °F. On exam, she had abdominal tenderness and was clinically hypovolemic. CT showed colonic wall thickening and edema, consistent with colitis (Fig. 23.1).

Colonic wall thickening and edema, consistent with colitis.

Differential Diagnosis

The differential for this patient's presentation of acute on chronic diarrhea is narrowed by her prior history; however, the challenge lies in distinguishing between one pathological process versus two distinct entities. Certainly, this presentation is highly suspicious for a concurrent recurrent CDI and persistent ICI colitis, but we must also recognize the possibility that one of these two pathologies may contribute more than the other. This ambiguity made the management more challenging.

Hospital Course and Follow Up

She was admitted to the hospital the following day for intravenous (IV) hydration. Her C. diff DNA and toxin were positive for which she was started on IV metronidazole 500 mg every 8 h and fidaxomicin 200 mg every 12 h. Her oral prednisone was increased from 40 mg daily to 50 mg daily for concurrent refractory ICI colitis. She continued this regimen for 7 days with persistent symptoms, and therefore received an endoscopically administered fecal microbiota transplantation (FMT) on day 8 for the purpose of clearance of C. diff component, so treatment for ICI colitis

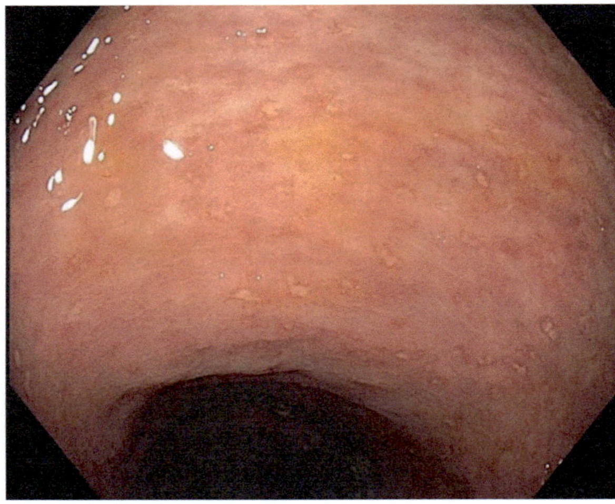

Fig. 23.2 Colonoscopy during first FMT. Inflammation characterized by congestion (edema), erosions, erythema and granularity was found in a continuous and circumferential pattern from the rectum to ascending colon. This was graded as Mayo Score 1 (mild, with erythema, decreased vascular pattern, mild friability)

could be safely escalated. The colonoscopy at the time of FMT showed congestion (edema), erosions, erythema and granularity in a continuous and circumferential pattern from the rectum to ascending colon (Fig. 23.2).

By the following day after FMT, her diarrhea, appetite, and energy levels improved dramatically. She was discharged with prednisone with taper. She remained asymptomatic with resolution of colitis on 3 months follow up colonoscopy. She was not restarted on atezolizumab but did receive palliative radiation therapy, 400 cGY in 2 fractions, 3 months later due to increased size and metabolism of anterior mediastinal lymph nodes.

Subsequently, she had another recurrent CDI (rCDI) as evidenced by recurrent watery diarrhea, positive C. diff toxin and DNA assays, and pseudomembrane formation on colonoscopy 11 months after receiving her first FMT. Of note, she received antimicrobial therapy 3 months prior to this second presentation for infectious diarrhea including metronidazole, ciprofloxacin, and azithromycin. She was started on fidaxomicin followed by bezlotoxumab, but her diarrhea persisted after this infusion. Accordingly, she underwent an additional FMT 9 days later with resolution of symptoms.

Her last follow up was 3 months after her second FMT for a colonoscopy, which demonstrated sustained remission from CDI and ICI colitis. Due to further progression of her underlying malignancy, she elected to pursue home hospice care 2 months later.

Case Summary

We present a case of a patient with low-grade B cell lymphoma on atezolizumab who presented with concurrent ICI colitis and recurrent CDI refractory to standard therapies. FMT provided rapid and significant improvement in symptoms with a

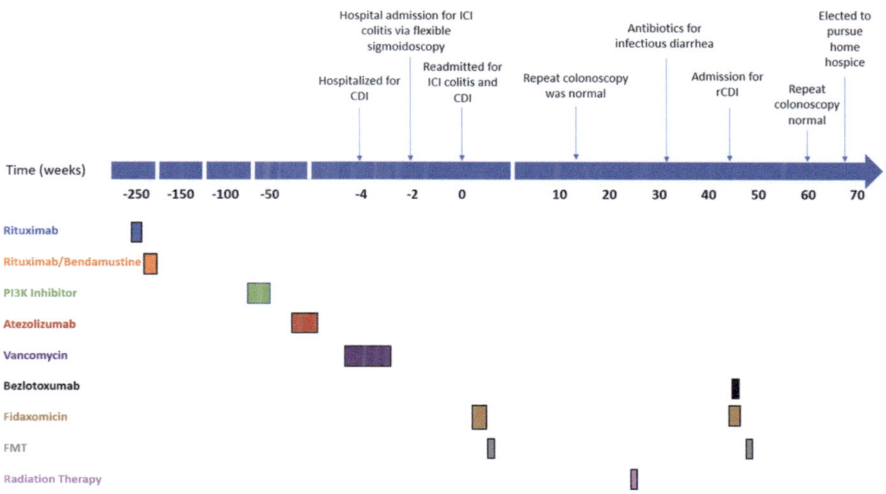

Fig. 23.3 Summary of events on timeline (Timepoint of 0 is the diagnosis of ICI colitis and rCDI)

sustained response as evidenced by repeat colonoscopies, which can be considered as combined or alternative treatment option in such challenging cases. Summary of events is depicted in Fig. 23.3.

Discussion

Our patient's experience illustrates the challenge of treating ICI colitis and CDI as routine treatment for one, immunosuppression, worsens progression of the other, infection [1]. Furthermore, there is an elevated risk of CDI in patients experiencing ICI colitis, and when present concurrently, the two pathologies increase severity of diarrhea [2]. While it is well-established that antibiotic use and proton pump inhibitor increases the risk of CDI, there is evidence that the severity of ICI colitis is increased with antibiotic therapy, especially after ICI initiation and those containing anerobic coverage [2, 3]. Our case highlights that judicious use of antibiotics is imperative in oncologic patients with a history of CDI, ICI colitis, or both.

FMT provides a unique opportunity to address both pathologies at the same time given the fundamental role the microbiome plays in each. Although further work is needed, several studies have demonstrated that certain microbiome profiles can either promote or inhibit the development of ICI colitis and CDI [4, 5]. Emerging evidence demonstrates that FMT is a promising treatment for CDI in the oncology population with an 84% response rate in a study of 19 patients with higher recurrence, 50%, among those who received antibiotics during or before FMT [6]. Similarly, a case series of 12 patients with ICI colitis receiving FMT revealed 92% of patients achieved clinical remission by the end of the study [7]. Our patient's case suggests FMT may provide an avenue to rapidly improve symptoms of two resilient pathologies that often antagonize each other. Clearance clearance of the refractory/recurrent CDI in the context of ICI colitis is critical to enable patient to receive more potent standard immunosuppressants safely when needed. Possible future directions include identifying microbial signatures within microbiomes that target Clostridioides difficile and ICI colitis simultaneously.

References

1. Avni T, Babitch T, Ben-Zvi H, Hijazi R, Ayada G, Atamna A, Bishara J. Clostridioides difficile infection in immunocompromised hospitalized patients is associated with a high recurrence rate. Int J Infect Dis. 2020;90:237–42.
2. Vasavada S, Panneerselvam K, Amin R, Varatharajalu K, Okhuysen PC, Oliva ICG, Wang J, Grivas P, Thomas AS, Wang Y. Clostridioides difficile infection in cancer patients receiving immune checkpoint inhibitors. Ann Gastroenterol. 2022;35(4):393.
3. Abu-Sbeih H, Herrera LN, Tang T, Altan M, Chaftari AMP, Okhuysen PC, Jenq RR, Wang Y. Impact of antibiotic therapy on the development and response to treatment of immune checkpoint inhibitor-mediated diarrhea and colitis. J Immunother Cancer. 2019;7:1–11.
4. Abu-Sbeih H, Wang Y. Gut microbiome and immune checkpoint inhibitor-induced enterocolitis. Dig Dis Sci. 2020;65:797–9.
5. Britton RA, Young VB. Role of the intestinal microbiota in resistance to colonization by Clostridium difficile. Gastroenterology. 2014;146(6):1547–53.
6. Ali H, Khurana S, Ma W, Peng Y, Jiang ZD, DuPont H, Zhang HC, Thomas AS, Okhuysen P, Wang Y. Safety and efficacy of fecal microbiota transplantation to treat and prevent recurrent Clostridioides difficile in cancer patients. J Cancer. 2021;12(21):6498.
7. Halsey TM, Thomas AS, Hayase T, Ma W, Abu-Sbeih H, Sun B, Parra ER, Jiang ZD, DuPont HL, Sanchez C, El-Himri R, Brown A, Flores I, McDaniel L, Ortega Turrubiates M, Hensel M, Pham D, Watowich SS, Hayase E, Chang CC, Jenq RR, Wang Y. Microbiome alteration via fecal microbiota transplantation is effective for refractory immune checkpoint inhibitor–induced colitis. Sci Transl Med. 2023;15(700):eabq4006.

Chapter 24
Immune Related Toxicities in Multiple Organs in a Patient with Preexisting Autoimmune Disease

Alice Saji, Omar Alhalabi, Shailender Bhatia, and Yinghong Wang

Abbreviations

AD	Autoimmune disorder
ALP	Alkaline phosphatase
ALT	Alanine transaminases
AST	Aspartate transferase
CT	Computed tomography
CRRT	Continuous renal replacement therapy
GI	Gastrointestinal
ICI	Immune checkpoint inhibitor
ICU	Intensive Care Unit
irAE	Immune related adverse events
PSC	Primary sclerosing cholangitis
UC	Ulcerative colitis

A. Saji · Y. Wang (✉)
Department of Gastroenterology, Hepatology & Nutrition, The University of Texas MD Anderson Cancer Center, Houston, TX, USA
e-mail: asaji@mdanderson.org; ywang59@mdanderson.org

O. Alhalabi
Department of Genitourinary Medical Oncology, The University of Texas MD Anderson Cancer Center, Houston, TX, USA
e-mail: OAlhalabi@mdanderson.org

S. Bhatia
Division of Hematology and Oncology, Fred Hutch Cancer Center, University of Washington, Seattle, WA, USA
e-mail: sbhatia@uw.edu

Y. Wang (ed.), *Challenging Cases in Immunotherapy Related Organ Toxicities*,
https://doi.org/10.1007/978-3-031-83533-9_24

Clinical Presentation and Clinical Course

This is a Caucasian male in his 50s with past medical history of multiple autoimmune disorders including ulcerative colitis (UC), ankylosing spondylitis, and iritis, and was treated with sulfasalazine, methotrexate, folic acid, and was most recently on etanercept. He was getting annual colonoscopies for 6 years and was diagnosed with renal cell carcinoma with metastasis to pancreas 6 months ago. He is status post right renal nephrectomy and then received pazopanib 800 mg/day for 5 months. Since he had progression of disease on pazopanib, he was started on cabozantinib 60 mg/day for 4 weeks and with continues progression of disease. His oncology team decided to start the patient on nivolumab. Patient had a colonoscopy at baseline prior to immune checkpoint inhibitor (ICI) which showed normal mucosa and pathology was negative for any active inflammation (Fig. 24.1). Patient was also cleared by rheumatology service for ankylosing spondylitis and arthritis based on the available lab results and images to proceed with immunotherapy and was okayed to discontinue etanercept. Patient was educated on potential flare of his known autoimmune diseases upon immunotherapy treatments.

Patient was admitted with altered mental status, abdominal pain, dysphagia and failure to thrive approximately after 2 weeks of first dose of nivolumab. CT brain was negative for metastasis disease and for any other acute changes. CT abdomen/pelvis on admission shows progression of metastatic disease in the liver (Fig. 24.2). Patient had mildly elevated liver enzymes (Grade 1) before starting the nivolumab, but rapidly worsened since admission, mainly aspartate transferases (AST) and bilirubin and alkaline phosphate (ALP) (Table 24.1). He also had renal insufficiency (creatinine 1.75 mg/dL) upon admission. Altered mental status was attributed to morphine and it was changed to hydromorphone. The increased AST (340 IU/L), alanine transaminases (ALT, 40 IU/L), hyperbilirubinemia (total 2.4 mg/dL, direct 1.6 mg/dL) raised the concern of immune related liver toxicity. Liver work up for

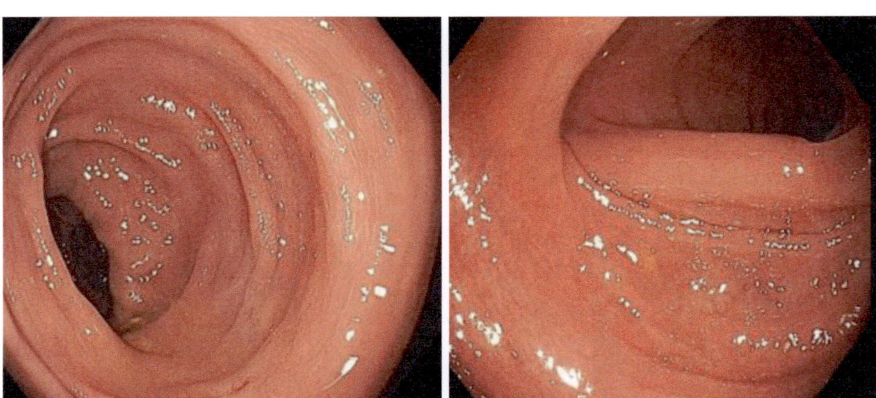

Fig. 24.1 Colonoscopy images. There is normal appearing mucosa throughout. No evidence of active inflammation, or mucosal scarring

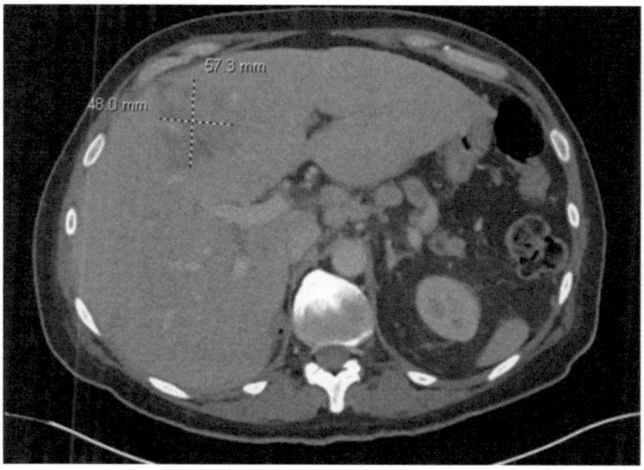

Fig. 24.2 CT abdomen/pelvis showed increased burden of liver metastasis

Table 24.1 Lab values

Value with normal reference range	At the time of first dose of Nivolumab	At the time of onset of symptoms	Value at the time patient was made comfort care
BUN (6–23 mg/dL)	19	**31 (H)**	**85 (H)**
Creatinine (0.67–1.17 mg/dL)	1.29	**1.75 (H)**	**3.22 (H)**
ALT (≤41 U/L)	**72 (H)**	**47 (H)**	**131 (H)**
AST (≤40 U/L)	**55 (H)**	**340 (H)**	**455 (H)**
ALP (40–129 U/L)	**291 (H)**	**349 (H)**	**488 (H)**
Bilirubin (direct) (≤0.3 mg/dL)	0.2	**1.6 (H)**	**5.3 (H)**
Bilirubin (indirect) (0.0–0.9 mg/dL)	0.6	0.8	0.6
Bilirubin Total (≤1.2, mg/dL)	0.8	**2.4 (H)**	**5.9 (H)**
INR (0.86–1.12)	1.14	**2.38 (H)**	**2.12 (H)**

BUN blood urea nitrogen, *ALT* alanine transaminases, *AST* aspartate transferase, *ALP* alkaline phosphatase, *INR* International normalized ratio, *mg/dL* milligram/Deciliter, *U/L* units/liter, *H* high

acute and chronic liver disease were negative and differential diagnosis included immunotherapy induced hepatitis versus progression of metastatic disease or both. With the known history of ulcerative colitis (UC) he was considered at the elevated risk of primary sclerosing cholangitis (PSC), but this was not seen on numerous images of biliary tree previously. A liver biopsy was recommended to confirm the diagnosis after holding the apixaban which he has been taking long term for his known history of chronic left portal vein thrombosis. With the concern of renal toxicity related to immunotherapy, nephrology consulting team recommended gentle hydration to treat the pre-renal condition and biopsy to clarify the immunotherapy related etiology given suboptimal response with conservative management. Primary oncology team started him on high dose steroids for possible immunotherapy induced multiple organ toxicities.

Clinical Outcome

Unfortunately, our patient's clinical condition progressively worsened with increased agitation, continuous deterioration of liver enzymes and renal function. Though he was off apixaban, his INR remained elevated and liver and renal biopsies were unable to be performed safely. Although liver metastasis hyper progression couldn't be excluded, his worsening liver and kidney function could be new onset of immune-related events especially in the context of existing history of two autoimmune diseases (ulcerative colitis and HLA B27+ arthritis). Despite there is a hypothetical predisposition of these adverse events, his UC and arthritis were both adequately managed pre-ICI and remained quiescent post ICI. Patient was subsequently transferred to intensive care unit (ICU) for continuous renal replacement therapy (CRRT) and his liver and renal dysfunction persisted despite 5 days of steroid. Patient's condition deteriorated quickly with multiorgan failure, and patient was made comfort care the next day and died in 2 days within the same hospital stay.

Summary of the Case

This is a patient with metastatic renal cell carcinoma as well as pre-existing multiple autoimmune disorders including ulcerative colitis, ankylosing spondylitis developed acute quick onset of multi-organ failure (neuro, liver, kidney) after one dose of nivolumab leading to hospital admission. Despite thorough work up, and prompt treatment of high dose steroids, patient continued to deteriorate rapidly and deceased within the same hospitalization. However, his pre-existing autoimmune disorders e.g. ulcerative colitis remained dormant without any recurrent activity, even though the gastrointestinal toxicity is supposed to be more common compared to other organ toxicities. Summary of the events was depicted in Fig. 24.3.

Discussion

There is existing evidence supporting the higher risk of immune related adverse events among cancer patients with known autoimmune disorders [1–3]. Given the lack of practice guideline, general consensus based on observation, hypothesis, and limited literature is that patients tend to have higher incidence of ICI related adverse events if they have active autoimmune disease status at baseline, and optimization of medical treatment to minimize its activity before ICI may reduce the risk of immune related adverse events [2]. There is no clear association between the specific pre-existing autoimmune disorders and post ICI toxicity organ involvement. It may present as new immune related adverse events or exacerbation of pre-existing condition with very aggressive disease course and fatal outcome. Among them, it

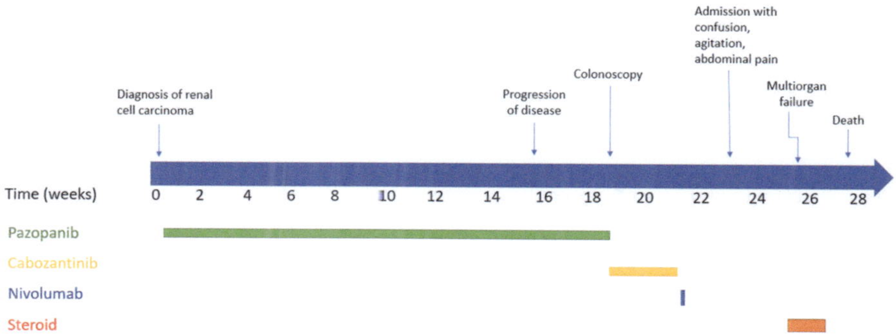

Fig. 24.3 Time line of the disease course (timepoint of 0 is the cancer diagnosis)

appears that patients with GI and rheumatology autoimmune disorders have higher incidence of flare up of pre-existing conditions, but patients with endocrine and neurologic autoimmune disorders have high incidence of adverse event involving new organ systems [3, 4]. Further, patients who required immunosuppressive therapy at the initiation of ICI for preexisting autoimmune disorders can have poorer outcome compared to those who were not on any therapy [5]. Management comprises prompt workup to confirm the diagnosis in the early phase of the disease course and initiates high dose of corticosteroids and other disease modifying drugs or immunosuppressant therapy to prevent detrimental result [3–5]. More retrospective and prospective studies are still critically needed to guide our clinical practice.

References

1. Machado AP, Shatila M, Liu C Wang J, Zhang HC, Thomas A, Wang Y. Immune-related adverse events after immune checkpoint inhibitor exposure in adult cancer patients with pre-existing autoimmune disease. J Cancer Res Clin Oncol. 2023;149:6341–50. https://doi.org/10.1007/s00432-023-04582-9.
2. Abdel-Wahab N, Shah M, Lopez-Olivo MA, Saurez-Almazor ME. Use of immune checkpoint inhibitors in the treatment of patients with cancer and preexisting autoimmune disease: a systematic review. Ann Intern Med 2018;168:121–30. https://doi.org/10.7326/M17-2073.
3. Abu-Sbeih H, Faleck DM, Ricciuti B, Mendelsohn RB, Naqah AR, Cohen J, Sellers MC, et al. Immune checkpoint inhibitor therapy in patients with preexisting inflammatory bowel disease. J Clin Oncol. 2019;38:576–83. https://doi.org/10.1200/JCO.19.01674.
4. Coureau M, Meert AP, Berghmans T, Grigoriu B. Efficacy and toxicity of immune-checkpoint inhibitors in patients with preexisting autoimmune disorders. Front Med. 2020;7:137. https://doi.org/10.3389/fmed.2020.00137.
5. Tison A, Quéré G, Misery L, Funck-Brentano E, Danlos FX, Routier E, Robert C, Loriot Y, et al. Safety and efficacy of immune checkpoint inhibitors in patients with cancer and preexisting autoimmune disease: a nationwide, multicenter cohort study. Arthritis Rheumatol. 2019;71(12):2100–11. Epub 2019 Oct 21. https://doi.org/10.1002/art.41068.

Chapter 25
Upper Gastrointestinal Toxicity Following Immune Checkpoint Inhibitor Therapy

Malek Shatila, Krishnavathana Varatharajalu, Mehnaz A. Shafi, Anusha S. Thomas, and Yinghong Wang

Abbreviations

BMI	Body mass index
CT	Computed tomography
ECOG	Eastern Cooperative Oncology Group performance status
FDG	Fludeoxyglucose-18
GI	Gastrointestinal
ICI	Immune checkpoint inhibitor
IV	Intravenous
PET	Positron emission tomography
TPN	Total parenteral nutrition

Clinical Presentation

This case is that of a Caucasian male in his late 70s (body mass index of 22.7, and Eastern Cooperative Oncology Group performance status of 2) with non-small cell lung cancer metastatic to the brain and liver. He had a history of gastroesophageal reflux disease controlled with lansoprazole at the time of commencement of immune checkpoint inhibitor (ICI) therapy. He was initially treated with carboplatin and

M. Shatila · K. Varatharajalu · M. A. Shafi · A. S. Thomas · Y. Wang (✉)
Department of Gastroenterology, Hepatology & Nutrition, The University of Texas MD Anderson Cancer Center, Houston, TX, USA
e-mail: MShatila@mdanderson.org; KVaratharajalu@mdanderson.org; mashafi@mdanderson.org; ASThomas1@mdanderson.org; ywang59@mdanderson.org

Y. Wang (ed.), *Challenging Cases in Immunotherapy Related Organ Toxicities*, https://doi.org/10.1007/978-3-031-83533-9_25

pemetrexed but was later switched to second-line immunotherapy with nivolumab and concurrent neuro-radiation due to disease progression.

Around 6 months after his first ICI infusion, he began to experience mild nausea and abdominal cramping that was attributed to his dietary habits. A positron emission tomography/computed tomography (PET/CT) scan conducted earlier in the month had shown diffuse fludeoxyglucose-18 (FDG) uptake in the stomach (Fig. 25.1) but given the mild clinical profile and its association with food, further evaluation or treatment was deferred. The patient continued nivolumab for two more doses before he presented to the emergency room 1 month later with progressively severe symptoms anorexia, abdominal cramping, intractable persistent nausea and several episodes of vomiting and weight loss of over 12 pounds (Table 25.1).

He was hospitalized and received intravenous (IV) pantoprazole therapy in addition to anti-nausea medication viz. prochlorperazine. He was placed on a gastroparetic diet (small frequent meals, soft, easy to digest foods, fortified beverages, and avoidance of gastric irritants). Curiously, he was empirically placed on broad spectrum antibiotics (cefepime and vancomycin) due to a considerably low blood pressure on admission with high suspicion for sepsis (Table 25.1). His upper endoscopy showed evidence of gastric and duodenal inflammation suggestive of ICI-induced inflammation (Fig. 25.2). His symptoms improved on the above medications and he was discharged.

Nivolumab was held on account of the upper gastrointestinal (GI) toxicity, but he was admitted to the hospital 1 month later for the same complaints as before. Prior supportive measures were no longer effective and he continued to lose weight. Intravenous methylprednisolone (50 mg daily) was started, and his nausea and vomiting quickly resolved. He was discharged on oral budesonide (9 mg) after a short three-day hospital stay. Upon discharge, the patient failed to continue budesonide as instructed (open capsule) and had an almost immediate recurrence of symptoms after his hospital discharge with daily vomiting and nausea. He was therefore switched to oral prednisone (50 mg daily) to control the inflammation and

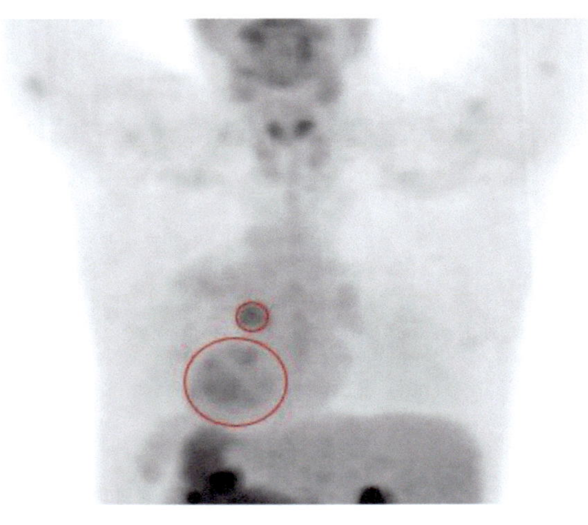

Fig. 25.1 Whole body PET/CT scan with FDG uptake in the stomach encircled in red

Table 25.1 Physical exam and laboratory findings at different timepoints along disease course

Timepoint	Immunotherapy initiation	Symptom onset	First hospitalization	Second hospitalization	Third hospitalization	One month after final discharge
Parameters						
Weight (kg)	62.8	59.4	56.6	**52.8 (L)**	**51.9 (L)**	55.6
Blood pressure[a] (mmHg/mmHg)	108/73	100/73	**84/58 (L)**	**88/61 (L)**	**98/65 (low of 81/52) (L)**	104/72
Sodium (mEq/L) Normal: 136–145 mEq/L	142	141	137	**133 (L)**	**133 (L)**	136
Potassium (mEq/L) Normal: 3.5–5.1 mEq/L	4.2	4.0	3.6	**3.3 (L)**	**2.8 (L)**	4.0
Chloride (mEq/L) Normal: 98–107 mEq/L	107	107	**110 (H)**	**110 (H)**	**110 (H)**	98
Creatinine (mg/dL) Normal: 0.67–1.17 mg/dL	0.92	0.98	0.74	0.74	**0.66 (L)**	0.91
Albumin (g/dL) Normal: 3.5–4.7 g/dL	4.1	**3.1 (L)**	**2.6 (L)**	**2.3 (L)**	**2.3 (L)**	3.6

[a]Patient had a chronically low blood pressure over the course of his immunotherapy with drops occurring during gastritis episodes. Interpretation—(L)—Low

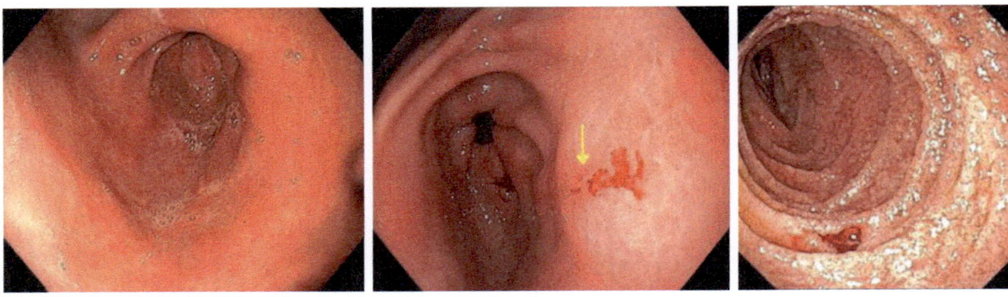

Fig. 25.2 Findings from upper endoscopy showing erythema of the gastric body (first image), a gastric erosion (second image) and granular mucosa in the duodenum (third image)

pre-prandial ondansetron and a scopolamine patch to control the severe nausea. This combination regimen was able to achieve resolution of his GI symptoms a month later. Open capsule budesonide was restarted while the prednisone was tapered down to ensure sustained resolution, but this was not enough to control the patient's symptoms—he had a recurrence necessitating a visit to the emergency department as soon as the prednisone was stopped, necessitating readmission for IV steroid therapy and eventual transition to oral prednisone.

Given the recalcitrant nature of his illness, a vedolizumab infusion was ordered to control his condition but was delayed due to issues with insurance. The patient's symptoms rapidly flared up within days of discharge, leading to another readmission for severe nausea and vomiting. He was also found to have severe hypotension and esophageal candidiasis. He was treated with both fluconazole and IV solumedrol without much improvement. Subsequently, he also developed adrenal insufficiency from his prolonged steroid use that necessitated the tapering of his steroid dose and the addition of fludrocortisone. Given the significant anorexia and loss of body fluids this patient had been experiencing across his disease course, he was profoundly malnourished and TPN was started. After a month in the hospital however his symptoms finally resolved, and he was able to be taken off TPN.

Vedolizumab was finally approved after this patient's difficult hospital course and he went on to receive three doses over the span of 2 months. The patient was weaned off prednisone during this period with no symptom recurrence and he was able to gain back all the weight he had lost after his harrowing disease course. A repeat upper endoscopy after his third and final dose of vedolizumab showed resolution of the previously noted inflammation, and staging PET scans conducted around this time revealed this patient's cancer to be in continued remission. The patient passed away years later due to non-cancer related cause. A timeline of this patient's disease course can be found in Fig. 25.3.

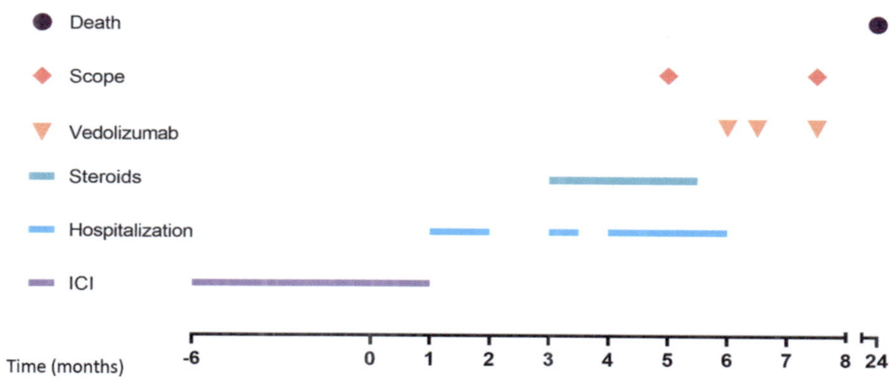

Fig. 25.3 Timeline of patients with disease course with 0 designating the time of symptom onset

Case Summary

This was the case of an elderly male with non-small cell lung cancer who developed severe anorexia, nausea, and vomiting with significant associated weight loss related to nivolumab. His initial episode resolved with intravenous acid suppression therapy and steroids, but he had multiple subsequent recurrences and hospitalizations on steroid taper. EGD demonstrated persistent moderate inflammation on multiple follow ups. Ultimately, the patient received vedolizumab and had complete resolution of his symptoms. Cancer therapy was not resumed given remission of his disease, and the patient passed away years later due to unrelated causes.

Discussion

Upper gastrointestinal inflammation from immune checkpoint inhibition is a relatively rare toxicity of these agents that occurs in around 4.1–5.4% of patients [1, 2]. It primarily manifests as gastritis as seen in this patient but may present as oral mucositis or esophagitis as well. Regardless, the inflammation typically extends to other parts of the GI tract, and up to 70% of patients having a concurrent enterocolitis with accompanying symptoms [2, 3].

The role of imaging in the assessment of ICI-gastritis remains unclear. Only one study so far has explored the potential utility of abdominal ultrasound to identify gastric inflammation and track clinical improvement, but its results are not generalizable [4]. Positron emission tomography has been suggested to have some value in predicting immune mediated colitis [5], but this has not been studied in gastritis. Our patient had FDG uptake in the stomach on his restaging PET scan around the time of symptom onset, but it is difficult to say whether this was a harbinger for future gastritis. One case report describes FDG uptake in the stomach accompanied by symptoms of gastritis, but this was later found to be caused by an ICI-related antitumor response in a metastatic lesion in the stomach rather than an immune-mediated toxicity [6]. While more research is needed in this regard, it serves to highlight the importance of upper endoscopy to evaluate the severity of ICI-gastritis and identify possible complications such as gastric hemorrhage or necrosis. Biopsies are critical as normal macroscopic findings may belie severe histological inflammation [1]. These should be taken from multiple locations as there can be contrasting pathology at different sites [1]. Signs of both active and chronic inflammation typical for checkpoint inhibitor toxicity may be seen on biopsy with increased neutrophils in the lamina propria, erosions and/or ulcerations in the epithelium, increased intraepithelial lymphocytes and plasma cells, and granulomatous inflammation [2, 7]. Eosinophilic gastritis has also been identified [8]. Other studies have found that periglandular gastric inflammation [9] and high numbers of apoptotic events [10] can help distinguish immune-mediated gastritis from other causes, especially in the absence of features such as endocrine cell hyperplasia and intestinal metaplasia [7].

The first-line treatment of ICI-gastritis involves acid suppression therapy with proton pump inhibitors. Steroids and biologic agents such as infliximab or vedolizumab are reserved for more severe or refractory cases [2], and endoscopic intervention with coagulation or hemostatic spray may be necessary in case of gastric bleeding [11]. Such treatments are effective at controlling symptoms, and up to 80% of cases achieve long-term symptom remission within 3 months of gastritis onset [12]. However, prolonged steroid use comes with the risk of various side effects including adrenal insufficiency, as seen in this patient. Around 15% of patients have disease recurrence despite immunosuppressive treatments, but long-term complications of this toxicity have yet to be seen [2].

References

1. Ungureanu I, Bonnet P, Julie C, Parlier D, Saiag P, Lamarque D, Emile J, Elisa F. Correlation between endoscopic appearance and histology in immune checkpoint inhibitors-induced gastritis. Virchows Arch. 2022;481:94–45.
2. Tang T, et al. Upper gastrointestinal symptoms and associated endoscopic and histological features in patients receiving immune checkpoint inhibitors. Scand J Gastroenterol. 2019;54(5):538–45.
3. Haryal A, et al. Immune checkpoint inhibitor gastritis is often associated with concomitant enterocolitis, which impacts the clinical course. Cancer. 2023;129(3):367–75.
4. Omotehara S, et al. A case of immune checkpoint inhibitor-associated gastroenteritis detected by ultrasonography. J Clin Ultrasound. 2021;49(6):605–9.
5. Lang N, et al. Clinical significance of signs of autoimmune colitis in (18)F-fluorodeoxyglucose positron emission tomography-computed tomography of 100 stage-IV melanoma patients. Immunotherapy. 2019;11(8):667–76.
6. Bello E, et al. Antitumor response to microscopic melanoma in the gastric mucosa mimicking ipilimumab-induced gastritis. J Immunother Cancer. 2019;7(1):41.
7. Johncilla M, et al. Morphological spectrum of immune check-point inhibitor therapy-associated gastritis. Histopathology. 2020;76(4):531–9.
8. Tsuji A, et al. A rare case of eosinophilic gastritis induced by nivolumab therapy for metastatic melanoma. Clin J Gastroenterol. 2022;15(5):876–80.

9. Zhang ML, et al. Immune-related adverse events in the gastrointestinal tract: diagnostic utility of upper gastrointestinal biopsies. Histopathology. 2020;76(2):233–43.
10. Placke JM, et al. Apoptotic gastritis in melanoma patients treated with PD-1-based immune checkpoint inhibition—clinical and histopathological findings including the diagnostic value of anti-Caspase-3 immunohistochemistry. Front Oncol. 2021;11:725549.
11. Earasi A, Figueroa E, Mehra P, Baray M, Crawford M, Hall R, Behm B. Immunotherapy-mediated hemorrhagic gastritis after Ipilimumab and Nivolumab therapy. Am J Gastroenterol. 2019;114:S1510–1.
12. de Malet A, et al. Evolution and recurrence of gastrointestinal immune-related adverse events induced by immune checkpoint inhibitors. Eur J Cancer. 2019;106:106–14.

Chapter 26
Immune Checkpoint Inhibitor Use in Patients with Pre-Existing Inflammatory Bowel Disease

David M. Faleck, Amitabh Srivastava, and Juliana Eng

Abbreviations

CTCAE	Common terminology criteria for adverse events
CTLA-4	Cytotoxic T-lymphocyte associated protein
IBD	Inflammatory bowel disease
ICI	Immune checkpoint inhibitor
irAE	Immune-related Adverse Event
irEC	ICI-related Enterocolitis
PD-(L)1	Programmed Cell Death Protein (Ligand)-1
UC	Ulcerative colitis

Clinical Presentation

A Caucasian woman in her 50 s with a 5-year history of ulcerative colitis (UC) and metastatic lung adenocarcinoma is evaluated for worsening colitis symptoms after receiving immune checkpoint inhibitor (ICI) therapy. She was diagnosed 5 years prior to presentation with left-sided UC after presenting with urgency, bloody and mucoid diarrhea, as well as erythema nodosum. She was treated with oral and rectal

D. M. Faleck (✉)
Gastroenterology, Hepatology and Nutrition Service, Memorial Sloan Kettering Cancer Center, New York, NY, USA
e-mail: faleckd@mskcc.org

A. Srivastava
Department of Pathology and Laboratory Medicine, Memorial Sloan Kettering Cancer Center, New York, NY, USA
e-mail: srivasa2@mskcc.org

J. Eng
Thoracic Oncology Service, Memorial Sloan Kettering Cancer Center, New York, NY, USA
e-mail: engj@mskcc.org

Y. Wang (ed.), *Challenging Cases in Immunotherapy Related Organ Toxicities*,
https://doi.org/10.1007/978-3-031-83533-9_26

mesalamine therapy with good response and maintained on oral mesalamine 4.8 g a day. Her baseline bowel habits during this time fluctuated between diarrhea and constipation. She reported an average of one flare-up a year, which was treated with short courses of rectal mesalamine. She had never required steroids or hospital admission for her UC. Her most recent colonoscopy was 1 year prior to presentation and revealed mild diverticulosis with no active colitis on endoscopy or histology.

Six months prior to presentation she was diagnosed with stage IV lung adenocarcinoma after presenting with right upper quadrant pain, and imaging was notable for multi-focal lower lobe lung masses. Further workup with PET/CT and MR spine and brain noted metastatic lesions in the bone, thoracic lymph nodes and brain. Bronchoscopy with biopsies revealed lung adenocarcinoma (PD-L1 60%, +KRAS G12A). After careful discussion given her pre-existing UC, the consensus among her thoracic oncologist, primary gastroenterologist, and the patient was to initiate pembrolizumab monotherapy while continuing her oral mesalamine for UC, as well as radiation therapy to her brain and bony lesions. She tolerated three cycles of pembrolizumab fairly well, though she noted erratic bowel habits throughout with alternating diarrhea and constipation. Her bowel pattern became progressively more consistent diarrhea after her third cycle. A restaging PET/CT after the fifth cycle noted mixed response and so pemetrexed and carboplatin were added to pembrolizumab (chemo-ICI).

Through the first two cycles of combined chemo-ICI, she noted progressively worsening diarrhea up to 4–6 bowel movements a day with rectal bleeding, consistent with Common Terminology Criteria for Adverse Events (CTCAE) grade 2 diarrhea and colitis, prompting gastroenterology referral (Fig. 26.1). Stool infection testing was negative for *C. difficile* and other gastrointestinal pathogens and a fecal calprotectin was 1097 μg/g (normal <50 μg/g) (Table 26.1). She was started on oral budesonide MMX extended release 9 mg daily for moderately active UC and an urgent flexible sigmoidoscopy revealed severe colitis, Mayo endoscopic score 3, in the rectum and sigmoid colon to the extent of the exam (Fig. 26.2). Biopsies showed severely active colitis, characterized by lymphoplasmacytic expansion of the lamina propria, cryptitis, focal ulceration, and architectural distortion. She was then initiated on vedolizumab, a monoclonal antibody against the $\alpha4\beta7$ integrin that mediates gut trafficking of activated lymphocytes.

Her colitis symptoms improved after one dose of vedolizumab with reduction to grade 1 symptoms. Her cancer was noted to be responding to the addition of chemotherapy and so she resumed dose-reduced chemo-ICI together with her second dose of vedolizumab 2 weeks from the first, but she had rapid worsening of her gastrointestinal symptoms with nausea, vomiting and bloody diarrhea which prompted hospital admission. Stool studies revealed a rotavirus infection and calprotectin >3000 μg/g. Upper endoscopy revealed only mild gastritis, and repeat sigmoidoscopy showed worsening colitis with deep ulcerations. Pathology was notable for moderately active colitis with negative viral studies. She was started on intravenous steroids and infliximab, an anti-TNF therapy, at a dose 5 mg/kg with clinical improvement and she was discharged on a prednisone taper. She continued infliximab induction dosing at weeks 2 and 6 and was tapered off prednisone over 5 weeks. A repeat sigmoidoscopy shortly before her week six dose of infliximab

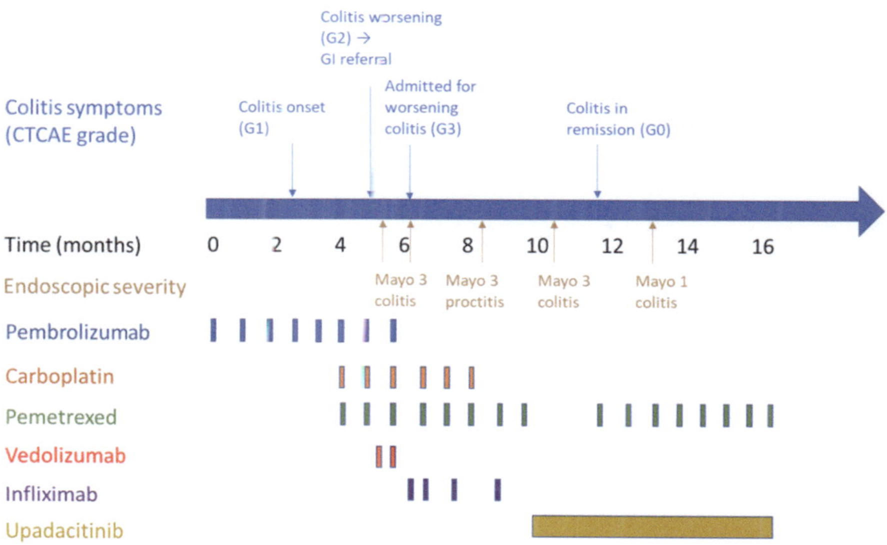

Fig. 26.1 Timeline of clinical presentation and management of ulcerative colitis flare on chemo-immunotherapy

Table 26.1 Lab values

Timepoint	Fecal Calprotectin (μg/g)
Colitis onset	1097
After vedolizumab × 2 doses + resuming chemotherapy	>3000
After infliximab × 2 doses	75
After resuming chemotherapy + infliximab booster	371
After 3 weeks on upadacitinib	<50
After 5 months on upadacitinib + chemotherapy	<50

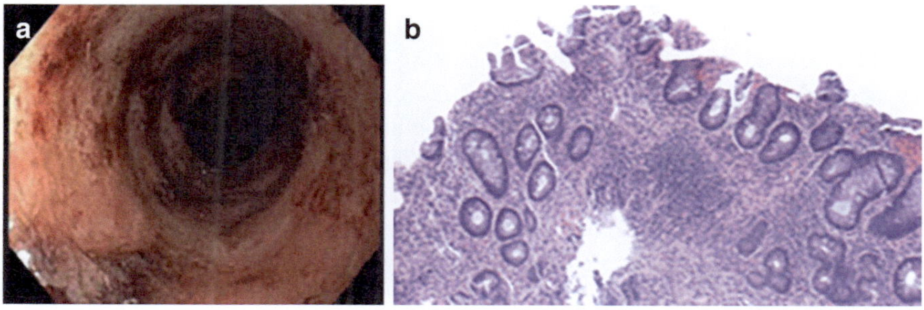

Fig. 26.2 Ulcerative colitis flare on chemo-immunotherapy with severe proctocolitis. (**a**) Baseline sigmoidoscopy demonstrating severe Mayo 3 colitis characterized by erythema, loss of vascularity and spontaneous bleeding. (**b**) Sigmoid biopsy demonstrating severe chronic active colitis with marked basal lymphoplasmacytosis and extensive surface erosion (hematoxylin and eosin stain, 40×)

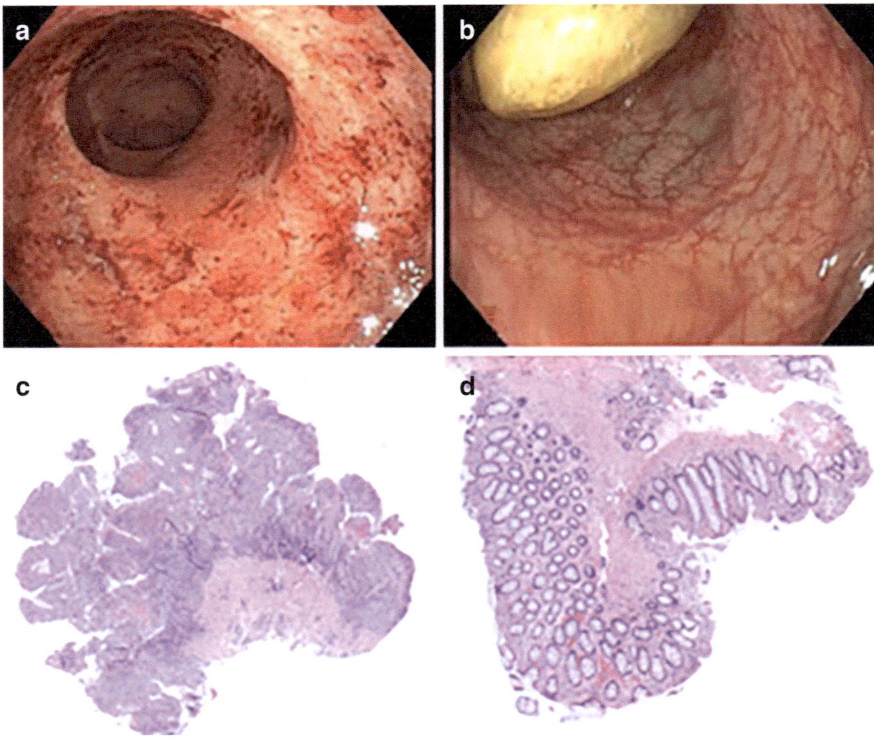

Fig. 26.3 Partial healing after two doses of infliximab with persistent severe proctitis and healing of the colon more proximally. (**a**, **b**) Sigmoidoscopy demonstrating persistent severe proctitis (erythema, loss of vascularity, spontaneous bleeding in the rectum, Mayo 3) (**a**), with complete healing of the mucosa in the sigmoid (Mayo 0) (**b**). (**c**, **d**) Rectum biopsy with severe chronic active proctitis with diffusal mucosal ulceration and prominent basal lymphoplasmacytosis (**c**). Sigmoid biopsy demonstrates colonic mucosa with mild regenerative epithelial changes, but the lamina propria is normal with no increase in inflammatory infiltrate (**d**). (**c** and **d**: hematoxylin and eosin stain, 20×)

revealed isolated Mayo 3 proctitis with healing of the colon more proximally, and repeat calprotectin was 75 μg/g (Fig. 26.3). Rectal mesalamine was added, and the decision was made to resume chemotherapy without ICI. Nonetheless, she experienced intermittent worsening of her colitis after this as well. Repeat calprotectin was 371 μg/g, budesonide rectal foam was added and she received a booster dose of escalated infliximab 10 mg/kg five weeks from the week 6 dose. She had no response to these interventions, and repeat sigmoidoscopy revealed new extension of severe colitis to the mid-sigmoid colon.

Options discussed at this point included a trial of an oral JAK inhibitor, an IL-12/23 inhibitor, or surgical management of her UC. After multi-disciplinary discussion with medical oncology, colorectal surgery and gastroenterology, she opted to pause chemotherapy and proceed with a trial of upadacitinib, an oral selective JAK1 inhibitor approved in 2022 for UC. Within 10 days of starting

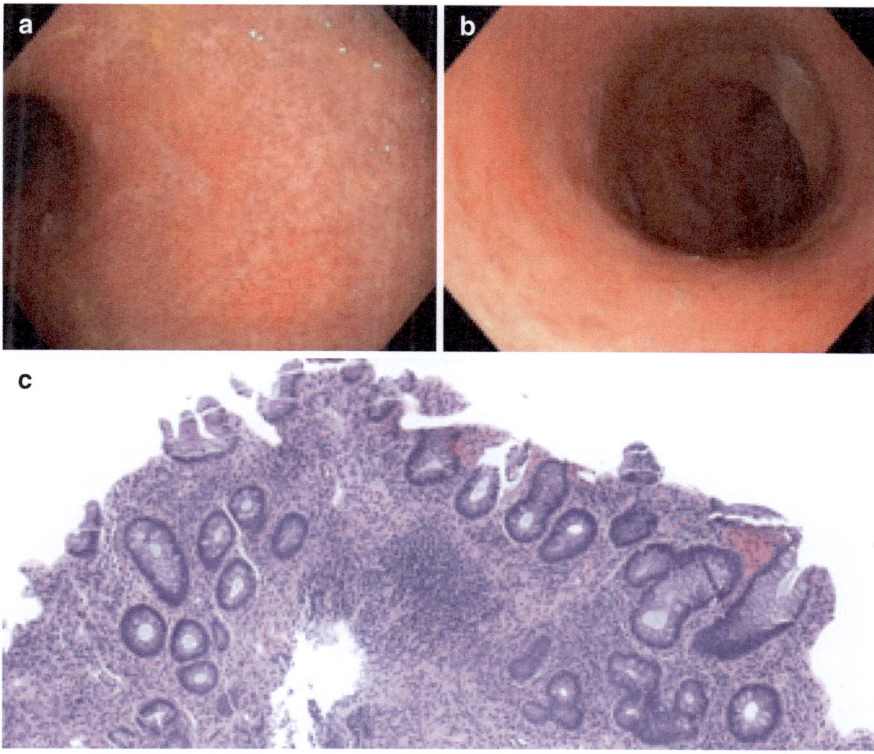

Fig. 26.4 Marked colitis healing after treatment with upadacitinib. (**a**, **b**) Sigmoidoscopy demonstrating mild erythema and altered vascularity in the rectum (**a**) and mid-sigmoid (**b**), Mayo 1. (**c**) Rectum biopsy with mild architectural disarray present with crypt branching and shortening along with mildly increased chronic inflammatory infiltrate in the lamina propria. (**c**: hematoxylin and eosin stain, 40×)

upadacitinib induction at 45 mg oral daily, she noted clinical improvement and her fecal calprotectin after 3 weeks of treatment normalized (<50 μg/g). Her PET/CT at this time showed continued cancer response. After completing the 8-week upadacitinib induction, she noted near complete remission of colitis. She was transitioned to low dose maintenance upadacitinib 15 mg daily as chemotherapy was restarted, which again triggered worsening of her colitis. Her colitis symptoms responded to increasing the upadacitinib maintenance dose to 30 mg daily and she continued on her chemotherapy regimen. A follow-up sigmoidoscopy 4 months after starting upadacitinib showed marked improvement in colitis with mild persistent Mayo 1 colitis (Fig. 26.4). At the most recent follow-up, she remains on pemetrexed and upadacitinib and is tolerating this well. Her most recent PET/CT shows concern of small volume cancer progression for which she is planned for a short interval follow-up.

Case Summary

A Caucasian female in her 50s with left sided UC previously managed effectively with mesalamine with deep remission, who was diagnosed with stage 4 lung adenocarcinoma. She was treated with pembrolizumab for five cycles with mixed response and slow worsening of her UC, despite mesalamine maintenance. Pemetrexed and carboplatin were added to pembrolizumab, which led to progressive worsening of her UC. On initial GI evaluation, she had a calprotectin >1000 μg/g and Mayo 3 colitis on sigmoidoscopy, consistent with severe colitis flare. The UC disease course was refractory to oral budesonide, had a transient response to vedolizumab induction × 2 doses that worsened with chemo resumption, a transient response to infliximab induction × 3 doses, but then relapsed after chemo resumption again, which was refractory to a booster dose of infliximab 10 mg/kg. Given her severe ongoing symptoms, she was started on upadacitinib while holding chemotherapy which led to clinical and biochemical remission with normalization of fecal calprotectin. She had mild worsening of symptoms after restarting chemotherapy that required maintenance dose adjustment of upadacitinib. Follow-up sigmoidoscopy showed mild, Mayo 1 colitis and her calprotectin remained <50 μg/g over 5+ months of treatment with pemetrexed plus upadacitinib. Her cancer has had a durable response over 12 months of follow-up, with the most recent scan showing possible low volume progression of disease that may require further adjustment of her cancer regimen.

Discussion

Immune checkpoint inhibitors (ICI), including anti-PD-(L)1 and anti-CTLA-4 therapies have revolutionized the management of advanced cancers yet are frequently associated with a range of immune-related adverse events (irAEs) that can affect various organ systems. Patients with pre-existing autoimmune conditions such as inflammatory bowel disease (IBD) may be uniquely susceptible to these immune-related side effects, which can be indistinguishable from a flare of their underlying disease [1–3]. Studies have found that in patients with pre-existing IBD, the risk of any grade colitis flare is 40%, with moderate-severe events occurring in approximately 20% [4, 5]. Risk factors for flare include the use of anti-CTLA-4 therapy, while the impact of IBD-related factors including disease activity and medication use at initiation of ICI therapy is less well understood due to small sample size in the studies to date. The additive impact of chemotherapy together with immunotherapy on the risk of colitis flares is not well understood, although previous studies have observed that cytotoxic chemotherapy alone is not associated with an increased risk of IBD flare [6].

The patient described here had a history of mild, left sided limited ulcerative colitis that was in biopsy-proven histologic remission on mesalamine a year prior to initiation of ICI. She was also maintained on mesalamine therapy through initiation of therapy. Nonetheless, she developed initially a mild-moderate worsening of symptoms on PD-1 therapy alone that was managed supportively, and then a severe exacerbation of her colitis after the addition of systemic chemotherapy to her ICI regimen. Her colitis was refractory to multiple lines of therapy commonly used for the management of both IBD and ICI-related enterocolitis (irEC), including oral + rectal corticosteroids, the anti-integrin therapy vedolizumab, and the anti-TNF agent infliximab including at escalated doses [7, 8]. Data on therapies for irEC refractory to both vedolizumab and anti-TNF therapy are limited, and include strategies such as use of the anti-IL12/23 agent ustekinumab [9], the oral non-selective JAK inhibitor tofacitinib [10], fecal microbiota transplant [11], and palliative surgery [12, 13].

Emerging data highlight the role of selective JAK1 inhibitors such as upadacitinib in the treatment of moderate-severe IBD [14, 15], and network meta-analyses have pointed to these therapies as the most effective to date in anti-TNF refractory patients [16, 17]. Safety concerns with JAK inhibitors include an elevated risk of infections including Herpes zoster, malignancies, cardiovascular events and thromboembolic disease, which have limited their use in the treatment of irEC to date [18, 19]. Nonetheless, given this patient's refractory colitis resulting from underlying IBD and exacerbation by immunotherapy and chemotherapy, using shared decision making the patient opted for initiation of JAK inhibitor rather than palliative colectomy, which led to marked clinical improvement in her colitis.

Limited data exist on the impact of immunosuppressive therapies on cancer outcomes. Baseline corticosteroid use of $\geq$10 mg of prednisone equivalent daily in patients with lung cancer initiating PD-1 therapy has been linked to decreased overall response rate, progression-free survival and overall survival [20]. The impact of immunosuppressants for irAEs on cancer outcomes remains controversial, with some studies observing a negative impact of corticosteroids [21, 22] or second-line immunosuppressives such as anti-TNF on cancer outcomes [23], while others have not observed a deleterious effect [24–26]. Studies focusing on the impact of baseline immunosuppressive use for patients with pre-existing autoimmune disease are lacking and will be key to address this knowledge gap.

In summary, this case highlights the complex care and multi-disciplinary expertise required to manage patients with underlying autoimmune disease such as IBD who are initiating immune checkpoint inhibitors. The incorporation of emerging knowledge and paradigms in the care of patients with autoimmune diseases and their thoughtful application to the management of patients with superimposed irAEs is critical. Integrated and close coordination between oncologists, medical and surgical subspecialists is key to optimize outcomes in patients with IBD treated with ICIs.

References

1. Haanen J, Ernstoff MS, Wang Y, Menzies AM, Puzanov I, Grivas P, et al. Autoimmune diseases and immune-checkpoint inhibitors for cancer therapy: review of the literature and personalized risk-based prevention strategy. Ann Oncol. 2020;31(6):724–44.
2. Pizuorno Machado A, Shatila M, Liu C, Wang J, Altan M, Zhang HC, et al. Immune-related adverse events after immune checkpoint inhibitor exposure in adult cancer patients with pre-existing autoimmune diseases. J Cancer Res Clin Oncol. 2023;149:6341.
3. Tison A, Garaud S, Chiche L, Cornec D, Kostine M. Immune-checkpoint inhibitor use in patients with cancer and pre-existing autoimmune diseases. Nat Rev Rheumatol. 2022;18(11):641–56.
4. Abu-Sbeih H, Faleck DM, Ricciuti B, Mendelsohn RB, Naqash AR, Cohen JV, et al. Immune checkpoint inhibitor therapy in patients with preexisting inflammatory bowel disease. J Clin Oncol. 2020;38(6):576–83.
5. Meserve J, Facciorusso A, Holmer AK, Annese V, Sandborn WJ, Singh S. Systematic review with meta-analysis: safety and tolerability of immune checkpoint inhibitors in patients with pre-existing inflammatory bowel diseases. Aliment Pharmacol Ther. 2021;53(3):374–82.
6. Axelrad JE, Fowler SA, Friedman S, Ananthakrishnan AN, Yajnik V. Effects of cancer treatment on inflammatory bowel disease remission and reactivation. Clin Gastroenterol Hepatol. 2012;10(9):1021–7 e1.
7. Harris JP, Postow MA, Faleck DM. Efficacy of infliximab dose escalation in patients with refractory immunotherapy-related colitis: a case series. Oncologist. 2022;27(4):e350–e2.
8. Zou F, Faleck D, Thomas A, Harris J, Satish D, Wang X, et al. Efficacy and safety of vedolizumab and infliximab treatment for immune-mediated diarrhea and colitis in patients with cancer: a two-center observational study. J Immunother Cancer. 2021;9(11):e003277.
9. Shirwaikar Thomas A, Lee SE, Shatila M, De Toni EN, Torok HP, Ben Khaled N, et al. IL12/23 blockade for refractory immune-mediated colitis: 2-Center experience. Am J Gastroenterol. 2023;118:1679.
10. Bishu S, Melia J, Sharfman W, Lao CD, Fecher LA, Higgins PDR. Efficacy and outcome of Tofacitinib in immune checkpoint inhibitor colitis. Gastroenterology. 2021;160(3):932–4 e3.
11. Halsey TM, Thomas AS, Hayase T, Ma W, Abu-Sbeih H, Sun B, et al. Microbiome alteration via fecal microbiota transplantation is effective for refractory immune checkpoint inhibitor-induced colitis. Sci Transl Med. 2023;15(700):eabq4006.
12. Baczewska N, Philippart M, Siplet J, Baurain JF, Stainier L, Laterre E, et al. Immune checkpoint inhibitor refractory colitis leading to total colectomy in a melanoma patient. Acta Gastroenterol Belg. 2023;86(2):371–3.
13. Steiger S, Marcucci V, Desai V, Zheng M, Parker G. Refractory fulminant colitis requiring surgical intervention in a patient with ulcerative colitis on Atezolizumab therapy for small cell lung cancer: an atypical case. Cureus. 2022;14(5):e25437.
14. Loftus EV Jr, Panes J, Lacerda AP, Peyrin-Biroulet L, D'Haens G, Panaccione R, et al. Upadacitinib induction and maintenance therapy for Crohn's disease. N Engl J Med. 2023;388(21):1966–80.
15. Danese S, Vermeire S, Zhou W, Pangan AL, Siffledeen J, Greenbloom S, et al. Upadacitinib as induction and maintenance therapy for moderately to severely active ulcerative colitis: results from three phase 3, multicentre, double-blind, randomised trials. Lancet. 2022;399(10341):2113–28.
16. Attauabi M, Dahl EK, Burisch J, Gubatan J, Nielsen OH, Seidelin JB. Comparative onset of effect of biologics and small molecules in moderate-to-severe ulcerative colitis: a systematic review and network meta-analysis. EClinicalMedicine. 2023;57:101866.
17. Burr NE, Gracie DJ, Black CJ, Ford AC. Efficacy of biological therapies and small molecules in moderate to severe ulcerative colitis: systematic review and network meta-analysis. Gut. 2021.

18. Ytterberg SR, Bhatt DL, Mikuls TR, Koch GG, Fleischmann R, Rivas JL, et al. Cardiovascular and cancer risk with Tofacitinib in rheumatoid arthritis. N Engl J Med. 2022;386(4):316–26.
19. Curtis JR, Yamaoka K, Chen YH, Bhatt DL, Gunay LM, Sugiyama N, et al. Malignancy risk with tofacitinib versus TNF inhibitors in rheumatoid arthritis: results from the open-label, randomised controlled ORAL surveillance trial. Ann Rheum Dis. 2023;82(3):331–43.
20. Arbour KC, Mezquita L, Long N, Rizvi H, Auclin E, Ni A, et al. Impact of baseline steroids on efficacy of programmed cell death-1 and programmed death-ligand 1 blockade in patients with non-small-cell lung cancer. J Clin Oncol. 2018;36(28):2872–8.
21. Bai X, Hu J, Betof Warner A, Quach HT, Cann CG, Zhang MZ, et al. Early use of high-dose glucocorticoid for the management of irAE is associated with poorer survival in patients with advanced melanoma treated with anti-PD-1 monotherapy. Clin Cancer Res. 2021;27(21):5993–6000.
22. Faje AT, Lawrence D, Flaherty K, Freedman C, Fadden R, Rubin K, et al. High-dose glucocorticoids for the treatment of ipilimumab-induced hypophysitis is associated with reduced survival in patients with melanoma. Cancer. 2018;124(18):3706–14.
23. van Not OJ, Verheijden RJ, van den Eertwegh AJM, Haanen J, Aarts MJB, van den Berkmortel F, et al. Association of Immune-Related Adverse Event Management with survival in patients with advanced melanoma. JAMA Oncol. 2022;8(12):1794–801.
24. Verheijden RJ, van Eijs MJM, May AM, van Wijk F, Suijkerbuijk KPM. Immunosuppression for immune-related adverse events during checkpoint inhibition: an intricate balance. NPJ Precis Oncol. 2023;7(1):41.
25. Lev-Ari S, Serzan M, Wu T, Ip A, Pascual L, Sinclaire B, et al. The impact of immunosuppressive agents on immune checkpoint inhibitor efficacy in patients with advanced melanoma: a real-world, multicenter, retrospective study. Cancer. 2023;129(12):1885–94.
26. Horvat TZ, Adel NG, Dang TO, Momtaz P, Postow MA, Callahan MK, et al. Immune-related adverse events, need for systemic immunosuppression, and effects on survival and time to treatment failure in patients with melanoma treated with Ipilimumab at memorial Sloan Kettering Cancer Center. J Clin Oncol. 2015;33(28):3193–8.

Chapter 27
Gastroparesis and Gastrointestinal Motility Dysfunction Following Immune Checkpoint Inhibitor Therapy

Matthew J. Townsend and Shilpa Grover

Abbreviations

ADL	Activities of daily living
ASCO	American Society of Clinical Oncology
CNS	Central Nervous System
EGD	Esophagogastroduodenoscopy
ESMO	European Society for Medical Oncology
NCS	nerve conduction study

Clinical Presentation

A Caucasian female patient in her 60s with metastatic non-small-cell lung cancer to liver and bone was treated with nivolumab after progression through multiple chemotherapy regimens. After four cycles of nivolumab, she presented with nausea and recurrent non-bloody emesis. Her medical history included hypertension, anxiety, hypothyroidism, and an appendectomy. Medications included atorvastatin, escitalopram, as-needed lorazepam, and lidocaine patches for chronic hip pain from bony metastases. Because of severe nausea and vomiting, she was unable to tolerate oral intake for 4 days prior to presentation. She denied abdominal pain, fevers or chills, diarrhea, or urinary symptoms. Neurologic exam noted preserved cranial nerves and

M. J. Townsend
Department of Internal Medicine, Duke University Medical Center, Durham, NC, USA
e-mail: matthew.townsend@duke.edu

S. Grover (✉)
Division of Gastroenterology, Hepatology, and Endoscopy, Brigham and Women's Hospital, Harvard Medical School, Boston, MA, USA
e-mail: sgrover@bwh.harvard.edu

Y. Wang (ed.), *Challenging Cases in Immunotherapy Related Organ Toxicities*,
https://doi.org/10.1007/978-3-031-83533-9_27

sensory/motor function of all extremities. Initial laboratory testing revealed a mild leukocytosis, chronic normocytic anemia, and stable electrolytes, bicarbonate, creatinine, and liver enzymes (Table 27.1). She was admitted for evaluation of acute severe nausea and vomiting and symptom management.

Esophagogastroduodenoscopy (EGD) revealed a normal-appearing stomach and duodenum but with significant gastroesophageal and duodenogastric reflux, and moderate erosive esophagitis (Los Angeles grade B) (Fig. 27.1); histopathology demonstrated mild active esophagitis without viral cytopathic changes, and no evidence of gastric inflammation. An abdominal radiograph showed no dilated or distended bowel loops to suggest bowel obstruction or severe ileus. Symptoms did not improve with twice-daily proton pump inhibitor administration. Repeat EGD at 6 weeks visualized interval resolution of esophagitis. Gastric emptying scintigraphy demonstrated delayed gastric emptying: retention was 84% at 90 min, 83% at 2 h, 65% at 3 h and 69% at 4 h (Fig. 27.2). Her gastroparesis was ascribed to most likely immune checkpoint inhibitor use.

Differential Diagnosis

While gastroparesis has been observed in association with immune checkpoint inhibitor use in a small case series [2], it is a rarely reported event; other causes of delayed gastric emptying and nausea must be considered. Immune checkpoint inhibitors can induce an inflammatory gastritis and/or enteritis which often similarly present with bloating, dyspepsia, and nausea; these conditions may be differentiated by endoscopic appearance and histology, and particularly in the case of enteritis, by diarrhea [3, 4]. Intestinal pseudo-obstruction, ileus, and constipation have also been described as gastrointestinal motility immune-related adverse events in patients on checkpoint inhibitor therapy [5–8]. Ileus or small bowel obstruction may likewise manifest with anorexia and persistent nausea. Workup should also include evaluation for hypo- or hyperthyroidism, diabetes mellitus or hyperglycemia, adrenal insufficiency, HIV, amyloidosis, scleroderma (Scl-70 antibody), antecedent viral illness, medications potentially contributory to gastrointestinal dysmotility (e.g., opioids, anticholinergics), and electrolyte or metabolic disturbances (e.g., hypokalemia, hypomagnesemia). If there is concern for concurrent polyneuropathy, a nerve conduction study (NCS) or electromyography could be considered. Paraneoplastic gastrointestinal dysmotility has been observed in association with antineuronal nuclear antibody type 1 (ANNA-1, aka anti-Hu) [9]. CNS involvement of malignancy may manifest as intractable nausea and vomiting without evidence of delayed gastric emptying.

Imaging and endoscopy aid in the diagnosis of immune checkpoint inhibitor-related gastroparesis and exclusion of alternative diagnoses. Scintigraphy is a sensitive, cost-effective study to confirm delayed gastric emptying of solids. Abdominal imaging may evaluate for ileus or anatomic cause of obstruction. EGD may visualize stasis of gastric contents and help rule out gastric outlet obstruction and

Table 27.1 Laboratory testing at the time of clinical presentations

Complete blood count	Metabolic panel	Miscellaneous tests
WBC 11.4 k/μL (H)	Na 140 mmol/L	TSH 2.18 uIU/mL
Hgb 9.8 g/dL (L)	K 3.5 mmol/L	Cortisol (9 am) 19.9 μg/dL
Platelets 250 k/μL	CO_2 25 mmol/L	Hemoglobin A1c 5.6%
	Cr 0.7 mg/dL	Mg 2.0 mg/dL
	Albumin 3.1 g/dL (L)	Lipase 13 U/L

Values are within normal limits except where denoted as lower (L) or higher (H) than reference range

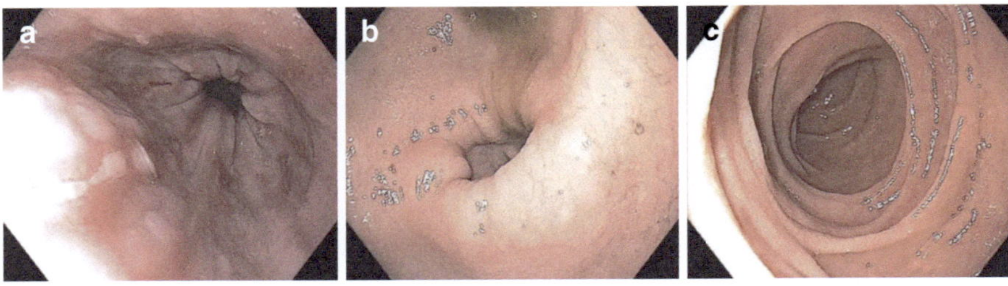

Fig. 27.1 Esophagogastroduodenoscopy for Nausea and Recurrent Emesis. (**a**) Moderate erosive esophagitis, with histopathologic correlate of mild active esophagitis. (**b**, **c**) Normal-appearing pylorus (**b**) and duodenum (**c**) with no inflammation endoscopically or on histopathology

Fig. 27.2 Delayed Gastric Emptying by Scintigraphy. Exam performed with standard 255-kcal, 2%-fat meal (Egg Beaters® 120 g, 2 slices of bread, jelly 30 g) [1]

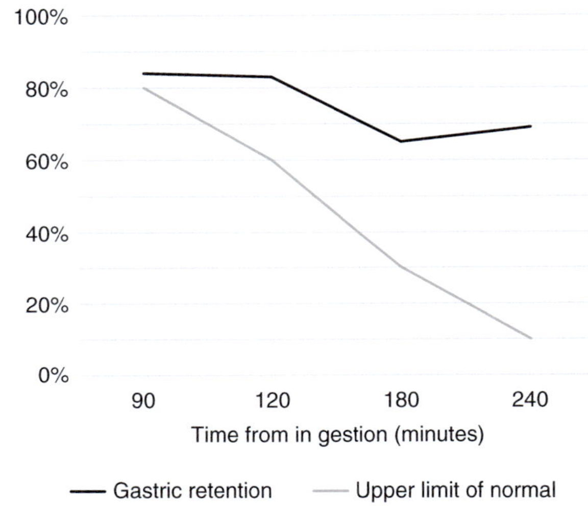

checkpoint inhibitor gastritis (with biopsies). The use of deep endoscopic biopsies has not been validated to assess for myenteric neuron involvement, though may be considered in comprehensive evaluation. As nausea, bloating, and abdominal pain are nonspecific and common with immune checkpoint inhibitor use and in the oncologic population, immunotherapy-associated gastroparesis is potentially underdiagnosed.

Management Options

While no specific consensus recommendations exist for gastrointestinal motility immune-related adverse events, the National Comprehensive Cancer Network (NCCN), American Society of Clinical Oncology (ASCO), and European Society for Medical Oncology (ESMO) offer guidelines on management of checkpoint inhibitor-related neuropathy which may underlie the issue [10–12]. ASCO 2021 guidelines recommend close monitoring of symptoms for Grade 1 autonomic neuropathy (no interference with function), and hold of checkpoint inhibitor therapy and observation or prednisone for Grade 2 neuropathy (moderate, some interference with ADLs); for Grade 3–4 neuropathy (severe, limiting self-care), hospitalization, high-dose intravenous steroids, and permanent discontinuation of checkpoint inhibitor therapy are warranted [11]. ESMO 2022 guidelines suggest oral or intravenous steroids even for Grade 2 neuropathy [10]. Both societies recommend a low threshold for neurology consultation for suspected immune-related neuropathies. The degree to which these recommendations apply to neuropathy limited to the gastrointestinal tract is unclear; outcomes after steroid treatment for ICI-related gastroparesis have not been reported. We favor a trial of promotility and antiemetic agents for symptomatic relief.

Follow Up and Outcome

Our patient presented with moderate symptoms which were managed with close inpatient monitoring, metoclopramide 10 mg thrice daily, as-needed antiemetics, and dietary modification to include small frequent meals (Fig. 27.3). She was also prescribed omeprazole 40 mg twice daily for concurrent esophagitis. Steroids were deferred given moderate, non-progressive symptoms without evidence of a widespread neuropathy or concurrent immune-related adverse event. Opioids and anticholinergic agents were avoided. The patient experienced clinical improvement with these interventions with improvement of nausea and emesis within 72 h. She was not rechallenged with nivolumab as she elected to transition to hospice care in discussion with her oncologist. She was continued on the above treatments for

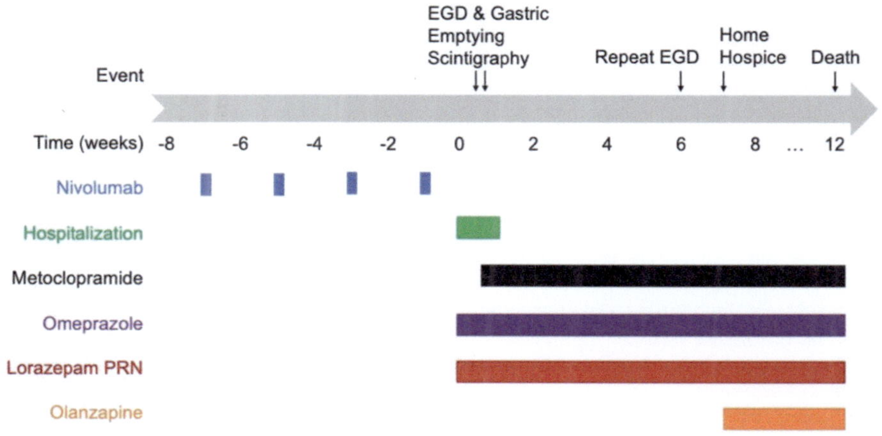

Fig. 27.3 Summary of time course of gastroparesis and gastrointestinal motility dysfunction following immune checkpoint inhibitor use

symptom control through time of enrollment in home hospice (6 weeks from hospitalization) and death (12 weeks from hospitalization) without symptom recurrence.

Case Summary and Discussion

Gastroparesis and other delayed gastrointestinal motility disorders are rare but clinically important toxicities of immune checkpoint inhibitor therapy. Work-up of suspected ICI-related enteric neuropathy and gastrointestinal motility dysfunction should include non-invasive measurement of gastric emptying, upper endoscopy, and the serologic workup above for more common endocrine, metabolic, obstructive, autoimmune and infiltrative mimics. Consensus recommendations for ICI-related gastrointestinal motility disorders are not available but society guidelines on diagnostics and treatment of ICI-related autonomic neuropathies may be relevant [11]. The moderate symptoms of our patient were responsive to prokinetic, anti-emetic pharmacotherapy and dietary modification; for more severe symptoms or where there is evidence of more generalized neuropathy, the therapeutic role of steroids remains to be clarified. Further characterization of ICI-related gastroparesis through larger cohorts, more widespread scintigraphy, and/or deep tissue biopsies for myenteric neuron involvement may refine this clinical entity.

This case was previously presented in lesser detail in Digestive Diseases and Sciences, Springer Nature [2].

References

1. Tougas G, Eaker EY, Abell TL, Abrahamsson H, Boivin M, Chen J, et al. Assessment of gastric emptying using a low fat meal: establishment of international control values. Am J Gastroenterol. 2000;95(6):1456–62.
2. Atieh J, Sack J, Thomas R, Rahma OE, Camilleri M, Grover S. Gastroparesis following immune checkpoint inhibitor therapy: a case series. Dig Dis Sci. 2021;66(6):1974–80.
3. Haryal A, Townsend MJ, Baskaran V, Srivoleti P, Giobbie-Hurder A, Sack JS, et al. Immune checkpoint inhibitor gastritis is often associated with concomitant enterocolitis, which impacts the clinical course. Cancer. 2023;129(3):367–75.
4. Tang T, Abu-Sbeih H, Luo W, Lum P, Qiao W, Bresalier RS, et al. Upper gastrointestinal symptoms and associated endoscopic and histological features in patients receiving immune checkpoint inhibitors. Scand J Gastroenterol. 2019;54(5):538–45.
5. Collins M, Soularue E, Marthey L, Carbonnel F. Management of patients with immune checkpoint inhibitor-induced enterocolitis: a systematic review. Clin Gastroenterol Hepatol. 2020;18(6):1393–403 e1.
6. Appelbaum J, Wells D, Hiatt JB, Steinbach G, Stewart FM, Thomas H, et al. Fatal enteric plexus neuropathy after one dose of ipilimumab plus nivolumab: a case report. J Immunother Cancer. 2018;6(1):82.
7. Besaw RJ, Smith MP, Zerillo JA, Bullock AJ. Chronic intestinal pseudo-obstruction in a patient with metastatic gastro-oesophageal junction cancer receiving treatment with pembrolizumab. BMJ Case Rep. 2019;12(12):e232388.

8. Bhatia S, Huber BR, Upton MP, Thompson JA. Inflammatory enteric neuropathy with severe constipation after ipilimumab treatment for melanoma: a case report. J Immunother. 2009;32(2):203–5.
9. Kashyap P, Farrugia G. Enteric autoantibodies and gut motility disorders. Gastroenterol Clin North Am. 2008;37(2):397–410, vi–vii.
10. Haanen J, Obeid M, Spain L, Carbonnel F, Wang Y, Robert C, et al. Management of toxicities from immunotherapy: ESMO clinical practice guideline for diagnosis, treatment and follow-up. Ann Oncol. 2022;33(12):1217–38.
11. Schneider BJ, Naidoo J, Santomasso BD, Lacchetti C, Adkins S, Anadkat M, et al. Management of immune-related adverse events in patients treated with immune checkpoint inhibitor therapy: ASCO guideline update. J Clin Oncol. 2021;39(36):4073–126.
12. Thompson JA, Schneider BJ, Brahmer J, Achufusi A, Armand P, Berkenstock MK, et al. Management of immunotherapy-related toxicities, version 1.2022, NCCN clinical practice guidelines in oncology. J Natl Compr Canc Netw. 2022;20(4):387–405.

Chapter 28
Celiac Disease in the Setting of Immune Checkpoint Inhibitor Therapy

Ayo Falade, Yousef Badran, and Michael Dougan

Clinical Presentation

A white male in his 70s with widespread metastatic melanoma diagnosed 4 months prior was started on first-line ipilimumab (3 mg/kg) and nivolumab (1 mg/kg) infused every 3 weeks. After cycle 2, he was found to have a partial response on staging scans. However, shortly after completing cycle two, he began to have loose stools. His symptoms slowly escalated, with his stool frequency increasing from his baseline of two solid bowel movements to 4–6 movements daily by the end of cycle 4. Aside from diarrhea, he denied dyspepsia, nausea, vomiting, abdominal cramping, or hematochezia. Stool infectious work up was negative including *Clostridioides difficile*. Given CTCAE grade 1–2 diarrhea, endoscopic evaluation was deferred. Between cycles 2 and 4, he also developed 1+ edema of the bilateral lower extremities. His edema steadily worsened over time, and he was found to have a steadily down-trending albumin. Upon presentation to the clinic for nivolumab maintenance therapy following induction, he described dyspnea on exertion. His exam revealed peri-orbital edema, ascites, and 3+ pitting edema of bilateral lower extremities.

His labs on presentation were notable for significant hypoalbuminemia (1.7 g/dL), hypophosphatemia (1.4 mg/dL), and rising transaminitis (ALT 65 U/L and AST 62 U/L). His alkaline phosphatase (ALKP) was 503 U/L. His remaining liver function tests were within normal limits (Table 28.1). He was admitted from the oncology clinic to the hospital for an expedited work-up of a presumed immune checkpoint inhibitor toxicity. Diagnostic testing during his admission included an

A. Falade
Massachusetts General Brigham Salem Hospital, Salem, MA, USA
e-mail: afalade@mgb.org

Y. Badran · M. Dougan (✉)
Division of Gastroenterology, Massachusetts General Hospital, Boston, MA, USA
e-mail: yousef.badran@mgh.harvard.edu; mldougan@partners.org

Y. Wang (ed.), *Challenging Cases in Immunotherapy Related Organ Toxicities*,
https://doi.org/10.1007/978-3-031-83533-9_28

Table 28.1 Highlighting the lab values on admission, discharge, and 3 months follow-up showing progressive improvement and resolution across the timeline

	On admission	On discharge	3 Months later
Albumin (g/dL)	**1.6**	**1.9**	4.0
ALK Phos (U/L)	**460**	**371**	68
ALT (U/L)	**54**	**61**	16
AST (U/L)	**44**	40	21
TTG IgA (U/mL)	**>100**	**16.9**	**4.4**
Magnesium (mg/dL)	**1.6**	**1.7**	1.8
Calcium (mg/dL)	**7.2**	**7.4**	9.3
LDH (U/L)	**237**	**217**	162

Normal lab values references provided below. Black bold fonts are abnormal values
Albumin [3.5–5.2 g/dL]; ALK Phos [40–130 U/L]; ALT [10–50 U/L]; AST [15–41 U/L]; TTG IgA [0.00–3.99 U/mL]; Magnesium [1.8–2.5 mg/dL]; Calcium [8.9–10.3]; LDH [98–192 U/L]

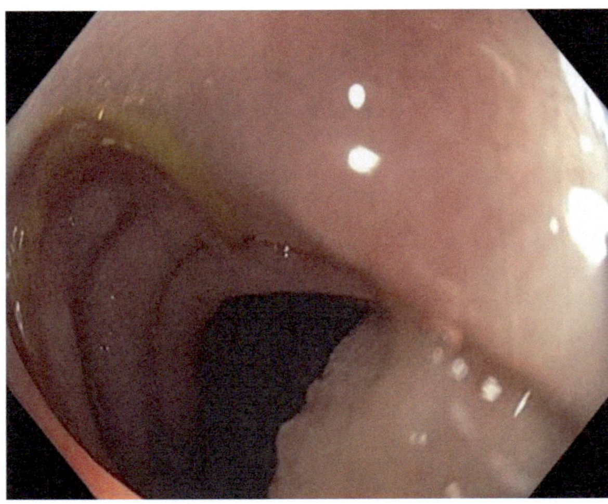

Fig. 28.1 Duodenal atrophy observed on endoscopy

upper endoscopy (Fig. 28.1), and colonoscopy with biopsy, and a CT chest, abdomen and pelvis.

Differential

On arrival, he was initially hypotensive, and a broad differential was considered for his anasarca and hemodynamic compromise, including sepsis, tumor progression, Budd-Chiari syndrome, nephritis with an evolving nephrotic syndrome, heart failure, endocrinopathies (including myxedema and adrenal insufficiency), and protein-losing enteropathy with potential concurrent hepatitis. Diagnostic work-up including viral hepatitis serologies, CMV serologies, and a urinalysis were negative for infection and proteinuria. The protein/urine creatinine ratio was within normal limits.

Further Work-Up

A CT imaging of the chest, abdomen and pelvis demonstrated continued control of his melanoma, but new bilateral ground glass opacities (GGOs), pleural effusions, and ascites were noted (Fig. 28.2). These findings suggest potential associated pulmonary and/or cardiac toxicities, as multiple irAEs are common in hospitalized patients, especially after treatment with dual immune checkpoint inhibitor (ICI) therapy. The cardiac work up was initiated accordingly. A Transthoracic Echocardiogram (TTE) demonstrated a normal ejection fraction. EKG and troponin levels were within normal limits, with an NT-proBNP of 9768 pg/mL. While hospitalized, his alkaline phosphatase (ALKP) continued to rise with a peak of 566 U/L, with ALT/AST peaking at 91 U/L and 71 U/L, respectively. Stool anti-alpha-1 antitrypsin returned negative. As part of the work up for a protein-losing enteropathy, an upper and lower endoscopy were performed with extensive biopsies. Diffuse mucosal atrophy was visualized throughout the duodenum and ileum, and the colon was normal. Duodenal biopsies demonstrated marked villous blunting, intraepithelial lymphocytosis, and expansion of lamina propria (Fig. 28.3). Subsequent work up on TTG IgA returned positive (>100 U/mL), confirming a celiac disease diagnosis.

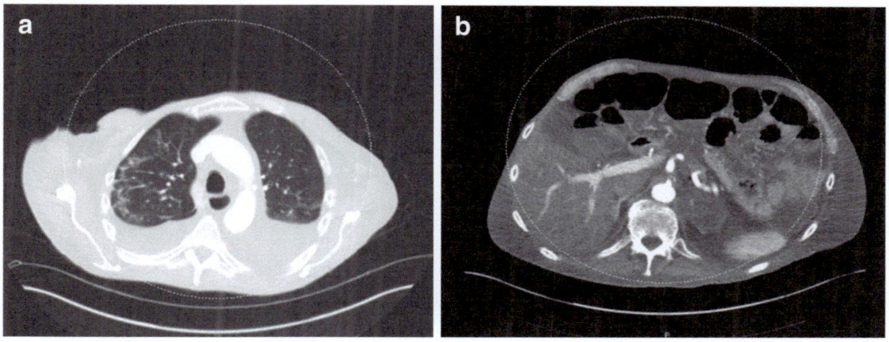

Fig. 28.2 (**a**) Axial contrast-enhanced computed tomography images of the chest and (**b**) upper abdomen with metastatic melanoma demonstrating patchy ground glass opacities, bilateral pleural effusions, ascites, and diffuse soft tissue edema

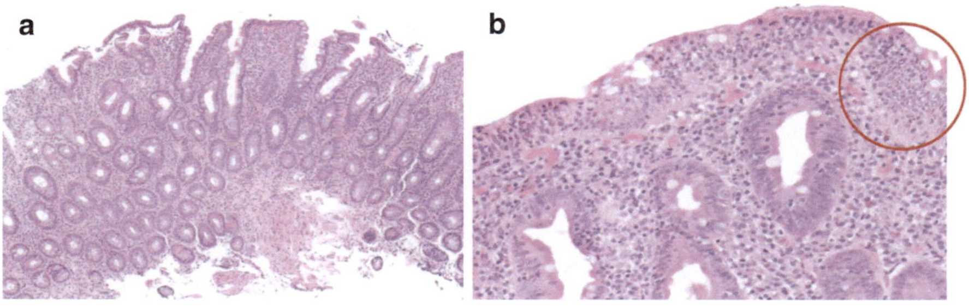

Fig. 28.3 (**a**) H&E-stained slide (10×) Duodenal biopsy demonstrating marked villous blunting, crypt hyperplasia and expansion of lamina propria by lymphocytes and plasma cells. (**b**) H&E-stained slide (10×) of duodenal biopsy highlights the marked intraepithelial lymphocytosis (circled) without evidence of epithelial injury or neutrophils. (Images are reproduced from [1])

Management Options

During the hospitalization, the patient received intravenous albumin (12.5 g) and furosemide (10 mg IV and 20 mg orally 2 days later), which improved his hypotension, bilateral lower extremity edema, and dyspnea. He was ultimately initiated on a gluten-free diet. No systemic immunosuppression was required.

Follow-Up and Outcome

His edema resolved by adhering to a gluten-free diet for several weeks. About 4 months later, his labs showed resolution of hypoalbuminemia, and a decline in TTG IgA levels (4.40 U/mL). His immunotherapy was held while recovering, and CT scans demonstrated continued disease control and resolution of prior GGOs most consistent with a resolved grade 1 pneumonitis. Unfortunately, his cancer progressed about 15 months after celiac diagnosis, and he received multiple lines of therapies including ICI and targeted therapy without response, and eventually passed away around 10 months after. Summary of the timeline events is shown in Fig. 28.4.

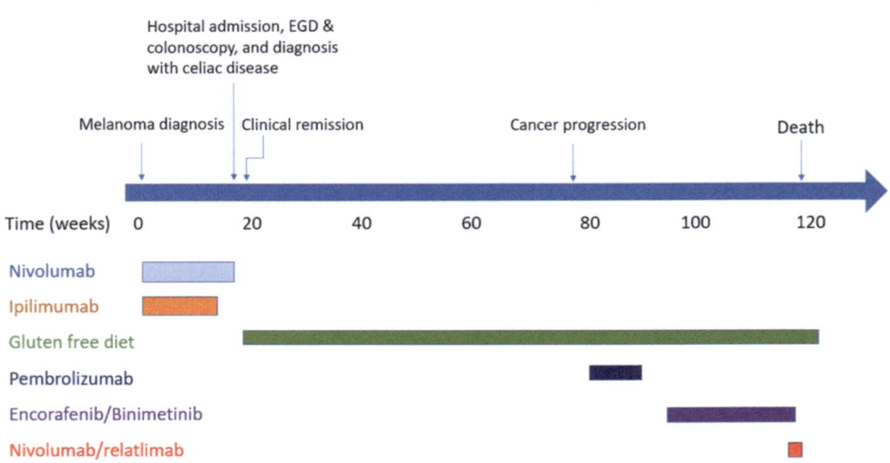

Fig. 28.4 Summarizing the series of events from diagnosis to clinical remission

Brief Summary

Here we present a case with widespread metastatic melanoma who developed rapid onset anasarca and transaminitis after initiating combination nivolumab/ipilimumab (PD-1/CTLA-4 inhibition). An extensive work-up included serologies returning positive for TTG IgA and endoscopy revealing duodenal mucosal atrophy with pathognomonic features confirming celiac disease. All symptoms resolved after initiation of a gluten-free diet without the addition of immunosuppression. The patient eventually passed away due to cancer progression.

Discussion

Immune checkpoint inhibitor-related celiac disease is a rare gastrointestinal immune-related adverse event thought to occur in about 1 percent of patients treated with immune checkpoint inhibitors [1, 2]. Patients usually manifest with diarrhea or abdominal pain, and the work-up demonstrates an elevated TTG IgA with endoscopic and histologic features characteristic of celiac disease. It remains unknown whether this entity represents new-onset celiac disease due to a breach in tolerance related to immune checkpoint inhibition or if it is unmasking of previously subclinical celiac disease.

The first line treatment is to initiate a gluten-free diet, to which the majority of patients respond without needing to stop the immune-checkpoint inhibitors. If this is insufficient to control symptoms, additional immunosuppression with systemic glucocorticoids or biologic therapy, including infliximab or vedolizumab, can be utilized.

References

1. Falade AS, Reynolds KL, Zubiri L, Deshpande V, Fintelmann FJ, Dougan M, et al. Case report: fulminant celiac disease with combination immune checkpoint therapy. Front Immunol. 2022;13:871452.
2. Badran YR, Shih A, Leet D, Mooradian MJ, Coromilas A, Chen J, et al. Immune checkpoint inhibitor-associated celiac disease. J Immunother Cancer. 2020;8(1):e000958.

Chapter 29
Non-Celiac Enteropathy Post Immune Checkpoint Inhibitor Therapy

Jessica El Halabi and Jessica Philpott

Abbreviations

CTCAE	Common terminology criteria for adverse events
CVID	Common variable immunodeficiency
ICI	Immune checkpoint inhibitor
IgA	Immunoglobulin A
IgG	Immunoglobulin G
IVIG	Intravenous immunoglobulin therapy
PD-1	Programmed cell death protein-1EGD: esophagogastroduodenoscopy

Clinical Presentation

A 64 year-old female with stage IV non-small cell lung adenocarcinoma presented with diarrhea and weight loss. She was diagnosed with lung cancer 2 years prior to this presentation, when she developed dyspnea, found to have large right pleural effusion and 2.7 × 1.9 cm right upper lobe para-mediastinal spiculated mass. She was initially treated with carboplatin, pemetrexed and pembrolizumab for four cycles. This was followed by maintenance pemetrexed and pembrolizumab for

J. El Halabi
Division of Gastroenterology and Hepatology, Department of Medicine, School of Medicine, Johns Hopkins University, Baltimore, MD, USA
e-mail: jelhala1@jhmi.edu

J. Philpott (✉)
Inflammatory Bowel Disease Center, Digestive Disease and Surgical Institute, Cleveland Clinic, Cleveland, OH, USA
e-mail: philpoj@ccf.org

Y. Wang (ed.), *Challenging Cases in Immunotherapy Related Organ Toxicities*,
https://doi.org/10.1007/978-3-031-83533-9_29

Table 29.1 Lab values and weight

	Initial onset of symptoms	Month 5 After repeat dose Pembrolizumab	Month 7	Month 10	Month 15	Month 22
Calprotectin mg/kg (nl <50)	117	583	1404	493	73	50
Lipase U/L (<160)		2089	30			
Albumin g/dL (nl 3.9–4.9)		3.7	3.7	3.4	4.0	4.0
Weight	59 kg (BMI 22)	55 kg (BMI 21)	53 kg (BMI 20.8)	45 kg (BMI 19.4)	55 kg (BMI 20.2)	56.7 kg (20.3)

27 cycles followed by ongoing maintenance pembrolizumab monotherapy. After 1 year of pembrolizumab treatment, she developed anemia (hemoglobin of 9.9 mg/dL normal range 11.5–15.5 mg/dL) which normalized with one iron infusion treatment.

Two months after being diagnosed with anemia, she developed CTCAE grade 2 diarrhea, 5–7 times per day with nocturnal episodes, dark brown in color, non-bloody and without any associated urgency or tenesmus. She was then evaluated for infectious etiology and celiac serology which were both negative. Other studies revealed low fecal elastase but normal fecal fat. Calprotectin was 117 mg/kg (normal range was <50 mg/kg) (Table 29.1). Further study included esophagogastroduodenoscopy (EGD) that was reported as normal mucosa. Histology showed chronic active gastritis with increased intraepithelial lymphocytes but no evidence of *H pylori,* and duodenal mucosa with patchy increased intraepithelial lymphocytes and associated villous blunting. Colonoscopy was significant for erythematous mucosa in the sigmoid and ascending colon with biopsies showing active colitis with increased intraepithelial lymphocytes.

The pembrolizumab was held and she was started on enteric coated budesonide 9 mg once daily and lipase-protease-amylase 36,000–114,000–180,000 units, resulting in more formed stools and decreased stool frequency. After achieving clinical remission of her GI symptoms, she received one additional dose of pembrolizumab. Within a week she developed epigastric pain and was found to have pancreatic edema on PET scan as well as an elevation of lipase level (2089 U/L), CRP 3.1 mg/dL, and calprotectin of 583 mg/kg. She was treated with prednisone 1 mg/kg once daily with improvement in symptom of pain, however, when her steroids were slowly tapered over 3 months, she developed progressive weight loss, loose stool (CTCAE grade 1) and her calprotectin was noted to further increase to 1404 mg/kg and she would report inability to eat whenever her dose was less than 20 mg of prednisone.

Given concern for ongoing intestinal inflammation, based on elevated calprotectin and steroid dependence, she was then started on vedolizumab. Despite receiving 3 doses, she continued to clinically worsen with ongoing weight loss and her

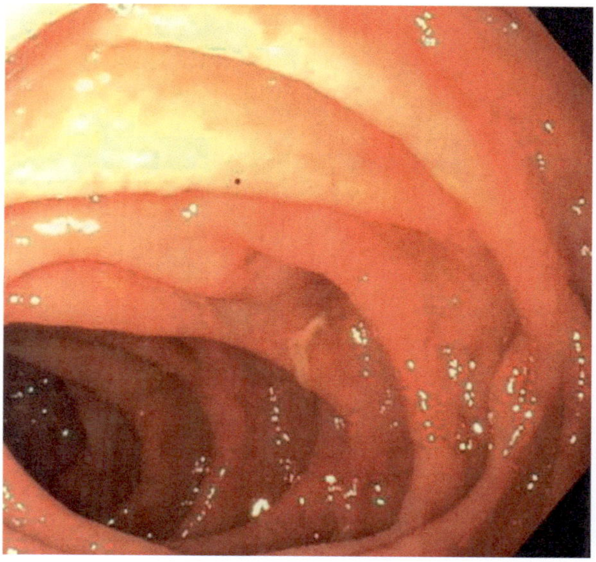

Fig. 29.1 Repeat duodenal images on week 9 after presentation with congestion, flattened villi and erosion

calprotectin level still remained elevated at 493 mg/kg. She then underwent a repeat EGD and flexible sigmoidoscopy. The EGD revealed stomach with patchy erythema, and duodenum with congestion, erosions, and variability in the visible villi (Fig. 29.1). Biopsies revealed chronic inactive gastritis, and persistent intraepithelial lymphocytosis and villous blunting in duodenum. The colon was normal both endoscopically and histologically. Additional lab assessment revealed a low IgG (252 mg/dL) (normal 700–1600 mg/dL), IgA (32 mg/dL) (normal 70–400 mg/dL) and elevated IgM level. Her repeat hematologic celiac evaluation was negative. The vedolizumab was stopped, given the resolution of colitis. She was referred to immunology given the abnormal lab findings and other work up was unrevealing for additional immune abnormalities, so she then began intravenous immunoglobulin therapy (IVIG).

Differential Diagnosis

The differential for enteropathy presenting in this patient include serologically negative sprue, autoimmune enteropathy, common variable immunodeficiency (CVID) and selective IgA deficiency related, Human Immunodeficiency Virus infection, and also Crohn's disease, vasculitis. This patient had not been assessed for CVID prior to diagnosis of lung cancer, but she had no clinical history suggestive of CVID or enteropathy and as such, the clinical course of diffuse GI inflammation initially, then pancreatitis suggests that her pathology was most likely related to immunotherapy adverse events. The refractory disease course of enteritis despite aggressive immunosuppressant treatments raised the concern of potential additional component of pathology e.g. hypogammaglobulinemia that may warrant different treatment.

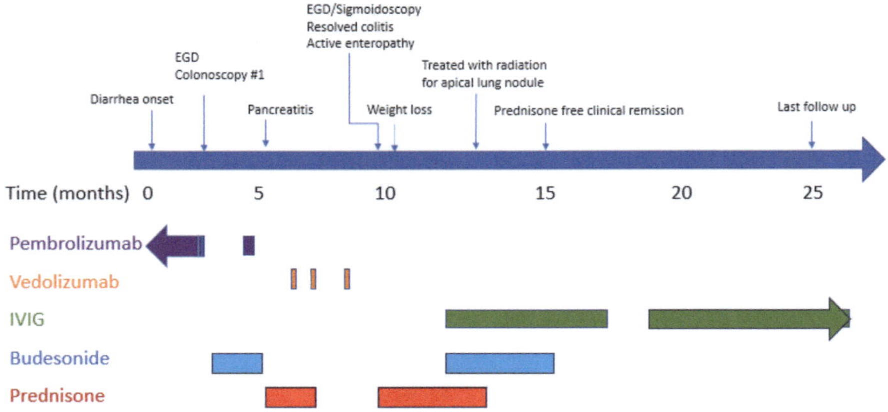

Fig. 29.2 Clinical course and timeline of the events. (Timepoint 0 is the development of GI symptoms)

Clinical Outcome

Within five months of starting IVIG and 9 months of last dose of pembrolizumab, she was at stable weight with normal bowel movements with ability to stop prednisone therapy and normalization of the calprotectin. When IVIG was stopped, her immunoglobulin levels fell which prompted her to restart IVIG treatment. She was also in process of tapering budesonide. She was maintained off systemic anticancer therapy with monitoring, other than radiation for a new lung apical nodule and continues to be stable at last evaluation 25 months after presentation with diarrhea (Fig. 29.2).

Summary of This Case

After several years of tolerating pembrolizumab therapy, this patient with metastatic lung cancer developed a series of gastrointestinal complications which included enterocolitis, and pancreatitis. Despite immunosuppressant treatment, the enteritis persisted leading to progressive weight loss and steroid dependency. IVIG treatment was successful to resolve the symptoms, achieve biochemical remission of enteritis, and cessation of steroid.

Discussion

Seronegative enteropathy is a rare entity and may be difficult to manage [1]. The full characterization and epidemiology of small bowel pathology as a complication of ICI is not fully known but is most commonly diagnosed with duodenal biopsies which could reveal intra-epithelial lymphocytes and neutrophil infiltration and blunting [2]. This presentation seems less common than colitis, but it may be underdiagnosed because the most common evaluation for patients with diarrhea is a colonoscopy or flexible sigmoidoscopy with small bowel biopsy less frequently performed.

Management of immunotherapy induced enteropathy mainly focus on the use of steroids and specifically budesonide, often administered as open capsule. Use of traditional biologics used for inflammatory bowel disease are reported [3], but in our experience have been disappointing. The management of immunodeficiency associated enteropathy is also not fully characterized in the literature, but in general IVIG is not necessarily effective to manage the intestinal complications [4]. With high complexity of the clinical disease course, the actual underlying etiology may never be confirmed. Fortunately, the treatment of both immunosuppressants and IVIG could provide support to the wide spectrum of the presentation and resolve the symptoms.

This case points out several points that are important to highlight. Importantly, when presentation of gastrointestinal complaints suspected to be ICI toxicity, providers should have low threshold for assessing the proximal small bowel for enteropathy via EGD and biopsy, as this may require different or additional management. This case also demonstrates that toxicity can have a delayed onset after years of therapy, and can have aggressive presentations. Finally, when patient had refractory disease course on standard treatment, assessing for alternative etiology such as immunoglobulin deficiency should be considered.

References

1. Leonard MM, Lebwohl B, Rubio-Tapia A, et al. AGA clinical practice update on the evaluation and management of seronegative enteropathies: expert review. Gastroenterology. 2021;160(1):437–44. https://doi.org/10.1053/j.gastro.2020.08.061.
2. Zhang ML, Neyaz A, Patil D, et al. Immune-related adverse events in the gastrointestinal tract: diagnostic utility of upper gastrointestinal biopsies. Histopathology. 2020;76(2):233–43. https://doi.org/10.1111/his.13963.
3. Sanders D, Webber D, Chatur N. Enteritis with immune checkpoint inhibitor use. CMAJ. 2019;191:E1106. https://doi.org/10.1503/cmaj.190244.
4. Agarwal S, Cunningham-Rundles C. Gastrointestinal manifestations and complications of primary immunodeficiency disorders. Immunol Allergy Clin North Am. 2019;39(1):81–94. https://doi.org/10.1016/j.iac.2018.08.006.

Chapter 30
Refractory Immune Checkpoint Inhibitor (ICI)-Mediated Colitis

Joseph Sleiman, Rhonda M. Brand, Reetesh Pai, Randall E. Brand, John Rhee, Marc Schwartz, and Diwakar Davar

Abbreviations

CRP	C-reactive protein
CS	Corticosteroids
CTCAE	Common Terminology Criteria for Adverse Events
ESR	Erythrocyte sedimentation rate
hgb	Hemoglobin

J. Sleiman · R. E. Brand · M. Schwartz
Division of Gastroenterology, Hepatology and Nutrition, University of Pittsburgh School of Medicine, Pittsburgh, PA, USA
e-mail: sleimanj@upmc.edu; brandre@upmc.edu; schwartzm@upmc.edu

R. M. Brand
Division of Gastroenterology, Hepatology and Nutrition, University of Pittsburgh School of Medicine, Pittsburgh, PA, USA

Magee Womens Research Institute and Foundation, Pittsburgh, PA, USA
e-mail: rmb91@pitt.edu

R. Pai
Department of Pathology, University of Pittsburgh, Pittsburgh, PA, USA
e-mail: pair@upmc.edu

J. Rhee
UPMC Hillman Cancer Center, University of Pittsburgh, Pittsburgh, PA, USA
e-mail: rheejc@upmc.edu

D. Davar (✉)
UPMC Hillman Cancer Center, University of Pittsburgh, Pittsburgh, PA, USA

Division of Hematology-Oncology, Department of Medicine, University of Pittsburgh, Pittsburgh, PA, USA
e-mail: davard@upmc.edu

Y. Wang (ed.), *Challenging Cases in Immunotherapy Related Organ Toxicities*, https://doi.org/10.1007/978-3-031-83533-9_30

ICI	Immune checkpoint inhibitors
imDC	Immune-mediated diarrhea and colitis
irAEs	Immune-related adverse events
JAK/STAT	Janus kinase/signal transducers and activators of transcription
MSI-H	Microsatellite instability-high
NCI	National Cancer Institute
UC	Ulcerative colitis

Clinical Presentations

A Caucasian female in 60s with a history of stage IIC mismatch repair-deficient/microsatellite instability-high (MSI-H) colon adenocarcinoma in the transverse colon developed recurrence in the liver and thoracic spine following definitive surgery (ileal resection with extended right hemicolectomy) and adjuvant capecitabine and oxaliplatin. Given MSI-H status, nivolumab and ipilimumab were initiated about 3 months after the initial cancer diagnosis based on the CheckMate-142 study results [1]. Following 2 cycles of combined immune checkpoint inhibitor (ICI) therapy by 1 month, she developed common terminology criteria of adverse events (CTCAE) Grade 2 nausea, Grade 2 anorexia, and Grade 2 mucoid non-bloody diarrhea, consistent with grade 2 immune-mediated diarrhea and colitis (imDC). She was admitted for further workup.

A CT scan showed rectosigmoid and descending colon mild thickening with surrounding hyperemia, which suggested colitis (Fig. 30.1). Enteric pathogens and C. difficile testing were negative. Her C-reactive protein (CRP) was 4.06 mg/dL, and erythrocyte sedimentation rate (ESR) was 32 mm/h. She had no leukocytosis (WBC 4.6 × 109 count/L) or anemia (Hgb 12.6 g/dL) (Table 30.1). A colonoscopy was performed on the second day of hospitalization, before initiation of any corticosteroids (CS). This showed inflammation and erythema in the entire colon consistent with endoscopic ulcerative colitis (UC) Mayo score 1, as well as ulcerations in the neo-terminal ileum (Fig. 30.2). Histopathology from the ileum and random colon revealed acute enteritis and colitis with features of villitis, cryptitis, mild architectural distortion, and prominent crypt apoptotic figures (Fig. 30.2). A cytomegalovirus stain was negative for inclusion bodies. Based on the above findings, the patient was treated with a course of weight-based CS at a dose closer to 1.7 mg prednisone/kg/day, with initial improvement of symptoms, and discharged with a prolonged taper over 8 weeks.

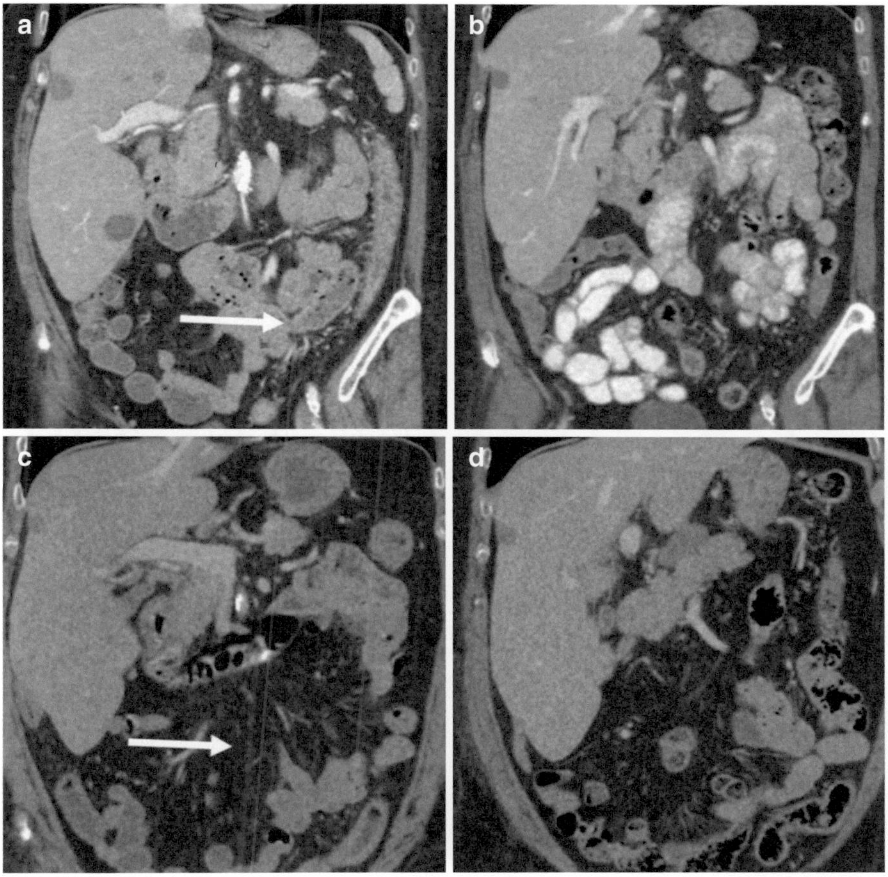

Fig. 30.1 CT abdomen and pelvis throughout the clinical presentation. (**a**) During the first imDC (after ipilimumab/nivolumab cycle 2), CT showed mildly thickened rectosigmoid and descending colon with surrounding hyperemia suggesting colitis; (**b**) During the recurrence while on nivolumab re-challenge, CT showed normal caliber of bowel without hyperemia. (**c**) As the patient had persistence of imDC despite infliximab and vedolizumab, CT showed that the left colon and rectum are mildly thickened with surrounding fat stranding compatible with proctocolitis. (**d**) After imDC response to tofacitinib therapy, the CT scan commented on previous colitis findings appearing to have improved in the interim with some probable residual inflammation in the left colon and the rectosigmoid

Table 30.1 Lab values at different timepoints of the disease course

	Normal reference of laboratory tests	First ICI colitis admission	First recurrence, 1-month outpatient follow-up	Second recurrence 8 months after index colitis, after 7 cycles of Nivolumab therapy	Second admission while on infliximab and nivolumab 3 months after the second recurrence
WBC (10^9 count/L)	3.8–10.6	4.6	4.8	6.9	8.5
Hemoglobin (g/dL)	11.6–14.6	12.6	13.1	13	10.7 (L)
CRP (mg/dL)	0.5–0.74	4.06 (H)	0.45		
ESR (mm/h)	0–40	32	7		
Fecal Lactoferrin (µg/mL)	<30 Normal				75.9 → 94.3 (H) on vedolizumab
Fecal Calprotectin (µg/g)	<50 Normal 51–120 Borderline >120 High				4840 → 1760 → 2830 (H) on vedolizumab
Stool cultures		Negative	Negative		Negative
C. diff 2-step testing		Negative	Negative		Negative

After a month of tapered prednisone to 30 mg twice daily (0.8 mg/kg/day), CRP was 0.45 mg/dL and ESR was 7 mm/h, yet the patient redeveloped severe diarrhea (20 loose stools daily with hematochezia) and abdominal discomfort with repeated negative infectious workup. This prompted the addition of infliximab at 10 mg/kg as well as prednisone escalation to 50 mg twice daily with subsequent resolution of symptoms. The patient was able to taper off CS by 80 days since CS initiation, and a second dose of infliximab was given on that last day given the concern of cancer progression based on follow-up imaging and the need for resumption of nivolumab monotherapy 2 months after.

Three months later, after 7 cycles of nivolumab treatment, the patient had a recurrence of hematochezia, 15–20 daily watery bowel movements, anorexia, and lightheadedness consistent with persistent imDC. A repeat outpatient colonoscopy showed severe diffuse colitis with mucosal friability, erosions, and bleeding. Prednisone was restarted at a dose of 80 mg daily, and two more doses of infliximab were administered in the following month. The patient was able to wean down her prednisone to 10 mg daily and had a reduction in her diarrhea burden, yet she continued to have hematochezia and abdominal discomfort. Upon re-hospitalization for severe dehydration, repeat imaging and endoscopy continued to show diffuse proctocolitis, so she was given $\alpha 4\beta 7$ integrin inhibitor vedolizumab 300 mg intravenously. Fecal calprotectin was followed which did not improve, remaining above 1000 µg/g (normal <50 µg/g). Timeline events are summarized in Fig. 30.3.

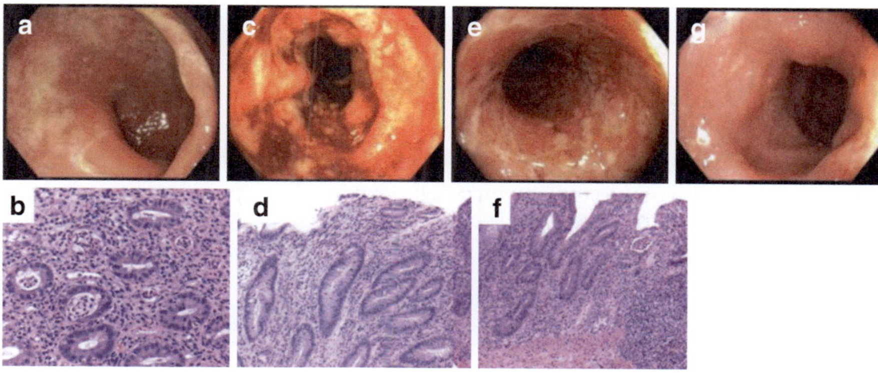

Fig. 30.2 Colonoscopic and histopathological evaluation throughout the clinical presentation. (**a** and **b**) During the first imDC (after ipilimumab/nivolumab cycle 2), colonoscopy showed a moderately inflamed neo-terminal ileum characterized by patchy ulceration and altered vascularity. The entire colon is mildly congested, erythematous, with decreased vascular pattern. Histopathology revealed acute enteritis and colitis, as evidenced by cryptitis, villitis, mild architectural distortion, and prominent crypt apoptotic bodies; (**c** and **d**) During the recurrence while on nivolumab rechallenge, flexible sigmoidoscopy showed a diffuse area of moderately hemorrhagic, ulcerated mucosa with loss of vascular patterns. Histopathology revealed colitis with subepithelial collagen and apoptotic bodies. (**e** and **f**) As the patient had persistence of imDC despite infliximab and vedolizumab, flexible sigmoidoscopy revealed a diffuse, severely erythematous mucosa with exudates, and friability was found in the rectum extending to the sigmoid colon. There was an area of luminal narrowing in the sigmoid colon. Histopathology showed colonic mucosa with acute and chronic colitis (cryptitis, crypt abscesses, lymphoplasmacytic expansion of the lamina propria, and mild crypt distortion) along with prominent crypt apoptotic figures. (**g**) After imDC response to tofacitinib therapy, the colonoscope revealed diffuse mildly erythematous and edematous mucosa with residual shallow ulcerations in the entire examined colon, much improved in comparison to the previous exam. No histopathology sample was collected

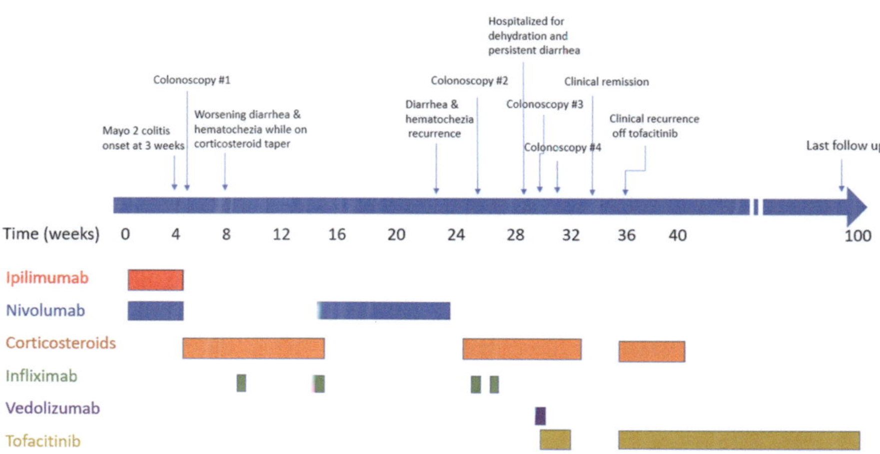

Fig. 30.3 Summary of timeline events (timepoint of 0 is the starting of ICI)

Differentials Diagnosis

At this stage, the differential for colitis included persistent imDC that is refractory to standard selective immunosuppressive therapy (SIT) such as infliximab and vedolizumab. Even though infectious colitis (Clostridioides difficile, cytomegalovirus infection, or other opportunistic infections) could complicate the disease course, and remained in the differential, however, this particular case never had an infection identified. There was low suspicion of an ischemic entity.

Management Options

In some refractory instances, colorectal surgery could be involved for the potential need for total colectomy, yet the patient, who did not have a toxic megacolon, was hoping for colon-preserving options. A literature review showed promise for fecal microbiota transplantation as an emerging treatment option, as well as the use of other SITs that are adapted from ulcerative colitis (UC) treatment. We opted for the latter with tofacitinib.

Follow-Up and Outcome

Tofacitinib 10 mg twice daily was initiated. Symptoms subsided within the third day, with diarrhea reduced to 3 times daily without hematochezia. A colonoscopy 1 week after initiation of tofacitinib revealed improved mucosal inflammation. Tofacitinib was continued as an outpatient therapy. The patient was also on a prednisone 90 mg daily dose with tapers of 10 mg weekly. She continued tofacitinib for 1 month and finished her prednisone taper a month later while maintaining imDC remission. A third recurrence of imDC occurred just a week after prednisone tapering while off tofacitinib maintenance treatment, and a CT scan again showed remnant thickening in the colon with loss of haustration and minimal vasa recta congestion, paralleling her chronic colitis symptomatology. Tofacitinib and prednisone were restarted with quick resolution of symptoms, and she has since been well-controlled on tofacitinib 10 mg twice daily after a 4-week prednisone taper. ICI was not restarted. A few months later, the dose was reduced to 5 mg twice daily, with persistent remission for more than 1 year. The patient did not develop other irAEs. 15 months later, she remains on observation without chemotherapy and with radiologically stable hepatic metastases. CEA has remained low. She remains on tofacitinib 5 mg twice daily and dicyclomine 10 mg twice daily with overall improvement in her bowel movements. Should she progress, the plan is to consider encorafenib (BRAF-targeted drug) with panitumumab (human monoclonal antibody EGFR antagonist).

Brief Summary

We presented a case of imDC who failed to respond clinically, biochemically, and immunohistochemically to corticosteroids, infliximab, and vedolizumab with sustainable effect. A trial of tofacitinib, a pan-JAK inhibitor, led to rapid clinical, biochemical, and immunohistochemical control of imDC. Tofacitinib treatment was continued indefinitely at a reduced dose given the chronic colitis evolution radiologically.

Discussion

ICIs' immune activating properties are known to produce a spectrum of autoimmune pathologies across several organs, collectively termed immune-related adverse events (irAEs). imDC is among the commonest irAEs, with rates of 6–20%, occurring more likely with anti-CTLA-4 or combination anti-PD-1/anti-CTLA-4 therapy [2]. A significant number of patients, roughly 3%, are refractory to mainstay therapies such as corticosteroids and biologics (or SIT) such as infliximab and vedolizumab; the management of these patients is unclear [3]. Fecal microbiota transplantation is one avenue for such patients [4], as are other biologic and small molecule therapies that are traditionally used in UC. Tofacitinib, an orally bioavailable small-molecule, is FDA-approved for the treatment of rheumatoid arthritis, psoriatic arthritis and UC. It acts on the Janus kinase/signal transducers and activators of transcription (JAK/STAT) signaling pathway, specifically JAK1/JAK3 with its dysregulation implicated in both inflammatory conditions and cancers [5]. Given the overlap in the clinical manifestations, as well as inflammatory pathways between UC and imDC, going as deep as changes in microbiome profiles [6], and even metabolomic pathways [7], the use of tofacitinib has been described in refractory imDC in recent case studies [8–12]. However, more understanding of the long-term safety of this therapy needs to be explored in future studies, specifically in terms of tumor response, given the critical roles of JAK/STAT signaling in mediating ICI efficacy [13, 14]. Nevertheless, in complicated refractory imDC cases, the use of tofacitinib may be considered with close monitoring, as it can achieve rapid and durable clinical response.

References

1. Andre T, Lonardi S, Wong KYM, et al. Nivolumab plus low-dose ipilimumab in previously treated patients with microsatellite instability-high/mismatch repair-deficient metastatic colorectal cancer: 4-year follow-up from CheckMate 142. Ann Oncol. 2022;33(10):1052–60. Epub 20220625.

2. Abu-Sbeih H, Ali FS, Wang Y. Immune-checkpoint inhibitors induced diarrhea and colitis: a review of incidence, pathogenesis and management. Curr Opin Gastroenterol. 2020;36(1):25–32.
3. Geukes Foppen MH, Rozeman EA, van Wilpe S, et al. Immune checkpoint inhibition-related colitis: symptoms, endoscopic features, histology and response to management. ESMO Open. 2018;3(1):e000278. PMCID: PMC5786923. Epub 20180113.
4. Fasanello MK, Robillard KT, Boland PM, et al. Use of fecal microbial transplantation for immune checkpoint inhibitor colitis. ACG Case Rep J. 2020;7(4):e00360. PMCID: PMC7224717. Epub 20200410.
5. O'Shea JJ, Schwartz DM, Villarino AV, et al. The JAK-STAT pathway: impact on human disease and therapeutic intervention. Annu Rev Med. 2015;66:311–28. PMCID: PMC5634336.
6. Sakai K, Sakurai T, De Velasco MA, et al. Intestinal microbiota and gene expression reveal similarity and dissimilarity between immune-mediated colitis and ulcerative colitis. Front Oncol. 2021;11:763468. PMCID: PMC8578892. Epub 20211027.
7. Sakurai T, De Velasco MA, Sakai K, et al. Integrative analysis of gut microbiome and host transcriptomes reveals associations between treatment outcomes and immunotherapy-induced colitis. Mol Oncol. 2022;16(7):1493–507. PMCID: PMC8978521. Epub 20210728.
8. Esfahani K, Hudson M, Batist G. Tofacitinib for refractory immune-related colitis from PD-1 therapy. N Engl J Med. 2020;382(24):2374–5.
9. Holmstroem RB, Dahl EK, Helms M, et al. Tofacitinib and faecal microbiota transplantation in treating checkpoint inhibitor-induced enterocolitis: case report. BMJ Open Gastroenterol. 2022;9(1):e000989. PMCID: PMC9806036.
10. Sasson SC, Slevin SM, Cheung VTF, et al. Interferon-gamma-producing CD8(+) tissue resident memory T cells are a targetable Hallmark of immune checkpoint inhibitor-colitis. Gastroenterology. 2021;161(4):1229–44 e9. PMCID: PMC8527886. Epub 20210617.
11. Bishu S, Melia J, Sharfman W, et al. Efficacy and outcome of Tofacitinib in immune checkpoint inhibitor colitis. Gastroenterology. 2021;160(3):932–4e3. Epub 20201021.
12. Sleiman J, Brand RM, Pai R, et al. Mirroring UC care pathways in refractory immune checkpoint inhibitor (ICI)-mediated colitis: distinct features and common pathways. Clin J Gastroenterol. 2023;16(5):680–4. https://doi.org/10.1007/s12328-023-01826-6.
13. Shin DS, Zaretsky JM, Escuin-Ordinas H, et al. Primary resistance to PD-1 blockade mediated by JAK1/2 mutations. Cancer Discov. 2017;7(2):188–201. PMCID: PMC5296316. Epub 20161130.
14. Zaretsky JM, Garcia-Diaz A, Shin DS, et al. Mutations associated with acquired resistance to PD-1 blockade in melanoma. N Engl J Med. 2016;375(9):819–29. PMCID: PMC5007206. Epub 20160713.

Part V
Hematology

Chapter 31
Autoimmune Hemolytic Anemia Post Immune Checkpoint Inhibitors

Blessie Elizabeth Nelson, Thein Hlaing Oo, and Cristhiam Rojas-Hernandez

Abbreviations

ADAMTS13	A disintegrin and metalloproteinase with thrombospondin type 1 motif, member 13
AIHA	Autoimmune hemolytic anemia
ALT	Alanine aminotransferase
AST	Aspartate aminotransferase
ATN	Acute tubular necrosis
DAT	Direct antiglobulin test
ECOG	Eastern Cooperative Oncology Group
GU	Genitourinary
HER2	Human epidermal growth factor receptor 2
Hgb	Hemoglobin
HUS	Hemolytic uremic syndrome
IHC	Immunohistochemistry
INF-gamma	Interferon gamma
ITP	Immune thrombocytopenic purpura
LDH	Lactate dehydrogenase
MSS	Microsatellite stable

B. E. Nelson
Department of General Oncology, The University of Texas MD Anderson Cancer Center, Houston, TX, USA
e-mail: BENelson1@mdanderson.org

T. H. Oo (✉) · C. Rojas-Hernandez (✉)
Section of Benign Hematology, The University of Texas MD Anderson Cancer Center, Houston, TX, USA
e-mail: thoo@mdanderson.org; CMRojas@mdanderson.org

Y. Wang (ed.), *Challenging Cases in Immunotherapy Related Organ Toxicities*,
https://doi.org/10.1007/978-3-031-83533-9_31

NGS	Next-generation sequencing
PD-1	Programmed cell death protein 1
PDL-1 CPS	Programmed death-ligand 1 combined positive score
RBCs	Red blood cells
TNF	Tumor necrosis factor

Case Presentation

This is an Asian male patient in 50s with metastatic gastric adenocarcinoma with metastasis to the abdominal lymph nodes and liver presented after progressing on three lines of therapies including FOLFOX, capecitabine, and irinotecan, paclitaxel and ramucirumab based therapies. His past medical history was significant for stage III chronic kidney disease and hypertension with ECOG (Eastern Cooperative Oncology Group) performance status of 1. His tumor histology was classified as moderately differentiated adenocarcinoma while it was HER2 (Human Epidermal Growth Factor Receptor 2) negative and MSS (Microsatellite Stable) by IHC (Immunohistochemistry) and PD-L1 CPS (Programmed Death-Ligand 1 Combined Positive Score) was 10%. On his tumor NGS (next-generation sequencing), he was found to have an *SRC* amplification and *TP53 R249W.* He enrolled in an early-phase clinical trial with a PD-1 (Programmed Cell Death Protein 1) and cytokine fusion bi-specific antibody.

Seven days after the infusion of the investigational agent, he presented to the emergency department with acute onset fatigue, generalized abdominal pain, and tea-colored and bloody urine production. His vitals were stable while his physical examination was pertinent for scleral icterus. A tabulated view of pertinent laboratory features is provided in Table 31.1 and trend of hemoglobin and total bilirubin levels are depicted in Fig. 31.1.

Table 31.1 Laboratory investigations performed in the case

Hemoglobin	LDH	Reticulocyte count %	Haptoglobin	Total bilirubin	Spherocytes	DAT	Super coombs
6.7 g/dL	3914 U/L	11.9%	N/A	3.9 mg/dL	Yes	Negative	Negative

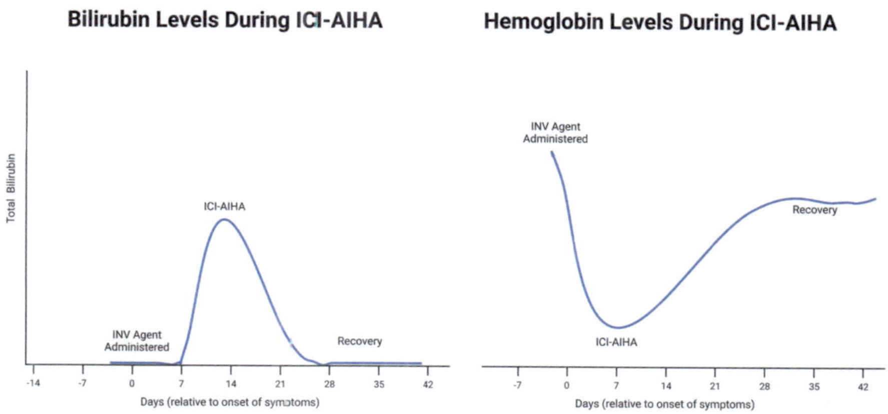

Fig. 31.1 Hemoglobin and bilirubin trend during ICI-AIHA management (INV: investigational; ICI-AIHA: immune checkpoint inhibitor autoimmune hemolytic anemia)

Evaluations and Diagnosis

From baseline hemoglobin (Hgb) of 9.6 g/dL before trial enrollment, his Hgb dropped to 6.7 g/dL, 1 week after receiving cycle 1 day 1 of the bispecific antibody. Concurrently, he also experienced mild thrombocytopenia (121 K/μL), grade 2 hyperbilirubinemia with predominant indirect bilirubinemia (total bilirubin: 3.9 mg/dL), grade 2 acute kidney injury (AKI with serum creatinine of 1.90 mg/dL from 1.18 mg/dL at baseline) with grade 2 AST (Aspartate Aminotransferase: 171 U/L) elevation and grade 1 ALT (Alanine Aminotransferase: 76 U/L) elevation. Notably, his reticulocyte index peaked at 11.9 and LDH (Lactate Dehydrogenase) peaked at 3914 U/L. Urinalysis revealed moderate blood and RBCs (Red Blood Cells) while urine microscopy revealed granular casts and RBCs as well. He underwent a bedside cystoscopy to assess for a GU (genitourinary) etiology for blood loss and no source was identified. Despite serial-packed RBC (Red Blood Cell) transfusions, he was found to have an inappropriate response in his Hgb levels. In light of this, a consultation with the benign hematology service was obtained. A peripheral blood smear of the patient's blood demonstrated microspherocytes, nucleated red blood cells, polychromasia, anisocytosis, and reticulocytosis, indicating RBC destruction and regenerative response with no schistocytes. A direct Coombs test was negative for IgG or C3 antibodies. Hence, a super-coombs test was performed where the eluate was negative while DAT (Direct Antiglobulin Test) Anti-IgG, Anti-C3b, Anti-C3d, and Anti-IgA were also negative. He also underwent extensive autoimmune workup, complement levels assessment, and protein electrophoresis which were unremarkable. His ADAMTS13 (A Disintegrin and Metalloproteinase with Thrombospondin Type 1 Motif, Member 13) activity was low at 41%. He was evaluated by the nephrology service for his AKI and was found to have non-oliguric ATN (Acute Tubular Necrosis) confirmed via renal biopsy. Other conditions such as HUS (Hemolytic Uremic Syndrome), ITP (Immune Thrombocytopenic Purpura) or immunotherapy mediated nephritis were ruled out. In light of the cytokine component of the investigational bi-specific antibody, he also underwent a cytokine level assessment where TNF-alpha (70 pg/mL), INF-gamma (6 pg/mL), IL-6 (50 pg/mL) levels were found to be elevated. Adopting a holistic perspective, the acute anemia presentation with inappropriate response to transfusion, peripheral blood smear with microspherocytosis and reticulocytosis and absence of schistocytes, indirect hyperbilirubinemia, elevated reticulocyte count and LDH with negative super-coombs testing, this led to the diagnosis of DAT negative autoimmune hemolytic anemia with extravascular hemolysis.

Treatment

He was started on prednisone at the dose of 1 mg/kg promptly and achieved favorable improvement in Hgb levels 2 weeks after initiation of steroids with continuous response over the next month. His prednisone regimen was slowly tapered over the next 3 months and experienced no further relapse and maintained his pretreatment Hgb baseline levels. In his interim restaging visit, he continued to experience stable cancer condition, but owing to grade 3 anemia likely related to the anti-PD-1/cytokine fusion bi-specific antibody, he was taken off the trial. He also developed concomitant immune-mediated hypoparathyroidism requiring elemental calcium and calcitonin to normalize his serum calcium level. Subsequently, he went on to participate in fifth-line therapy with an alternate non-immunotherapy/cytokine-based early-phase clinical trial successfully. Table 31.2 provides a brief overview of the characteristics and management recommendation of selected challenging case. A timeline of this case is depicted in Fig. 31.2.

Table 31.2 Characteristics of selected challenging case in hematological immune-related adverse events

Condition	Incidence	Onset	Lab testing	Treatment guidelines	Relapse rate	Recurrence rate with rechallenge
DAT-negative AIHA	Less than 1%	4–10 weeks	• CBC; CMP • Peripheral blood smear • Infectious panel testing • Haptoglobin, LDH, reticulocyte count • Coagulation panel • Review medication history • Autoimmune workup • Serum and urine protein electrophoresis • Bone marrow biopsy not required unless concomitant cytopenias noted • DAT testing • Super-Coombs testing	• Ascertain diagnosis by ICI-AIHA criteria • Grade 1 (Hgb <10 g/dL): can continue ICI without IST • Grade 2 (Hgb 8–10 mg/dL): prednisone 0.5–1 mg/kg • Discontinue ICI for grade 3–4 toxicities (Hgb <8 g/dL): prednisone 1–2 mg/kg; FA; pRBCs • Second line treatment if no recovery of Hgb noted	20–40%	50%

DAT: direct antiglobulin test; AIHA: autoimmune hemolytic anemia; IST: immunosuppressive therapy; CBC: complete blood count; CMP: comprehensive metabolic panel; ICI: immune checkpoint inhibitor; LDH: lactate dehydrogenase; pRBC: packed red blood cells

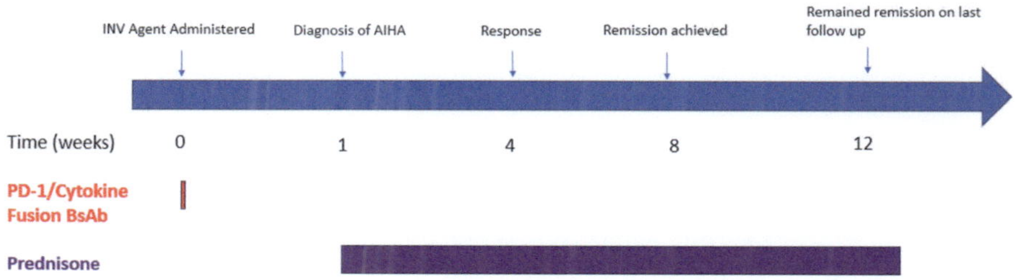

Fig. 31.2 Timeline of clinical events of ICI-AIHA (INV: investigational; ICI-AIHA: immune checkpoint inhibitor autoimmune hemolytic anemia; PD-1/cytokine fusion BsAb: programmed cell death protein 1 and cytokine fusion bi-specific antibody)

Summary

This is a case with metastatic gastric adenocarcinoma encountered severe hemolytic anemia during an early-phase clinical trial with a PD-1 and cytokine fusion bi-specific antibody. These events manifested as acute DAT negative hemolytic anemia, necessitating prompt intervention. The administration of corticosteroid resulted in a complete resolution, enabling the patient to proceed with participation in a subsequent fifth-line therapy trial. The successful management of the adverse events underscores the significance of vigilant monitoring, timely diagnosis, and appropriate therapeutic strategies especially in the context of clinical trials with limited knowledge on safety. The patient's positive response to prednisone not only addressed the DAT negative hemolytic anemia but also facilitated a seamless transition to another early-phase clinical trial. Summary of the timeline events is shown in Fig. 31.2.

Discussion

In this particular case, we highlighted how a DAT-negative AIHA can masquerade as acute anemia with extravascular hemolysis. Although classically associated with DAT positivity, there is growing evidence that ICI-mediated AIHA can also present as a DAT-negative entity. In the seminal work conducted by Leaf et al. where for the first time, DAT-negative AIHA cases were included, they identified 14 cases of ICI-mediated AIHA where 5 patients (38%) had DAT-negative AIHA. The authors note the possibility that DAT-negative AIHA is a separate disorder where it is conceivable that macrophages directly phagocytose red blood cells (RBCs) without the requirement for antibodies, similar to the clearance of damaged RBCs by macrophages. This process may be a result of immune activation induced by ICIs, where macrophages, which themselves express PD-1, engulf the RBCs [1–3]. When dealing with drug-mediated AIHA, distinguishing it from other ICI-mediated AIHA is important, as drug-mediated AIHA causes autoantibody-mediated RBC binding mediated by a hapten causing the annihilation of RBCs via complement activation [4]. Therefore, in the criteria for immune checkpoint inhibitor-associated autoimmune hemolytic anemia (ICI-AIHA), the necessity for a positive DAT is not obligatory. This acknowledges the existence of cases where DAT may be negative, highlighting the potential for under diagnosis and the need for increased detection methods. Notably, the investigational agent also had a cytokine component along with an anti-PD-1 bi-specific antibody where there is a dearth of evidence in mediating AIHA. However, it's unclear what role this could have played in the clinical picture. Nelson et al. reviewed the incidence of ICI-mediated AIHA in the setting of early-phase clinical trials where two cases were identified elicited by anti-PD-1 and anti-PD-L1 therapies respectively. The median time to occurrence was 4–6 weeks while recovery time was between 8 and 20 weeks with 1 patient receiving rechallenge with no recurrence of ICI-mediated AIHA [5].

When it comes to rechallenge, evidence is scarce on retreatment set in the background of a low prevalence of ICI-mediated AIHA. However, in the study by Leaf et al., 7/14 (50%) were rechallenged with ICI, with only one patient who developed AIHA recurrence. Although no predictive risk factors for AIHA recurrence have been determined, it should be mentioned in a temporal correlation, among the patients included in the Leaf et al. study, 4/14 patients (29%), 2/9 patients (22%) from Delanoy et al. study and 1/2 patients (50%) from Nelson et al. had a pre-existing lymphoproliferative disorder before ICI exposure leading to AIHA [3, 5, 6]. This observation suggests that individuals with pre-existing immune dysfunction may have a higher susceptibility to developing ICI-associated autoimmune hemolytic anemia.

The consensus clinical practice guideline by the American Society of Clinical Oncology (ASCO) recommends complete cessation of ICIs if the hemoglobin drops less than 8.0 g/dL although it does not take into account, the patient's pre-treatment baseline values [7]. Management strategies involve the initiation of corticosteroids, such as prednisone at a dose of 0.5–2 mg/kg daily with an emphasis on the slow taper to avoid relapses along with packed RBC transfusions if symptomatic. For non-responders to corticosteroids, second-line agents such as rituximab, intravenous immunoglobulin (IVIG), cyclosporine, or mycophenolic acid are recommended [7–9]. Similar consensus guidelines have been drafted by ESMO (European Society for Medical Oncology) and SITC (Society for Immunotherapy of Cancer) [10, 11]. Wilson et al. examined the rate of response of hematologic-irAEs to immunosuppressive therapy and found that the average proportional response rate and heterogeneity index (I^2) to immunosuppression was around 68% proportional response ($I^2 = 0\%$) [12].

An extended DAT panel called Super-Coombs can be utilized to identify specific antibodies and markers, including IgA or IgM antibodies. A false negative DAT can result secondary to methodology. Sparse detection or deficient cross-link of reagent of IgG on the cell surface or IgA or IgM mediated AIHA may fail the sensitivity limit of regular DAT testing. Additionally, washing steps during DAT processing may remove low-affinity IgG molecules. Conventional diagnostic DAT primarily captures IgG and complement, resulting in reduced sensitivity for detecting other classes of antibodies. Performing the Super-Coombs panel overcomes these limitations and provides a comprehensive assessment of antibodies and markers involved in DAT-negative AIHA. It enables a more thorough evaluation, facilitating accurate diagnosis and appropriate management of the condition [3, 13]. There are currently no validated biomarkers to predict or prognosticate H-irAEs and patient outcomes.

Conclusion

In conclusion, the hematological toxicities associated with ICI therapy present significant challenges in clinical practice, particularly in cases of DAT-negative autoimmune hemolytic anemia, immune thrombocytopenic purpura, and autoimmune neutropenia. These rare and complex conditions underscore the intricate interplay between the immune system and hematopoietic cells, necessitating a multidisciplinary approach for optimal management. As our understanding of the underlying mechanisms evolves, tailored strategies encompassing immunomodulatory agents, supportive care measures, and close monitoring are crucial for achieving favorable outcomes in these challenging cases.Authors' Disclosures of Potential Conflicts of InterestAuthors claimed no disclosures.

References

1. de Back DZ, Kostova EB, van Kraaij M, van den Berg TK, Van Bruggen R. Of macrophages and red blood cells; a complex love story. Front Physiol. 2014;5:9.
2. Huang X, Venet F, Wang YL, Lepape A, Yuan Z, Chen Y, et al. PD-1 expression by macrophages plays a pathologic role in altering microbial clearance and the innate inflammatory response to sepsis. Proc Natl Acad Sci. 2009;106(15):6303–8.
3. Leaf RK, Ferreri C, Rangachari D, Mier J, Witteles W, Ansstas G, et al. Clinical and laboratory features of autoimmune hemolytic anemia associated with immune checkpoint inhibitors. Am J Hematol. 2019;94(5):563–74. https://doi.org/10.1002/ajh.25448.
4. Hwang SR, Saliba AN, Wolanskyj-Spinner AP. Immunotherapy-associated autoimmune hemolytic anemia. Hematol Oncol Clin North Am. 2022;36(2):365–80. https://doi.org/10.1016/j.hoc.2021.11.002.
5. Nelson BE, Ejezie CL, Stephen BA, Nardo M, Campbell E, Gong J, et al. Spectrum of immune checkpoint inhibitor anemias: results from a single center, early-phase clinical trials case series experience. J Hematol. 2022;11(3):113–20.
6. Delanoy N, Michot J-M, Comont T, Kramkimel N, Lazarovici J, Dupont R, et al. Haematological immune-related adverse events induced by anti-PD-1 or anti-PD-L1 immunotherapy: a descriptive observational study. Lancet Haematol. 2019;6(1):e48–57.
7. Brahmer JR, Lacchetti C, Schneider BJ, Atkins MB, Brassil KJ, Caterino JM, et al. Management of immune-related adverse events in patients treated with immune checkpoint inhibitor therapy: American Society of Clinical Oncology Clinical Practice Guideline. J Clin Oncol. 2018;36(17):1714.
8. Kroll MH, Rojas-Hernandez C, Yee C. Hematologic complications of immune checkpoint inhibitors. Blood. 2022;139(25):3594–604. https://doi.org/10.1182/blood.2020009016.
9. Oo TH, Rojas-Hernandez CM. Hematology. In: Wang Y, editor. Managing immunotherapy related organ toxicities: a practical guide. Cham: Springer International Publishing; 2022. p. 97–117.
10. Haanen J, Carbonnel F, Robert C, Kerr KM, Peters S, Larkin J, et al. Management of toxicities from immunotherapy: ESMO Clinical Practice Guidelines for diagnosis, treatment and follow-up. Ann Oncol. 2017;28(Suppl 4):iv119–42. https://doi.org/10.1093/annonc/mdx225.
11. Brahmer JR, Abu-Sbeih H, Ascierto PA, Brufsky J, Cappelli LC, Cortazar FB, et al. Society for Immunotherapy of Cancer (SITC) clinical practice guideline on immune checkpoint inhibitor-related adverse events. J Immunother Cancer. 2021;9(6):e002435. https://doi.org/10.1136/jitc-2021-002435.
12. Wilson NR, Lockhart JR, Garcia-Perdomo HA, Oo TH, Rojas-Hernandez CM. Management and outcomes of hematological immune-related adverse events: systematic review and meta-analysis. J Immunother. 2022;45(1):13–24. https://doi.org/10.1097/cji.0000000000000390.
13. Rodberg K. DAT-negative autoimmune hemolytic anemia. Hematol Oncol Clin North Am. 2022;36(2):307–13. https://doi.org/10.1016/j.hoc.2021.11.004.

Chapter 32
Immune Thrombocytopenic Purpura Post Immune Checkpoint Inhibitor Therapy

Thein Hlaing Oo, Francisco Vega, and Cristhiam Rojas-Hernandez

Abbreviations

ICI	Immune checkpoint inhibitor
ITP	Immune thrombocytopenic purpura
PD-1	Programmed cell death protein 1

Clinical Presentation

A Caucasian male patient in his 70s developed osteomyelitis of the right thumb and underwent excision. The pathology revealed squamous cell carcinoma with positive surgical margin. Two months later, he underwent amputation of joint of finger with neurectomy and direct closure of the right thumb. About 4 months later, he underwent radical resection of the soft tissue mass from right thumb for a local recurrence. Then 6 months later, he developed another recurrence and metastatic lymphadenopathy in the right axilla. With progressive disease, patient was subsequently started on 3-weekly cemiplimab (PD-1 monoclonal antibody) for three doses within the following 3 months and underwent right thumb tumor excision. However, he was found to have multiple lung nodules, and enlarging mediastinal lymphadenopathy after systemic treatment. His past medical history also included

T. H. Oo (✉) · C. Rojas-Hernandez
Section of Benign Hematology, The University of Texas M.D. Anderson Cancer Center, Houston, TX, USA
e-mail: thoo@mdanderson.org; CMRojas@mdanderson.org

F. Vega
Department of Hematopathology, The University of Texas M.D. Anderson Cancer Center, Houston, TX, USA
e-mail: FVega@mdanderson.org

Y. Wang (ed.), *Challenging Cases in Immunotherapy Related Organ Toxicities*,
https://doi.org/10.1007/978-3-031-83533-9_32

Table 32.1 Lab values

Tests	Values	Reference range
WBC	5.8	4,0–11.0 × 10^9/L
Hb	13.0	14.0–18.0 g/dL
Platelet	2	140–440 × 10^9/L
Neutrophil	54.1	42–66%
Lymphocyte	24.3	24–44%
Monocyte	13.9	2–7%
Eosinophil	6.8	1–4%
Prothrombin time	13.8	11.5–13.9 s
Partial thromboplastic time	35.4	24.7–36.8 s
Fibrinogen	379	214–503 mg/dL
Viral serology		
Hepatitis B	Negative	Negative
Hepatitis C	Negative	Negative
HIV	Negative	Negative

HIV human immunodeficiency virus

deep vein thrombosis, hyperlipidemia, hypertension, obstructive sleep apnea, osteomyelitis, and renal stones.

Twenty-one weeks after the first cemiplimab administration, he presented to the oncology clinic with skin bruises. Complete blood count (CBC) showed severe isolated thrombocytopenia (2 × 10^9/L). The physical examination was unremarkable except multiple petechiae and purpura of the skin and tight upper extremity lymphedema. Blood smear review revealed normochromic normocytic erythrocytes, normal leukocyte morphology and profound thrombocytopenia. Initial investigations were described in Table 32.1. Bone marrow biopsy revealed 40–60% cellularity, progressively maturing trilineage hematopoiesis, and megakaryocytic hyperplasia (Figs. 32.1 and 32.2). The overall clinical picture was consistent with immune checkpoint inhibitor (ICI)-induced immune thrombocytopenic purpura (ITP). For ITP treatment, intravenous dexamethasone 40 mg daily for 4 days was started. Platelet count was 14 × 10^9/L the day after completion of high-dose dexamethasone, however, dropped to 9 × 10^9/L the next day. At that point, intravenous immune globulin 1 g/kg for 2 days was administered raising the platelet count to 25 × 10^9/L. He received one dose of subcutaneous romiplostim 4 μg/kg the next day. Then, he started eltrombopag 50 mg once daily. Two months later, he received radiotherapy to the right axilla with 6 doses of weekly cisplatin.

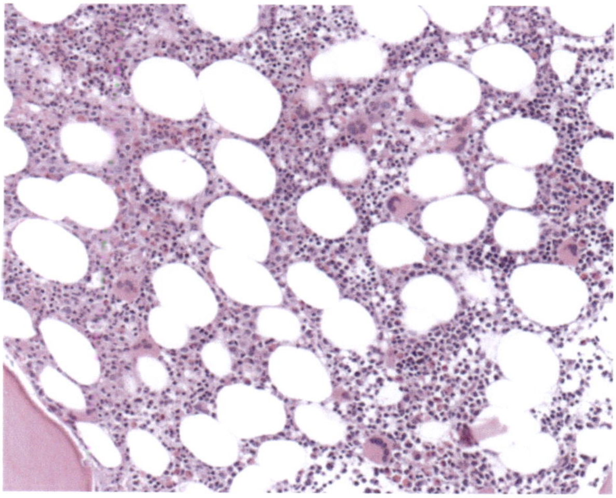

Fig. 32.1 Bone marrow core biopsy (hematoxylin and eosin) ×20, showing trilineage hematopoiesis and megakaryocytic hyperplasia

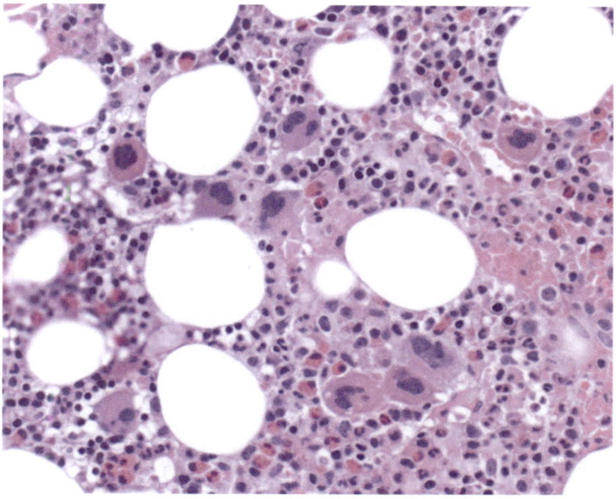

Fig. 32.2 Bone marrow core biopsy (hematoxylin and eosin) ×40, showing megakaryocytic hyperplasia. Megakaryocytes are morphologically unremarkable

Follow Up and Outcome

Two months after completion of radiotherapy, he came to the Hematology clinic for follow-up. He was well and the platelet count was 275 × 10^9/L. Eltrombopag was reduced to 25 mg once daily. However, he was found to have low platelet again 6 months later (platelet count of 1 × 10^9/L), consistent with relapsed ITP. Oral dexamethasone 40 mg daily for 4 days was restarted and eltrombopag was increased to 50 mg daily. Since the platelet count was slow to rise, he was given one dose of IVIG 1 g/kg and romiplostim 4 mg/kg weekly was started. Six months later, his ITP is in remission while on weekly administration of romiplostim. The timeline of clinical events is summarized in Fig. 32.3 (timepoint of 0 is ITP diagnosis).

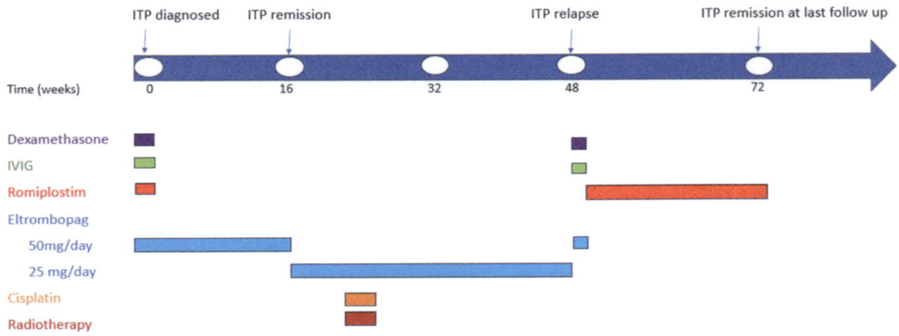

Fig. 32.3 Timeline of clinical events of ITP. Timepoint of 0 is the ITP diagnosis

Discussion

Usually, patients with ITP present with isolated thrombocytopenia (platelet count <100 × 10^9/L). It is a diagnosis of exclusion. Peripheral blood smear showed isolated thrombocytopenia with no other abnormalities (no schistocytes, dyspoietic changes, immature white blood cells). Large or giant platelets may be seen on the blood smear in some patients. The bone marrow biopsy may be necessary to exclude other causes of thrombocytopenia [1].

In terms of management strategy, the American Society of Clinical Oncology clinical practice guidelines suggest continuing ICI with close follow-up if the patient has grade I toxicity. If the platelet count is between 50 and 75 × 10^9/L (grade 2 toxicity), ICI should be held until the platelet count comes back up above 75 × 10^9/L. Steroids (e.g. prednisone 0.5–2 mg/kg/day for 2–4 weeks) followed by tapering over the next 4–6 weeks should be considered. For grade 3 (25–50 × 10^9/L) or grade 4 (<25 × 10^9/L) toxicity, hematology consultation should be obtained. Additional therapeutic options including IVIG, rituximab, and thrombopoietin mimetics (e.g. eltrombopag, romiplostim, avatrombopag) can be considered. In grade 3 and 4 toxicities, ICIs should be permanently discontinued if ITP gets worse or does not improve with therapy [2–8].

The outcome of treatment of ICI-induced ITP is usually good. About 71% of patients responded to steroids (57% complete response and 14% partial response). The remainder required additional therapies [9]. In our practice, we usually follow up the patients every 1–2 weeks during the induction phase. Once the platelet count is satisfactory, they can be followed up every 3–4 weeks and then 3–6 monthly thereafter.

References

1. Cooper N, Ghanima W. Immune thrombocytopenia. N Engl J Med. 2019;381(10):945–55. https://doi.org/10.1056/NEJMcp1810479.
2. Brahmer JR, Lacchetti C, Schneider BJ, Atkins MB, Brassil KJ, Caterino JM, et al. Management of immune-related adverse events in patients treated with immune checkpoint inhibitor therapy: American Society of Clinical Oncology clinical practice guideline. J Clin Oncol. 2018;36(17):1714–68. https://doi.org/10.1200/JCO.2017.77.6385.
3. Cheng Y, Wong RS, Soo YOL, Chui CH, Lau FY, Chan NP, et al. Initial treatment of immune thrombocytopenic purpura with high-dose dexamethasone. N Engl J Med. 2003;349(9):831–6. https://doi.org/10.1056/NEJMoa030254.
4. Blanchette V, Imbach P, Andrew M, Adams M, McMillan J, Wang E, et al. Randomized trial of intravenous immunoglobulin G, intravenous anti-D, and oral prednisone in childhood acute immune thrombocytopenic purpura. Lancet. 1994;344(8924):703–7. https://doi.org/10.1016/s0140-6736(94)92205-5.
5. Godeau B, Porcher R, Fain O, Lefrère F, Fenaux P, Cheze S, et al. Rituximab efficacy and safety in adult splenectomy candidates with chronic immune thrombocytopenic purpura: results of a prospective multicenter phase 2 study. Blood. 2008;112(4):999–1004. https://doi.org/10.1182/blood-2008-01-131029.
6. Cheng G, Saleh MN, Marcher C, Vasey S, Mayer B, Aivado M, et al. Eltrombopag for management of chronic immune thrombocytopenia (RAISE): a 6-month, randomised, phase 3 study. Lancet. 2011;377(9763):393–402. https://doi.org/10.1016/S0140-6736(10)60959-2.
7. Kuter DJ, Rummel M, Boccia R, Macik BG, Pabinger I, Selleslag D, et al. Romiplostim or standard of care in patients with immune thrombocytopenia. N Engl J Med. 2010;363(20):1889–99. https://doi.org/10.1056/NEJMoa1002625.
8. Bussel JB, Kuter DJ, Aledort LM, Kessler CM, Cuker A, Pendergrass KB, et al. A randomized trial of avatrombopag, an investigational thrombopoietin-receptor agonist, in persistent and chronic immune thrombocytopenia. Blood. 2014;123(25):3887–94. https://doi.org/10.1182/blood-2013-07-514398.
9. Michot J, Lazarovici J, Tieu A, Champiat S, Voison A, Ebbo M, et al. Haematological immune-related adverse events with immune checkpoint inhibitors, how to manage? Eur J Cancer. 2019;122:72–90. https://doi.org/10.1016/j.ejca.2019.07.014.

Part VI
Hepatology

Chapter 33
Hepatobiliary Toxicity Secondary to Immune Checkpoint Inhibitor Therapy: Early Tocilizumab Treatment to Decouple Steroid Dependency

Hao Chi Zhang, Sean Ngo, Deyali Chatterjee, Ethan Miller, Amado J. Zurita, and Lan Wang

Abbreviations

ALP	Alkaline phosphatase
ALT	Alanine aminotransferase
ANA	Anti-nuclear antibody
AST	Aspartate aminotransferase
DILI	Drug-induced liver injury
GGT	Gamma-glutamyl transferase
H&E	Hematoxylin and eosin
ICI	Immune checkpoint inhibitor
IgG	Immunoglobulin G
IMCH	Immune-mediated cholangiohepatitis
IMH	Immune-mediated hepatobiliary toxicity

H. C. Zhang (✉) · E. Miller · L. Wang
Department of Gastroenterology, Hepatology & Nutrition, The University of Texas MD Anderson Cancer Center, Houston, TX, USA
e-mail: hzhang20@mdanderson.org; emiller1@mdanderson.org; lwang25@mdanderson.org

S. Ngo
McGovern Medical School at The University of Texas Health Science Center at Houston, Houston, TX, USA
e-mail: sean.b.ngo@uth.tmc.edu

D. Chatterjee
Department of Pathology, The University of Texas MD Anderson Cancer Center, Houston, TX, USA
e-mail: dchatterjee@mdanderson.org

A. J. Zurita
Department of Genitourinary Medical Oncology, The University of Texas MD Anderson Cancer Center, Houston, TX, USA
e-mail: azurita@mdanderson.org

Y. Wang (ed.), *Challenging Cases in Immunotherapy Related Organ Toxicities*, https://doi.org/10.1007/978-3-031-83533-9_33

irAE	Immune-related adverse event
IV	Intravenous
LE	Liver enzymes
TCZ	Tocilizumab

Clinical Presentation

This is a male in 50s who presented with new-onset liver enzyme elevations. He has a history of obesity and type II diabetes mellitus (hemoglobin A1c of 6.6%) but no prior established liver disease. The patient also has a history of clear cell renal cell carcinoma for which he had received cabozantinib and two cycles of combination immune checkpoint inhibitor (ICI) therapy with ipilimumab and nivolumab. At a follow-up visit approximately 3 weeks after his second dose of ipilimumab and nivolumab, the patient's levels of alanine aminotransferase (ALT) had increased to 155 U/L, aspartate aminotransferase (AST) had increased to 166, and alkaline phosphatase (ALP) had increased to 430 U/L. Ipilimumab and nivolumab were held, and cabozantinib was discontinued to remove it as a confounding cause of possible drug-induced liver injury (DILI). Ursodiol was empirically started 10 days later to curtail the cholestatic effects, pending further investigation.

Evaluation

Laboratory studies indicated anti-nuclear antibody (ANA) titer of 1:320, positive anti-smooth muscle antibody, normal immunoglobulin G (IgG) level, and negative anti-mitochondrial antibody. Parenchymal liver biopsy obtained 3 weeks after this initial rise in liver enzymes revealed acute hepatitis with moderate portal chronic inflammation, including mild bile duct epithelial injury, as well as foci of lobular inflammation, predominantly in zone 3. There was scattered non-zonal minimal/mild macrovesicular steatosis, up to 5% (Fig. 33.1a, b). There was no underlying fibrosis, no diastase resistant cytoplasmic globules on PASD stain to suggest alpha-1 antitrypsin deficiency, and no abnormal iron accumulation on iron stain. The composite clinical picture was deemed compatible with immune-mediated cholangiohepatitis (IMCH) secondary to combination ICI therapy.

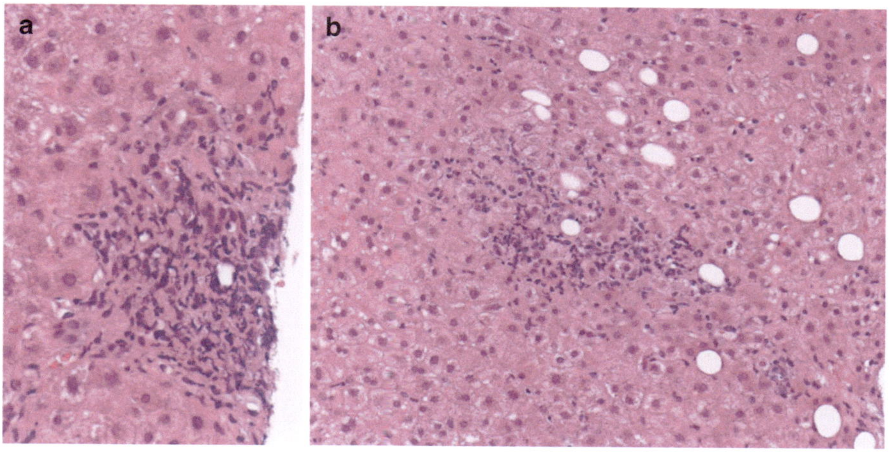

Fig. 33.1 (**a**) First diagnostic liver biopsy (H&E, ×200): acute hepatitis pattern of injury, with moderate portal chronic inflammation including focal interface activity; bile ducts show mild epithelial injury. (**b**) First diagnostic liver biopsy (H&E, ×100): Foci of zone 3 lobular inflammation; background mild non-zonal steatosis (5%)

Treatment and Disease Course

The patient was started on induction steroids with oral budesonide 9 mg/day for 10 days and resumed cabozantinib. Nine days later, however, ALT increased to 1563 U/L, AST increased to 1282 U/L, and ALP improved to 176 U/L without developing acute liver synthetic dysfunction (Table 33.1, Fig. 33.2a, b). Cabozantinib was again discontinued. The patient was admitted for inpatient care with transition to systemic corticosteroids. Intravenous (IV) methylprednisolone was initiated at 60 mg/day which curtailed further ALT increase. After 3 days, the ALT level improved to 725 U/L and then to 567 U/L a day later. Due to uncontrolled hyperglycemia (glucose >300 mg/dL) while on IV systemic steroids and to limit dependence on steroids, IV tocilizumab (TCZ) was given once (8 mg/kg), with immediate tapering of steroids across the next 3 weeks. By the end of this course, ALT had improved to 63 U/L, and shortly after, the patient resumed immunotherapy, receiving three more doses of nivolumab. Four months after TCZ was given, laboratory results revealed that the patient had continued to sustain steroid-free biochemical normalization of ALT despite having resumed nivolumab.

The patient's cancer disease was still progressing despite resuming nivolumab. Cabozantinib was resumed, but it was held again after a week due to ALT being elevated to 241 U/L and AST to 255 U/L (Table 33.2, Fig. 33.2a, c). A week after that, the patient presented to the hospital with a fever of 102.9 °F with ALT elevated to 1273 U/L and AST to 1118 U/L with normal total bilirubin (Table 33.2). Acute infectious work-up was negative and repeated liver biopsy showed marked centrilobular and bridging necrosis (Fig. 33.3a, b). The clinical picture could not exclude the possibility of recurrent IMCH. His hemoglobin A1c was 6.8%. Due to his prior

Table 33.1 Pertinent labs from first episode of immune-mediated cholangiohepatitis

	Baseline before ICMH	Initial peak ALT	1 day before TCZ	Day of TCZ	1 day after TCZ	30 days after TCZ	41 days after TCZ	127 days after TCZ
ALT (ref: ≤41 U/L)	16 U/L	**1563 U/L**	**725 U/L**	**567 U/L**	**388 U/L**	**67 U/L**	**47 U/L**	14 U/L
AST (ref: ≤40 U/L)	10 U/L	**1282 U/L**	**197 U/L**	**102 U/L**	**65 U/L**	**45 U/L**	36 U/L	20 U/L
ALP (ref: 40–129 U/L)	46 U/L	**176 U/L**	121 U/L	111 U/L	99 U/L	40 U/L	44 U/L	57 U/L
Direct bilirubin (ref: ≤0.3 mg/dL)	<0.2 mg/dL	0.3 mg/dL	0.2 mg/dL	0.2 mg/dL	0.2 mg/dL	–	<0.2 mg/dL	<0.2 mg/dL
INR (ref: 0.89–1.10)	–	1.13	1.22	1.2	–	1.1	–	–
CRP (ref: ≤10.00 mg/L)	–	37.33 mg/L	–	–	–	0.07 mg/L	–	–

U units, *L* liter, *mg* milligrams, *dL* deciliter, *ALT* alanine aminotransferase, *AST* aspartate aminotransferase, *ALP* alkaline phosphatase, *INR* international normalized ratio, *CRP* C-reactive protein
Abnormal values are **bolded** in the table

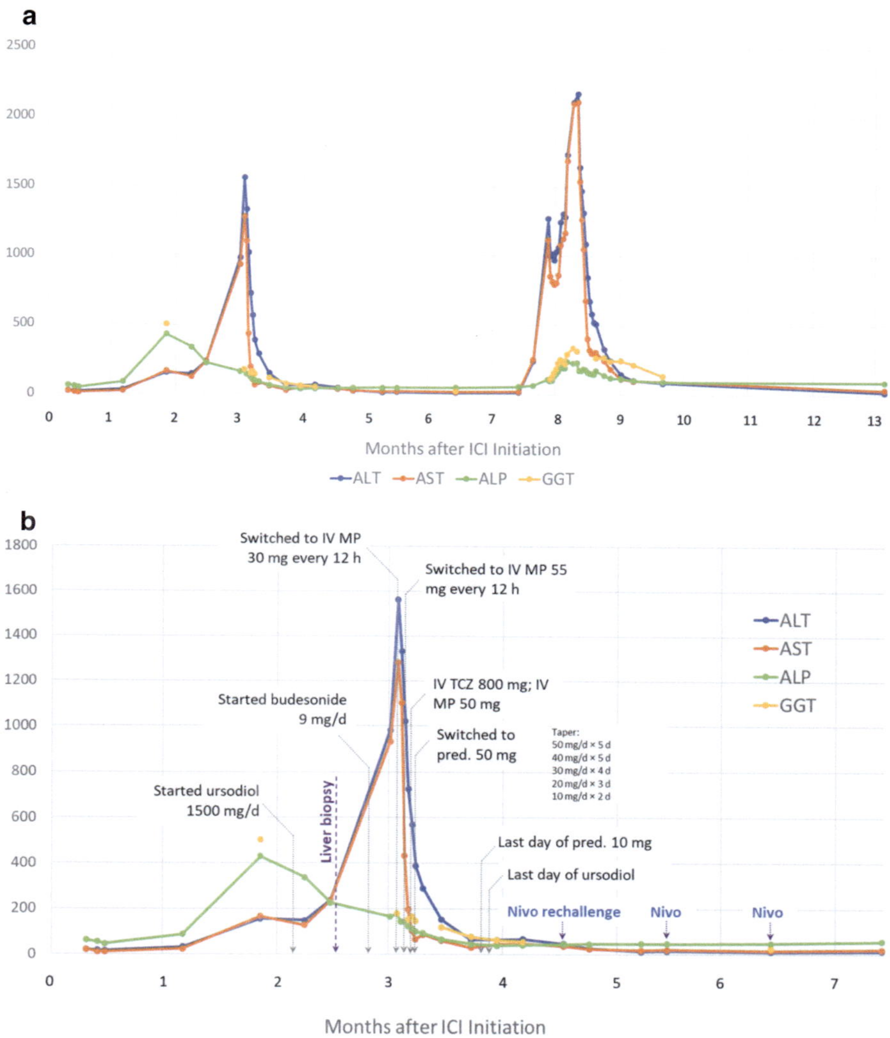

Fig. 33.2 (**a**) Overall chronological trend of liver biochemistries. (**b**) Zoomed-in view of liver biochemistries and medication administration during the first episode of immune-mediated cholangiohepatitis. (**c**) Zoomed-in view of liver biochemistries and medication administration during the second episode of immune-mediated cholangiohepatitis

favorable response to tocilizumab and in favor of avoiding systemic steroids in the setting of diabetes, monotherapy IV tocilizumab (8 mg/kg) was administered once again, and he was discharged from the hospital.

Six days after discharge, however, the patient was readmitted for continued elevation of ALT to 2170 U/L, AST to 2110 U/L, and direct bilirubin to 5.0 mg/dL (Table 33.2, Fig. 33.2a, c). Given further negative workup for other possible etiologies, the proximity to recent tocilizumab administration, and a third biopsy showing

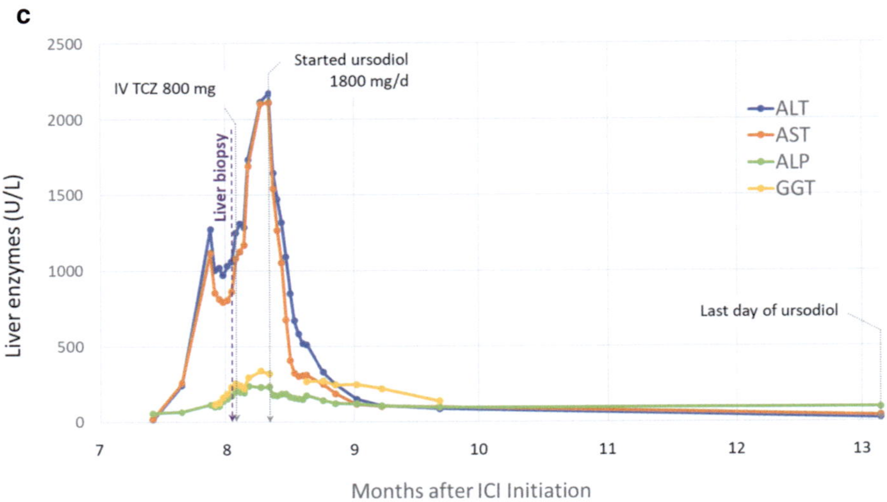

Fig. 33.2 (continued)

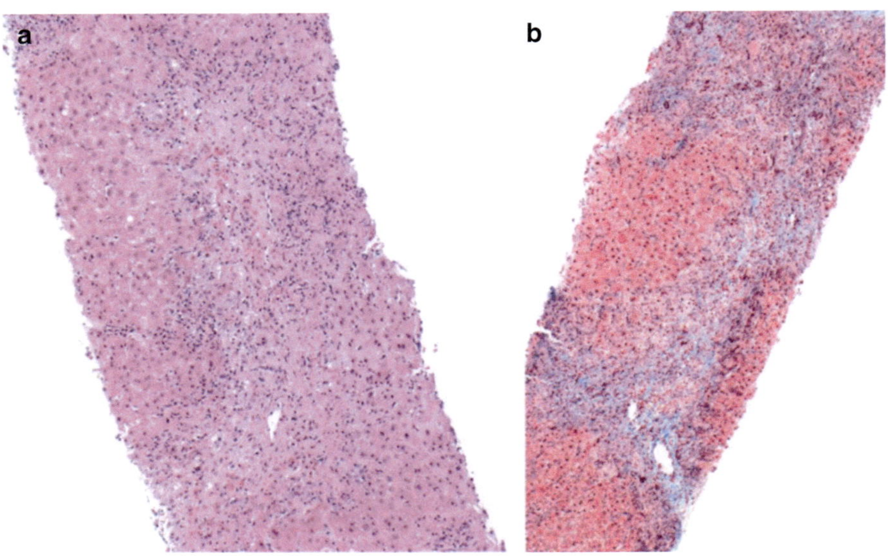

Fig. 33.3 (**a**) Second diagnostic liver biopsy (H&E, ×40): immune-mediated marked centrilobular and bridging necrosis. (**b**) Second diagnostic liver biopsy (Trichrome, ×20): corresponding trichrome stain revealing no underlying fibrosis

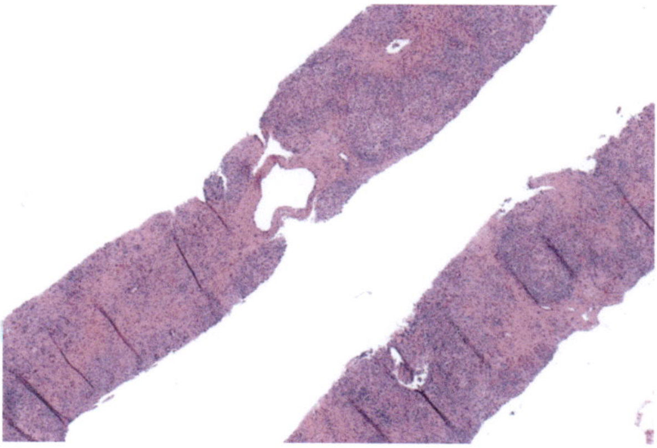

Fig. 33.4 Third diagnostic liver biopsy (H&E, ×40): submassive hepatocellular necrosis. Biopsy shows parenchymal collapse with extensive perivenular dropout and consequent portal and central approximation

submassive hepatocellular necrosis (Fig. 33.4), the patient was observed for diagnosis of suspected drug-induced liver injury (DILI) secondary to tocilizumab as opposed to a resurgent immune-mediated event. The patient was discharged once again with close liver biochemical lab monitoring three times a week over the next 2 weeks. On day 48 after the second dose of tocilizumab, the patient's ALT had improved to 85 U/L. On day 84 after, the ALT normalized to 26 U/L (<40 U/L) with AST of 46 U/L and normal ALP level (<120 U/L) (Table 33.2). And on day 93 after, ALT remained normal (at 27 U/L) with repeat testing for GGT also showing normalization (at 21 U/L, *N* = 8–61 U/L), effectively attaining biochemical remission of IMCH.

Table 33.2 Pertinent labs from second episode of immune-mediated cholangiohepatitis

	Initial onset of second episode (14 days before TCZ)	Initial peak ALT (7 days before TCZ)	Day of TCZ	Second peak ALT (7 days after TCZ)	14 days after TCZ	48 days after TCZ	84 days after TCZ	93 days after TCZ
ALT (ref: ≤41 U/L)	**241 U/L**	**1273 U/L**	**1308 U/L**	**2170 U/L**	**582 U/L**	**85 U/L**	26 U/L	27 U/L
AST (ref: ≤40 U/L)	**255 U/L**	**1118 U/L**	**1126 U/L**	**2110 U/L**	**300 U/L**	**97 U/L**	**46 U/L**	–
ALP (ref: 40–129 U/L)	65 U/L	112 U/L	**195 U/L**	**231 U/L**	**151 U/L**	95 U/L	95 U/L	–
Direct bilirubin (ref: ≤0.3 mg/dL)	<0.2 mg/dL	**0.5 mg/dL**	**0.8 mg/dL**	**5.0 mg/dL**	**5.5 mg/dL**	**2.6 mg/dL**	**1.5 mg/dL**	–
INR (ref: 0.89–1.10)	–	–	–	**1.51**	**1.38**	**1.30**	–	–
CRP (ref: ≤10.00 mg/L)	–	**229.48 mg/L**	–	6.28 mg/L	–	1.63	–	–

U units, *L* liter, *mg* milligrams, *dL* deciliter, *ALT* alanine aminotransferase, *AST* aspartate aminotransferase, *ALP* alkaline phosphatase, *INR* international normalized ratio, *CRP* C-reactive protein
Abnormal values are bolded in the table

Clinical Outcome

Across several weeks after his last hospital admission, the patient's liver enzymes trended towards biochemical normalization as mentioned (Table 33.2, Fig. 33.2a, c). Given the patient's two episodes of high-grade recurrent IMCH with suspected superimposed tocilizumab-induced DILI, the patient was advised against resuming ICI treatment. The decision was made on the basis that the patient had a repeat episode of IMCH (or recurrent IMCH) requiring complex management. His oncologist shifted his treatment to a combination of everolimus and lenvatinib, with treatment for his metastatic renal cell carcinoma still ongoing at his most recent follow up 14 months after his initial dose of immunotherapy.

Summary of the Case

A patient with a pre-existing medical diagnosis of obesity and diabetes who was treated with combination ICI therapy with ipilimumab and nivolumab, in addition to cabozantinib, then developed severe IMCH. The patient was started on ursodiol initially and then oral budesonide (accounting for diabetes history). Because budesonide was deemed inadequate to induce remission, IV steroids were promptly initiated at the expense of anticipated hyperglycemia as an adverse effect, but with the intention to bridge the patient directly to IV tocilizumab. Tocilizumab acted as a steroid-sparing strategy to decouple the treatment from steroids while still attaining biochemical remission. This attenuated the patient's hyperglycemia issues by allowing for a rapid steroid taper over only 3 weeks. His liver enzymes achieved biochemical remission, and the patient was restarted on nivolumab and then cabozantinib. After additional nivolumab cycles in remission from IMCH, he developed recurrence of ICI-related cholangiohepatitis. Tocilizumab was used again without concurrent use of steroids. A significant, but transient elevation of liver enzymes was seen due to a suspected tocilizumab drug-induced liver injury. The patient did not develop acute liver failure. Through observation only, his liver enzymes eventually returned to baseline, and the patient successfully attained biochemical remission again. Summary of timeline events is shown in Fig. 33.5.

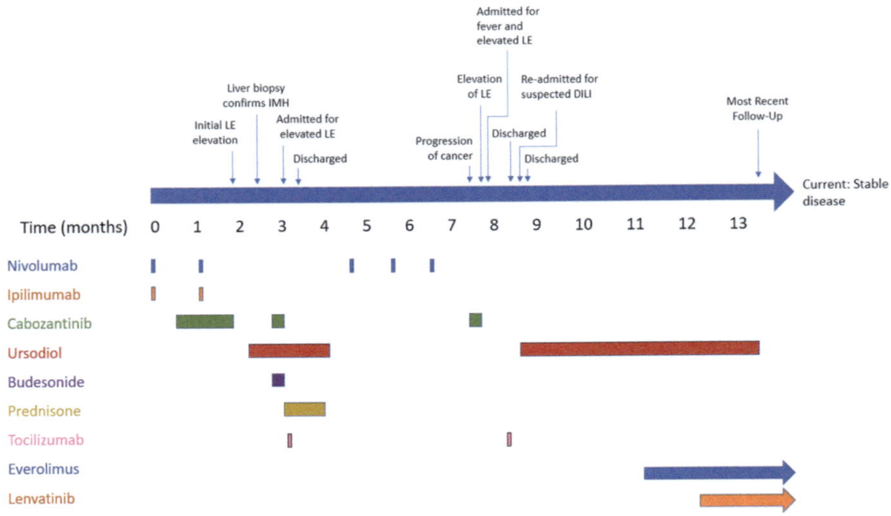

Fig. 33.5 Clinical course and timeline of events (timepoint 0 is the initiation of ICI)

Discussion

The initial diagnosis of IMCH was established by the overall clinical picture with the understanding of how immune-mediated liver injury behaves, and the histologic analysis from liver biopsy. In addition to ICI, some patients may be on adjunctive cancer treatments with other agent(s) that could cause DILI. For instance, cabozantinib-related DILI is not uncommon, either [1]. Therefore, when acute liver injury was identified, cabozantinib, as a confounder of the DILI analysis, was discontinued, with the expectation that cabozantinib-related DILI does not require steroids to promote biochemical remission, and the associated liver injury should be short-lived. Cholestatic DILI from cabozantinib is considered rare, whereas cholangiohepatitis phenotypes of immune-mediated hepatobiliary toxicity (IMH) is already well-recognized and likely more common in patients exposed to anti-PD-1/L1 agents [1]. A normal total serum IgG level in the acute hepatitis phase also would tend to disfavor idiopathic autoimmune hepatitis.

Currently society guidelines endorse the treatment for high-grade immune related adverse events (irAEs) like IMH with high-dose corticosteroids (CS) [2]. In patients who develop hyperglycemia or have comorbidities that disfavor or limit the use of systemic CSs (such as pre-existing diabetes or recent infections), it may be medically beneficial to minimize the exposure and duration of the patient's steroid course. As such, oral budesonide, given its limited systemic effects, was favored as the induction steroid before attempt at prescribing systemic CS [3–6]. Tocilizumab is an IL-6 receptor antagonist that has been shown to be effective in treating several types of irAEs, and in a few select cases, can treat IMH without relying on steroids for the immunosuppressive phase [7–17].

In this case, oral budesonide was deemed insufficient to attain initial biochemical improvement in liver enzymes. In an ongoing effort to minimize exposure to systemic CS, the risks and benefits of starting IV steroids were reviewed with the patient. The patient's steroid was transitioned directly to IV methylprednisolone inpatient, to determine if this could curtail further increases in the liver enzymes, thereby halting or slowing down the progression of liver injury. Whether the liver enzymes improved or not after initiation of IV steroids, the strategy was to bridge the patient to IV tocilizumab in order to "decouple" the patient's dependency on steroids to attain biochemical remission in the first place, akin to other methods of biologic treatment for other conditions like inflammatory bowel disease or immune-mediated colitis. In both clinical experience and published case reports, a single dose of IV tocilizumab can be sufficient [7–17]. After administration of tocilizumab, a much shorter steroid taper over 3 weeks (instead of the typical 4–6 weeks) was possible, even without first waiting for the ALT to achieve near-normal values. This strategy allowed the patient to recover from significant hyperglycemia episodes while on systemic CS and obviated the need to introduce other adjuncts such as mycophenolate mofetil, azathioprine, or tacrolimus, which generally still rely on concurrent steroids.

One potential adverse effect of tocilizumab is drug-induced liver injury [18]. Elevations in liver enzymes from tocilizumab-related DILI can be variable, and several cases have shown that these abnormal biochemical changes are typically transient and short-lived, returning to normal within 2–6 weeks [18, 19]. As such, the clinician should be aware that if tocilizumab is used to treat select cases of IMH, that paradoxical elevations in liver enzymes can occur within the first few weeks of tocilizumab administration. This can introduce a similar confounding element of another culprit towards DILI which would require weighing the relative likelihood of a resurgent immune response for IMH. Other potential adverse events from tocilizumab treatment may include leukopenia, opportunistic infections, and hyperlipidemia.

The patient did not exhibit tocilizumab-related DILI during the first episode of administration. If the new liver enzyme peak after the second tocilizumab administration were truly associated with tocilizumab-related DILI, one would regard it as an idiosyncratic DILI. Due to a higher confidence for tocilizumab-related DILI instead of resurgent IMH, the former entity was selected as the working diagnosis, which favored observation without immunosuppression. The expectation then would be that the therapeutic effects of tocilizumab would be observed within 4 weeks with net decrement of ALT from its peak during that time. Steroids were not prescribed at all during this phase, in favor of observation. The patient's liver injury (from both initial IMH and superimposed DILI from tocilizumab) gradually and spontaneously resolved, without progression to liver failure.

This clinical case also showcases another behavior of IMH that is unpredictable. For instance, after successful recovery from the first IMH episode (CTCAE grade 4, IMCH phenotype), the patient was rechallenged with nivolumab. This decision was made on the basis that collective published data estimates about two-thirds to three-fourths of patients do not suffer from a second episode of IMH after ICI resumption even after recovery from high-grade IMH [20–23]. While further longitudinal studies are necessary to characterize the behavior, the patient's resumption of ICI allowed him to receive three additional doses of nivolumab before a second IMH episode.

Conclusion

Understanding of the biochemical behavior and reported histologic features of IMH/IMCH can aid the clinician in its diagnosis. Tocilizumab may be a viable treatment option to mitigate the typical duration of exposure to systemic corticosteroids in the treatment of IMH/IMCH or its heterogeneous phenotypes. This offers an early steroid-sparing strategy that could obviate the need to introduce agents like mycophenolate mofetil. DILI associated with tocilizumab should be taken into consideration when administering the medication to treat IMH, but tocilizumab's adverse effects on the liver often resolve spontaneously over the course of less than 2 weeks.

References

1. Cabozantinib. In: LiverTox: clinical and research information on drug-induced liver injury. National Institute of Diabetes and Digestive and Kidney Diseases; 2012. [Updated 2017 Jan 4]. http://www.ncbi.nlm.nih.gov/books/NBK548279/.
2. Schneider BJ, Naidoo J, Santomasso BD, et al. Management of immune-related adverse events in patients treated with immune checkpoint inhibitor therapy: ASCO guideline update. J Clin Oncol. 2021;39(36):4073–126. https://doi.org/10.1200/JCO.21.01440.
3. Eleftheriotis G, Skopelitis E. Immune-checkpoint inhibitor-associated grade 3 hepatotoxicity managed with enteric-coated budesonide monotherapy: a case report. Medicine (Baltimore). 2022;101(31):e29473. https://doi.org/10.1097/MD.0000000000029473.
4. Zhang HC, Wang L, Wang Y, Miller E. S2722 budesonide as an alternative steroid agent, in combination with adjunctive agents, for the treatment of immune checkpoint inhibitor-mediated cholangiohepatitis: a case study. Am J Gastroenterol. 2021;116:S1139. https://doi.org/10.14309/01.ajg.0000784420.59476.c6.
5. Manns MP, Woynarowski M, Kreisel W, et al. Budesonide induces remission more effectively than prednisone in a controlled trial of patients with autoimmune hepatitis. Gastroenterology. 2010;139(4):1198–206. https://doi.org/10.1053/j.gastro.2010.06.046.
6. Machado A, Wang L, Miller E, Wang Y, Zhang HC. Tu1570 exploring clinical outcomes in immune checkpoint inhibitor-mediated hepatobiliary toxicity managed with oral budesonide: an introduction to novel strategies. Gastroenterology. 2023;164(6):S-1418–9. https://doi.org/10.1016/S0016-5085(23)04305-6.
7. Stroud CR, Hegde A, Cherry C, et al. Tocilizumab for the management of immune mediated adverse events secondary to PD-1 blockade. J Oncol Pharm Pract. 2019;25(3):551–7. https://doi.org/10.1177/1078155217745144.
8. Campochiaro C, Farina N, Tomelleri A, et al. Tocilizumab for the treatment of immune-related adverse events: a systematic literature review and a multicentre case series. Eur J Intern Med. 2021;93:87–94. https://doi.org/10.1016/j.ejim.2021.07.016.

9. Moi L, Bouchaab H, Mederos N, et al. Personalized cytokine-directed therapy with tocilizumab for refractory immune checkpoint inhibitor-related cholangiohepatitis. J Thorac Oncol. 2021;16(2):318–26. https://doi.org/10.1016/j.jtho.2020.09.007.
10. Reddy CA, Schneider BJ, Brackett LM, Tai AW. Nivolumab-induced large-duct cholangiopathy treated with ursodeoxycholic acid and tocilizumab. Immunotherapy. 2019;11(18):1527–31. https://doi.org/10.2217/imt-2019-0121.
11. Zhang HC, Eyada M, Taggart M, et al. S2724 clinical presentation, treatment strategies, and chronic sequelae of immune checkpoint inhibitor-mediated cholangiopathy: a case study. Am J Gastroenterol. 2021;116:S1140. https://doi.org/10.14309/01.ajg.0000784428.93302.00.
12. Dimitriou F, Hogan SA, Cheng PF, Dummer R, Menzies AM, Long GV. IL-6 blockade for prophylaxis and management of immune-related adverse events (irAEs) with anti-PD-1 based immunotherapy. J Clin Oncol. 2021;39(15 Suppl):9553. https://doi.org/10.1200/JCO.2021.39.15_suppl.9553.
13. Zhang HC, Miller ED, Wang L. S2913 tocilizumab as an effective steroid-sparing agent for the treatment of recurrent and steroid-dependent immune checkpoint inhibitor-mediated hepatotoxicity: a case study and insight into pathophysiology. Am J Gastroenterol. 2022;117(10S):e1896. https://doi.org/10.14309/01.ajg.0000868292.46390.96.
14. Zhang HC, Eyada M, Miller ED, Wang LS. Tocilizumab as an alternative treatment strategy for immunotherapy-mediated hepatobiliary toxicity: addressing an urgent unmet need. Poster presented at: AASLD The Liver Meeting, 2021; virtual.
15. Zhang HC, Miller ED, Wang L. A0541—early use of tocilizumab as an effective steroid-sparing strategy for the treatment of immune checkpoint inhibitor-mediated cholangiopathy: building foundations for personalized management. Poster presented at: American College of Gastroenterology 2022 annual scientific meeting abstracts, Oct 23, 2022; Charlotte, NC.
16. Lyles L, Farmer R, Abougergi M. A potential new use for tocilizumab: refractory checkpoint inhibitor hepatitis. ACG Case Rep J. 2023;10(9):e01162. https://doi.org/10.14309/crj.0000000000001162.
17. Ali SB, Vembar P, Sukumaran S, Gunawardane D, Hughes T, Smith A. Tocilizumab in grade 4 hepatitis secondary to immune checkpoint inhibitor: a case report and review of the literature. Immunotherapy. 2023;15(14):1125–32. https://doi.org/10.2217/imt-2023-0085.
18. Tocilizumab. In: LiverTox: clinical and research information on drug-induced liver injury. National Institute of Diabetes and Digestive and Kidney Diseases; 2012. http://www.ncbi.nlm.nih.gov/books/NBK548243/. Accessed 20 Oct 2023.
19. Muhović D, Bojović J, Bulatović A, et al. First case of drug-induced liver injury associated with the use of tocilizumab in a patient with COVID-19. Liver Int. 2020;40(8):1901–5. https://doi.org/10.1111/liv.14516.
20. Pollack MH, Betof A, Dearden H, et al. Safety of resuming anti-PD-1 in patients with immune-related adverse events (irAEs) during combined anti-CTLA-4 and anti-PD1 in metastatic melanoma. Ann Oncol. 2018;29(1):250–5. https://doi.org/10.1093/annonc/mdx642.
21. Miller ED, Abu-Sbeih H, Styskel B, et al. Clinical characteristics and adverse impact of hepatotoxicity due to immune checkpoint inhibitors. Am J Gastroenterol. 2020;115(2):251–61. https://doi.org/10.14309/ajg.0000000000000398.
22. Li M, Sack JS, Rahma OE, Hodi FS, Zucker SD, Grover S. Outcomes after resumption of immune checkpoint inhibitor therapy after high-grade immune-mediated hepatitis. Cancer. 2020;126(23):5088–97. https://doi.org/10.1002/cncr.33165.
23. Riveiro-Barciela M, Barreira-Díaz A, Callejo-Pérez A, et al. Retreatment with immune checkpoint inhibitors after a severe immune-related hepatitis: results from a prospective multicenter study. Clin Gastroenterol Hepatol. 2023;21(3):732–40. https://doi.org/10.1016/j.cgh.2022.03.050.

Chapter 34
Cholangiohepatitis with Extrahepatic Cholangiopathy and Cholecystitis Secondary to Immune Checkpoint Inhibitor Therapy

Hao Chi Zhang, Andres Urias Rivera, Ethan Miller, Yun Shin Chun, Celia Robinson Ledet, and Lan Wang

Abbreviations

ALP	Alkaline phosphatase
ALT	Alanine aminotransferase
AST	Aspartate aminotransferase
CBD	Common bile duct
CT	Computed tomography
CTCAE	Common Terminology Criteria for Adverse Events
ERCP	Endoscopic retrograde cholangiopancreatography
GI	Gastrointestinal
ICI	Immune checkpoint inhibitor
IMCH	Immune-mediated cholangiohepatitis
IMCp	Immune-mediated cholangiopathy
IMH	Immune-mediated hepatobiliary toxicity
irAE	Immune-related adverse event
MRCP	Magnetic resonance cholangiopancreatography

H. C. Zhang (✉) · E. Miller · L. Wang
Department of Gastroenterology, Hepatology & Nutrition, University of Texas MD Anderson Cancer Center, Houston, TX, USA
e-mail: hzhang20@mdanderson.org; emiller1@mdanderson.org; lwang25@mdanderson.org

A. U. Rivera
Department of General Internal Medicine, Baylor College of Medicine, Houston, TX, USA
e-mail: andres.uriasrivera@bcm.edu

Y. S. Chun · C. R. Ledet
Division of Surgery, Department of Surgical Oncology, University of Texas MD Anderson Cancer Center, Houston, TX, USA
e-mail: yschun@mdanderson.org; crobinson3@mdanderson.org

Y. Wang (ed.), *Challenging Cases in Immunotherapy Related Organ Toxicities*,
https://doi.org/10.1007/978-3-031-83533-9_34

PBC	Primary biliary cholangitis
PSC	Primary sclerosing cholangitis
ULN	Upper level of normal

Clinical Presentation

This is a male patient in his 70s with prediabetes who presented with abnormal liver enzymes after treatment with pembrolizumab. A year prior, he was diagnosed with locally advanced urothelial carcinoma. He had no underlying liver disease, with baseline ALT, AST, and ALP levels within normal limits. He was treated with four cycles of neoadjuvant carboplatin and gemcitabine, followed by three cycles of pembrolizumab. Radical nephroureterectomy was attempted but was aborted due to extensive local invasion limiting separation of organs. He was admitted to the hospital for new-onset right upper quadrant pain within a week of the last dose of pembrolizumab. CT imaging reported questionable neoplastic infiltration of the porta hepatis and general prominence of the intrahepatic and extrahepatic biliary tree without any obstructing lesions of the common bile duct (CBD). MRCP showed biliary obstruction at the distal CBD without definite cause and probable cholelithiasis. He underwent ERCP 2 days into that admission that revealed biliary sludge but no biliary stricture. The day after ERCP, labs showed mild, mixed pattern elevation of liver enzymes. A week after the ERCP, he was started on a prednisone 50 mg/day, with subsequent 6-week taper for concern of IMH, but no serological work up was done. Endoscopic ultrasound 12 weeks after the last dose pembrolizumab was normal, and the AST and ALT normalized but ALP remained elevated. Around this time, he received one cycle of enfortumab vedotin, which was stopped due to lack of response. Between week 12 and 22 after the last dose of pembrolizumab, ALT and ALP increased to CTCAE grade 2, with R factor 0.5, suggesting cholestatic-predominant pattern. Viral hepatitis infections were excluded. Anti-nuclear antibody, anti-mitochondrial antibody, and anti-liver kidney microsome type 1 antibody were negative. Serum total IgG level was not elevated with normal serum total IgM level; IgG4 subclass level was within normal limits.

On the basis that the patient may have had a history of choledocholithiasis, an elective cholecystectomy was attempted, which revealed a white, firm, contracted gallbladder which caused anatomical distortion leading to inability to demarcate the cystic duct (Fig. 34.1); the cholecystectomy was aborted. Intraoperative gallbladder biopsy showed scant crushed epithelium, fibrosis, and necrosis but no malignancy.

Evaluation, Diagnosis and Treatment

Twenty-two weeks after the last pembrolizumab dose, parenchymal liver biopsy was performed to determine if there was an underlying immune-mediated process. The histology from liver biopsy showed cholestatic hepatitis with portal and lobular

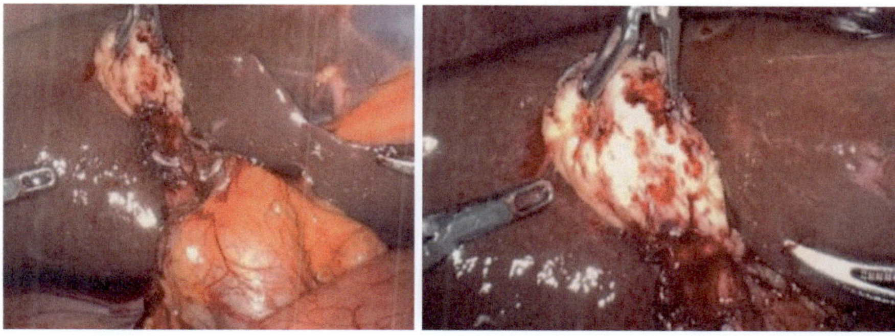

Fig. 34.1 Intra-operative photographs revealing a white, firm contracted gallbladder, with inability to demarcate the cystic duct and common bile duct; due to distortion of the extrahepatic biliary anatomy, cholecystectomy was aborted

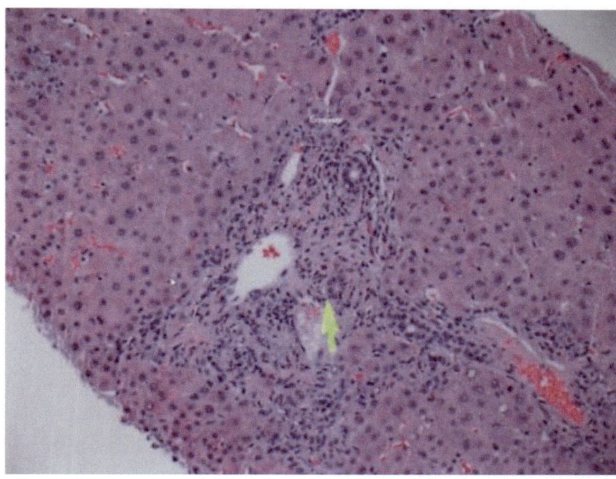

Fig. 34.2 Histologic evaluation (hematoxylin & eosin, ×100 magnification) from liver biopsy, showing chronic cholestatic hepatitis with portal and moderate lobular inflammation, bile duct injury (arrow), bile ductular proliferation, moderate cholestasis, and scattered hepatocyte necrosis; no significant fibrosis seen

inflammation, bile duct injury, and hepatocyte necrosis (Fig. 34.2). The features were not compatible with PBC or PSC. He was diagnosed with immune-mediated cholangiohepatitis (IMCH) with predominance of cholangiopathy on the basis of his extrahepatic biliary pathology. Oral budesonide (induction dose of 9 mg/day), azathioprine (as an early adjunctive immunomodulator therapy), and ursodiol were prescribed. Two weeks after liver biopsy, subcutaneous tocilizumab (TCZ) 162 mg was administered once. Budesonide was tapered to completion because treatment of IMH/IMCH no longer relied on steroids after tocilizumab was given, and azathioprine adjunct was also discontinued. The patient's AST and ALT levels normalized in 4 weeks after TCZ; however, ALP remained elevated, so ursodiol was continued indefinitely. Repeat MRCP showed intrahepatic biliary ductal dilation, ductal thickening and enhancement, and common bile duct dilation with a new stricture at the distal CBD. ERCP found one benign moderate biliary stricture at the distal CBD, and a plastic CBD stent was placed (Fig. 34.3).

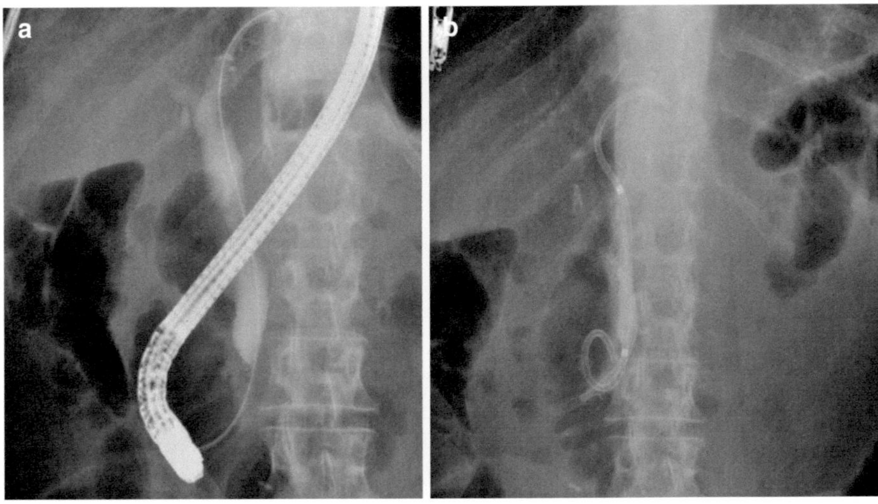

Fig. 34.3 Fluoroscopic images from ERCP performed after finding a CBD stricture on MRCP. Upper EUS performed immediately prior to this ERCP demonstrated minimal hyperechoic material compatible with biliary sludge with CBD diameter of 7 mm and CBD wall of 2 mm thickness. (**a**) Initial cholangiogram on ERCP demonstrating distal CBD stricture; the stricture was deemed benign. (**b**) Fluoroscopic image after placement of a 10 Fr × 7 cm plastic biliary stent, with a full external pigtail and full internal pigtail, in the CBD, and a second straight 10 Fr × 6 cm plastic biliary stent placed alongside the first stent

Clinical Outcome

His AST and ALT levels remained in biochemical remission, while his elevated ALP level stabilized, mostly <180 U/L until last checked, which was 1.5 years after the TCZ administration (Fig. 34.4). After completion of budesonide/azathioprine, ursodiol was continued long-term for persistent elevation of ALP. Multiple serial ERCPs for plastic biliary stent placement were performed for biliary sludge and for the unresolved distal CBD stricture. He had recurrent right upper quadrant pain, but given his advanced cancer and abnormal biliary anatomy, cholecystectomy was deferred. He restarted enfortumab vedotin for one cycle, but ultimately, the patient passed away from progression of his malignancy about 3 months later.

Summary of the Case

A patient with locally advanced urothelial carcinoma treated with gemcitabine, carboplatin, and pembrolizumab, developed a mixed biochemical pattern of liver injury with predominantly cholangiopathic disease, treated with budesonide induction bridged into early administration of tocilizumab to achieve steroid-free biochemical remission (Fig. 34.5). The patient had a concurrent diagnosis of cholecystitis

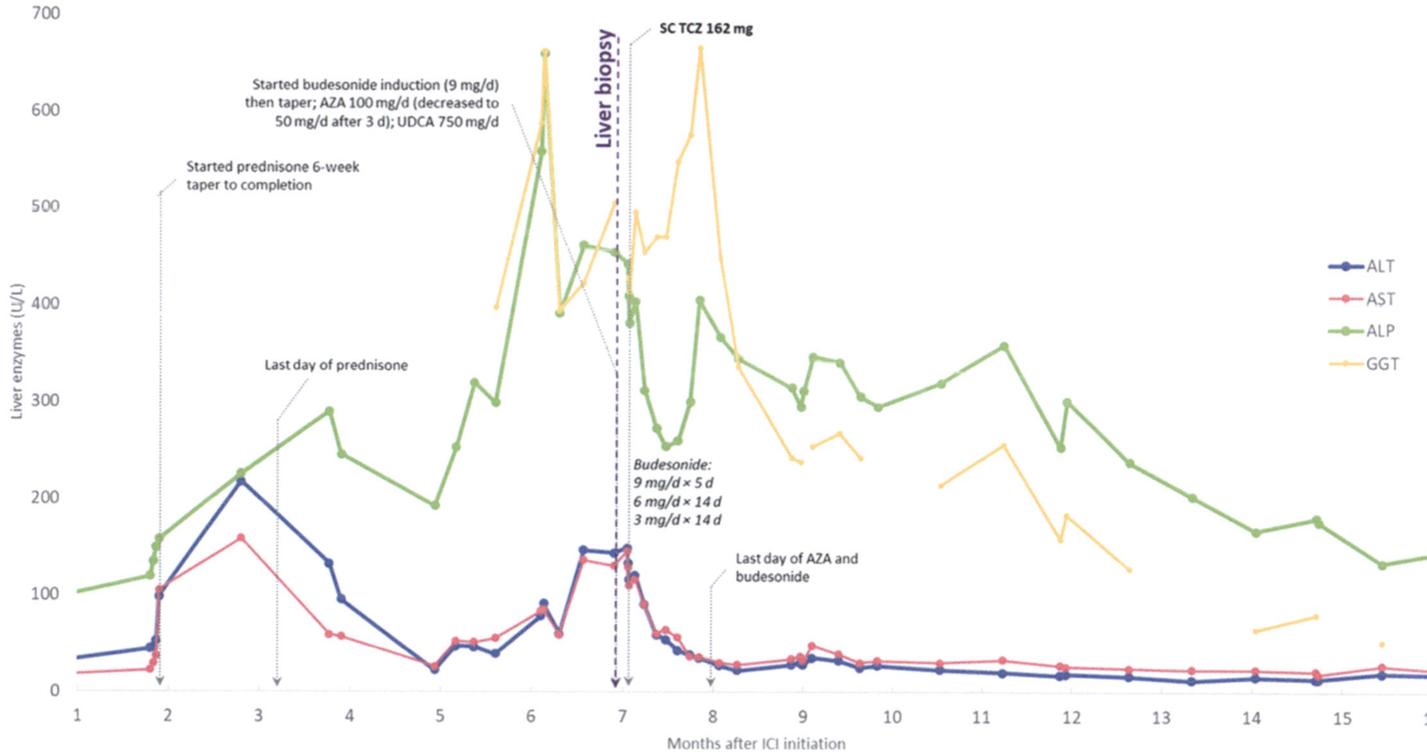

Fig. 34.4 Timeline of liver biochemical tests and associated treatments in weeks after last dose of pembrolizumab. *EUS* endoscopic ultrasound, *CCY* cholecystectomy, *MRI/MRCP* magnetic resonance imaging/magnetic resonance cholangiopancreatography, *ERCP* endoscopic retrograde cholangiopancreatography, *CBD* common bile duct, *ALT* alanine aminotransferase, *AST* aspartate aminotransferase, *ALP* alkaline phosphatase, *GGT* gamma-glutamyl transferase, *AZA* azathioprine, *UDCA* ursodeoxycholic acid, *SC* subcutaneous, *TCZ* tocilizumab

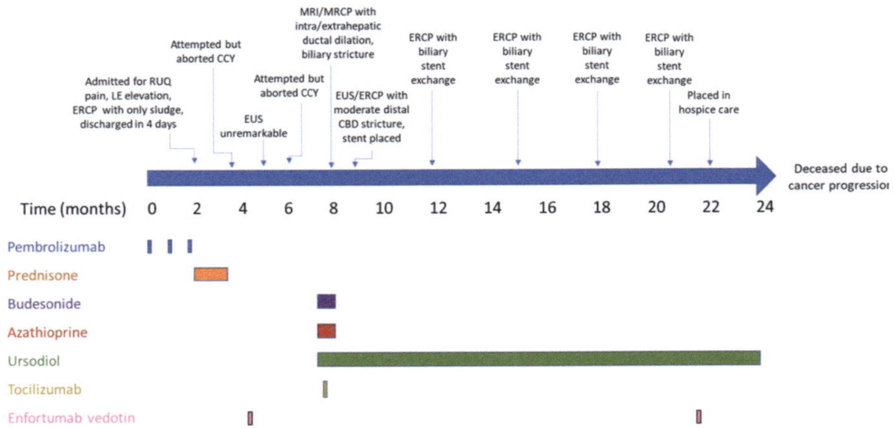

Fig. 34.5 Timeline of significant events and medication administration. *LE* liver enzyme, *CCY* cholecystectomy, *EUS* endoscopic ultrasound, *MRI/MRCP* magnetic resonance imaging/magnetic resonance cholangiopancreatography, *ERCP* endoscopic retrograde cholangiopancreatography, *CBD* common bile duct

deemed to be an irAE from ICI, wherein the intraoperative findings revealed extensive local fibrosis and distortion of anatomy preventing successful cholecystectomy. Liver biopsy was consistent with IMCH with predominance of cholangiopathy. Treatment of the patient's IMCH included a brief course of budesonide, azathioprine, ursodiol, and one dose of subcutaneous TCZ, yielding normalization of AST and ALT, and stabilization of ALP <200 U/L within a month. Ursodiol was continued long-term to control the cholestatic injury. The patient later developed distal CBD stricture, as a sequelae of IMCH, requiring biliary stent placement/exchanges. Unfortunately, he continued to decline due to cancer progression and passed away 15 months after TCZ was given.

Discussion

A recent retrospective study characterizing the clinical patterns of IMH revealed that mixed pattern of liver injury (or IMCH) may account for about 25% of IMH cases, and the cholestatic-predominant pattern of liver injury is comparable in incidence (37%) to that of hepatocellular predominant injury (38%) [1]. Cholangiocytes express PD-L1, which binds to PD-1 on activated T cells, and this interaction may offer a hypothetical reason for ICI-mediated cholangiopathies frequently reported in association with anti-PD-1/L1 agents [2]. IMCp often presents as a significant elevation of bilirubin relative to hepatic enzymes, which is more significant in large-duct cholangitis than small-duct cholangitis [3, 4]. Both intrahepatic and extrahepatic biliary duct involvement have been described. In a case series of 13 patients with IMCp, 77% of them had an R factor <2 [5]. Routine analysis of the R factor in cases of suspected immune-mediated hepatobiliary toxicity with ALP >1.5× upper limit of normal (equivalent to about 180 U/L in general) can aid in detection for possible cholangiopathic phenotypes. The CTCAE v5.0 threshold for grade 2 toxicity is an ALP value crossing 2.5× ULN. This threshold may lead to delayed diagnosis of cholestatic-predominant pattern of liver injury; other cholestatic liver diseases like PBC can already be diagnosed even before the ALP exceeds 2.5× ULN. Gamma-glutamyl transferase (GGT) should also be tested together with ALP to differentiate from bone-related ALP elevations. Initial blood laboratory studies should include testing for anti-nuclear antibody, serum total IgG level, anti-mitochondrial antibody, serum total IgM level, and IgG4 subclass level. A liver biopsy can also help clarify the diagnosis by demonstrating at least histologic bile duct injury and exclude other established diseases like IgG4-related disease, PBC, PSC, or vanishing bile duct syndrome.

There are no society guidelines on how to diagnose and treat IMCH or cholangiopathic phenotypes. Because ALP is not part of the standard liver injury assessment based on current society guidelines, IMCp may be under-recognized, and published cases often feature morbid sequelae that have already developed after failing standard immunosuppression therapy with steroids. This patient's diagnosis of IMCp was arguably delayed due to lack of familiarity with the significance of persistent ALP elevations >1.5× ULN because IMCp has not yet become a well-recognized entity in the medical community. Patients with IMCp can be difficult to treat, with one systematic review showing only 11.5% having good response to steroids [6]. Although steroids can be used to initially treat IMCp, aggressive escalation to alternative treatments such as tocilizumab is important to mitigate progression to biliary sequelae that might arise [7]. In addition, about half of patients with IMCp may relapse during steroid taper [3, 5], which makes tocilizumab an appealing option as a steroid-sparing strategy, without relying on an adjunct like mycophenolate mofetil or tacrolimus which may not allow early reduction in daily steroid doses. Case reports and a recent case series have shown that the ALT level generally exhibits net improvement by 20 days from the initial tocilizumab administration [8, 9].

The decision to utilize budesonide instead of a systemic corticosteroid (CS) like prednisone or methylprednisolone derives from standard-of-care practices in treating idiopathic autoimmune hepatitis. Budesonide as a first-line treatment is associated fewer adverse events than systemic CS, including risk of infection such as acute bacterial cholangitis for which our patient was at risk. In addition, budesonide was used with the anticipation of bridging to tocilizumab. In this manner, only a brief course of steroids was necessary for the induction phase in order to curtail further liver inflammation before administration of tocilizumab.

Choledocholithiasis and IMCp can occur simultaneously when extrahepatic biliary strictures form. These two entities are not mutually exclusive, as a new CBD stricture, for instance, may predispose to further cholestasis, formation of biliary sludge, and development of clinically significant bile stones or biliary obstruction from pre-existing cholelithiasis. As use of anti-PD-1/L1 agents expands, IMCp may become increasingly common, and prompt treatment of IMCp is of paramount importance. The clinician should be aware that when unusual or advanced features of cholangiopathy occur (significant intra- or extrahepatic biliary manifestations or biliary stricture or vanishing bile duct syndrome), no known available treatments (including tocilizumab) may reverse these sequelae. Clinically significant cases, including those with acute biliary symptoms, bacterial cholangitis, or stalling of cholestatic biochemical labs in ALP and direct bilirubin elevations, may warrant additional evaluation with MRCP or even urgent ERCP to address the biliary stricture and to exclude a malignant lesion causing biliary obstruction. Tocilizumab as an anti-IL-6 receptor antagonist may have the ability to reverse hepatocellular liver injury (the hepatitic component of IMH) on the basis of the physiologic intersection of IL-6 pathways with liver regeneration [8–10], The application of tocilizumab has been described in case reports involving steroid-refractory IMCH/IMCp. It is important for the clinician to recognize that, despite efforts to escalate the treatment to tocilizumab, severe involving steroid-refractory IMCH/IMCp cholangiopathic disease could become permanent if it has already developed. This patient required multiple serial ERCPs for biliary stent exchanges without resolution of the biliary stricture. Prompt immunosuppression and early adjunct initiation of ursodiol (13–15 mg/kg/day) may be important in cases of IMCp. However, research studies are needed to ascertain whether early aggressive treatment (with agents other than steroids) would reduce the likelihood of developing chronic sequelae.

The featured clinical case also raises the possibility of the diagnosis of ICI-associated cholecystitis, a rarely reported entity, for which the gross manifestations precluded surgical cholecystectomy, which is otherwise the traditional management for acute calculous cholecystitis. Due to limited knowledge about the optimal treatment for ICI-associated cholecystitis (whether calculous or acalculous subtypes) and clinical outcomes, further research and clinical reporting are necessary [11–15].

Conclusion

Cases of IMCp could be potentially overlooked or under-recognized because ALP is not featured in the current society guidelines' assessments for liver toxicity. Although the bilirubin level is part of the irAE assessment, IMCp cases are *not* always associated with hyperbilirubinemia, and interpretation of bilirubin can be complex since it can include a differential of acute liver synthetic dysfunction if the ALP is normal or cholestatic liver injury or infiltrative liver disease if the ALP and GGT are both elevated. Therefore, the analysis per guidelines of the ALT, AST, and total bilirubin, without ALP and GGT, do not allow for early detection of cholestatic phenotypes. Although steroids can be used to initially treat IMCp to curtail further hepatobiliary injury, aggressive escalation to alternative treatments such as tocilizumab is important to mitigate progression to biliary sequelae that might arise. As use of anti-PD-1/L1 agents expand, the incidence of IMCp may increase, so prompt identification of the diagnosis and tailored treatment are of paramount importance.

References

1. Hountondji L, Ferreira De Matos C, Lebossé F, Quantin X, Lesage C, Palassin P, Rivet V, Faure S, Pageaux GP, Assenat É, Alric L, Zahhaf A, Larrey D, Witkowski Durand Viel P, Riviere B, Janick S, Dalle S, Maria ATJ, Comont T, Meunier L. Clinical pattern of checkpoint inhibitor-induced liver injury in a multicentre cohort. JHEP Rep. 2023;5(6):100719. https://doi.org/10.1016/j.jhepr.2023.100719.
2. Syal G, Fausther M, Dranoff JA. Advances in cholangiocyte immunobiology. Am J Physiol Gastrointest Liver Physiol. 2012;303(10):G1077–86. https://doi.org/10.1152/ajpgi.00227.2012.
3. Berry P, Kotha S, Zen Y, Papa S, El Menabawey T, Webster G, Joshi D, Heneghan M. Immune checkpoint inhibitor-related cholangiopathy: novel clinicopathological description of a multicentre cohort. Liver Int. 2023;43(1):147–54. https://doi.org/10.1111/liv.15340. Epub 2022 Jun 23. PMID: 35704341.
4. Pi B, Wang J, Tong Y, Yang Q, Lv F, Yu Y. Immune-related cholangitis induced by immune checkpoint inhibitors: a systematic review of clinical features and management. Eur J Gastroenterol Hepatol. 2021;33(1S Suppl 1):e858–67. https://doi.org/10.1097/MEG.0000000000002280.
5. Eyada M, Taggart MW, Wang LS, Miller ED, Zhang HC. Su327 diagnosis and characteristics of immune checkpoint inhibitor-mediated cholangiopathy: a case series. Gastroenterology. 2021;160(6):S-851–2. https://doi.org/10.1016/S0016-5085(21)02763-3.
6. Onoyama T, Takeda Y, Yamashita T, Hamamoto W, Sakamoto Y, Koda H, et al. Programmed cell death-1 inhibitor-related sclerosing cholangitis: a systematic review. World J Gastroenterol. 2020;26(3):353.
7. Moi L, et al. Personalized cytokine-directed therapy with tocilizumab for refractory immune checkpoint inhibitor-related cholangiohepatitis. J Thorac Oncol. 2021;16(2):318–26. https://doi.org/10.1016/j.jtho.2020.09.007 Epub 2020 Sep 19. PMID: 32956849.
8. Reddy CA, et al. Nivolumab-induced large-duct cholangiopathy treated with ursodeoxycholic acid and tocilizumab. Immunotherapy. 2019;11(18):1527–31. https://doi.org/10.2217/imt-2019-0121. Epub 2019 Dec 2. PMID: 31789069.
9. Stroud CR, et al. Tocilizumab for the management of immune mediated adverse events secondary to PD-1 blockade. J Oncol Pharm Pract. 2019;25(3):551–7. https://doi.org/10.1177/1078155217745144. Epub 2017 Dec 5. PMID: 29207939.
10. Zhang HC, et al. P1868—Extrahepatic biliary sequelae in immune checkpoint inhibitor-mediated cholangiohepatitis: urgent unmet need for early effective treatment. In: ACG 2021 annual scientific meeting abstracts, vol. 116. Las Vegas, NV: American College of Gastroenterology; 2021. p. S1139. https://doi.org/10.14309/01.ajg.0000784424.97540.d9.
11. Abu-Sbeih H, Tran CN, Ge PS, Bhutani MS, Alasadi M, Naing A, Jazaeri AA, Wang Y. Case series of cancer patients who developed cholecystitis related to immune checkpoint inhibitor treatment. J Immunother Cancer 2019;7(1):118. https://doi.org/10.1186/s40425-019-0604-2.
12. Ravella B, Pirzada S, Brinkman M, Khaiser A. P2904—what made the gallbladder angry? A case of ipilimumab and nivolumab induced acute cholecystitis. In: ACG 2023 annual scientific meeting abstracts. Vancouver, BC: American College of Gastroenterology; 2023.
13. Cho JH, Sun JM, Lee SH, Ahn JS, Park K, Ahn MJ. Late-onset cholecystitis with cholangitis after avelumab treatment in non-small cell lung cancer. J Thorac Oncol. 2018;13(3):e34–6. https://doi.org/10.1016/j.jtho.2017.10.007.
14. Fouchard M, Jantzem H, Quere G, Descourt R, Robinet G, Poureau PG. Three cases of immune cholangitis related to anti-programmed cell death and programmed cell death ligand agents for the treatment of non-small cell lung cancer. Eur J Cancer. 2019;115:107–10. https://doi.org/10.1016/j.ejca.2019.04.022.
15. Kawakami H, Tanizaki J, Tanaka K, Haratani K, Hayashi H, Takeda M, Kamata K, Takenaka M, Kimura M, Chikugo T, Sato T, Kudo M, Ito A, Nakagawa K. Imaging and clinicopathological features of nivolumab-related cholangitis in patients with non-small cell lung cancer. Investig New Drugs. 2017;35(4):529–36. https://doi.org/10.1007/s10637-017-0453-0.

Chapter 35
Immune Checkpoint Inhibitor-Mediated Hepatotoxicity: Personalized Management Based on Evolving Biochemical Behaviors

Hao Chi Zhang, Jay Shah, Asif Rashid, Ethan Miller, Pavlos Msaouel, and Lan Wang

Abbrevviations

ALP	Alkaline phosphatase
ALT	Alanine aminotransferase
AST	Aspartate aminotransferase
CS	Corticosteroids
H&E	Hematoxylin and eosin
ICI	Immune checkpoint inhibitor
IgA	Immunoglobulin A
IgG	Immunoglobulin G
IgM	Immunoglobulin M
IMH	Immune-mediated hepatobiliary toxicity
INR	International normalized ratio
IV	Intravenous
MP	Methylprednisolone

H. C. Zhang (✉) · E. Miller · L. Wang
Department of Gastroenterology, Hepatology & Nutrition, The University of Texas MD Anderson Cancer Center, Houston, TX, USA
e-mail: hzhang20@mdanderson.org; emiller1@mdanderson.org; lwang25@mdanderson.org

J. Shah
Department of Internal Medicine, Baylor College of Medicine, Houston, TX, USA
e-mail: Jay.Shah@bcm.edu

A. Rashid
Department of Pathology, The University of Texas MD Anderson Cancer Center, Houston, TX, USA
e-mail: arashid@mdanderson.org

P. Msaouel
Department of Genitourinary Medical Oncology, Division of Cancer Medicine, The University of Texas MD Anderson Cancer Center, Houston, TX, USA
e-mail: pmsaouel@mdanderson.org

Y. Wang (ed.), *Challenging Cases in Immunotherapy Related Organ Toxicities*,
https://doi.org/10.1007/978-3-031-83533-9_35

MRCP	Magnetic resonance cholangiopancreatography
MRI	Magnetic resonance imaging
TCZ	Tocilizumab

Clinical Presentation

A man in his fifth decade of life with a history of obesity, Gilbert syndrome, and clear cell renal cell carcinoma, was treated with left nephrectomy and two cycles of combination ICI with ipilimumab and nivolumab. He was evaluated for new-onset acute elevations in his liver enzyme values. He had no prior history of established liver disease, was taking supplemental turmeric, black seed oil, and multivitamins, and consumed three cans of beer per month.

At baseline prior to acute liver injury, his liver enzymes included an ALT level of 38 U/L, AST of 22 U/L, and ALP of 103 U/L (Table 35.1). He received his first cycle of ipilimumab/nivolumab without any subsequent lab abnormalities initially. Three weeks after the second cycle of ipilimumab/nivolumab, he presented for evaluation after developing nausea and fatigue (Fig. 35.1).

Laboratory workup was notable for an ALT of 3266 U/L, AST of 1955 U/L, ALP of 209 U/L, and a total bilirubin of 2.8 (Fig. 35.1; Table 35.1). He reported no new medications or other potential drug culprits. He did not exhibit signs of acute liver failure, with a stable INR and normal mental status. Serologic work-up for liver disease was unrevealing, as the patient did not have lab work consistent with acute viral hepatitis. Antinuclear antibody, anti-smooth muscle antibody, and serum total IgG and IgM levels were within normal limits. Abdominal MRI/MRCP showed periportal edema without obstruction or biliary ductal dilation. To confirm the diagnosis of IMH, a liver biopsy was performed for which the histology demonstrated portal/lobular mononuclear inflammation with interface activity, zone 3 necrosis, hepatocyte dropout, and mixed steatosis (5%) (Fig. 35.2). These histologic features were considered unlikely due to idiopathic autoimmune hepatitis. The composite clinical impression was a diagnosis most compatible with IMH.

Clinical Outcome

After 10 days of observation without immunosuppression, the patient's ALT level improved to 579 U/L, but soon rose to 1210 U/L on day 14 of observation (Fig. 35.1; Table 35.1). The patient was admitted for induction steroids with IV methylprednisolone (MP). After receiving induction IV MP of 93.75 mg, followed by 60 mg/day and then transitioning to oral prednisone of 60 mg/day, the ALT level improved to 368 U/L after the first 4 days of steroids, but the ALT subsequently rose again to 976 U/L after 12 days, during the steroid-induction phase, even without a steroid taper. During this time, he exhibited no signs of acute liver failure, but he did suffer from hyperglycemic episodes as a result of systemic corticosteroids.

Table 35.1 Lab values

Laboratory parameters	Baseline before IMH	Initial onset of IMH	Nadir during observation	Peak after observation	1 day before TCZ	10 days after TCZ	33 days after TCZ	154 days after TCZ
ALT (N ≤41 U/L)	38	3266	579	1210	760	78	39	39
AST (N ≤40 U/L)	22	1955	267	558	175	22	28	22
ALP (N = 40–129 U/L)	103	209	168	183	183	147	101	84
Direct bilirubin (N ≤0.3 mg/dL)	0.3	1.3	1.5	1.2	0.8	0.7	0.4	0.2
INR (N = 0.87–1.12)	0.99	1.47	1.06	1.09	1.13	–	1.01	–
CRP (N ≤10.00 mg/dL)	0.98	7.65	–	6.59	0.49	–	–	–

Liver biochemical lab trends with respect to initial clinical presentation and tocilizumab treatment. The patient developed CTCAE (Common Terminology Criteria for Adverse Events) grade 4 liver injury without acute liver failure. After a single infusion of IV tocilizumab was administered, the patient completed an accelerated steroid taper with oral prednisone from 60 to 10 mg/day, across a total of 23 days. Patient exhibited biochemical remission (baseline liver enzymes) only 33 days after tocilizumab treatment, without need for ongoing steroids. *ALT* alanine aminotransferase, *AST* aspartate aminotransferase, *ALP* alkaline phosphatase, *INR* international normalization ratio, *d* days, *TCZ* tocilizumab

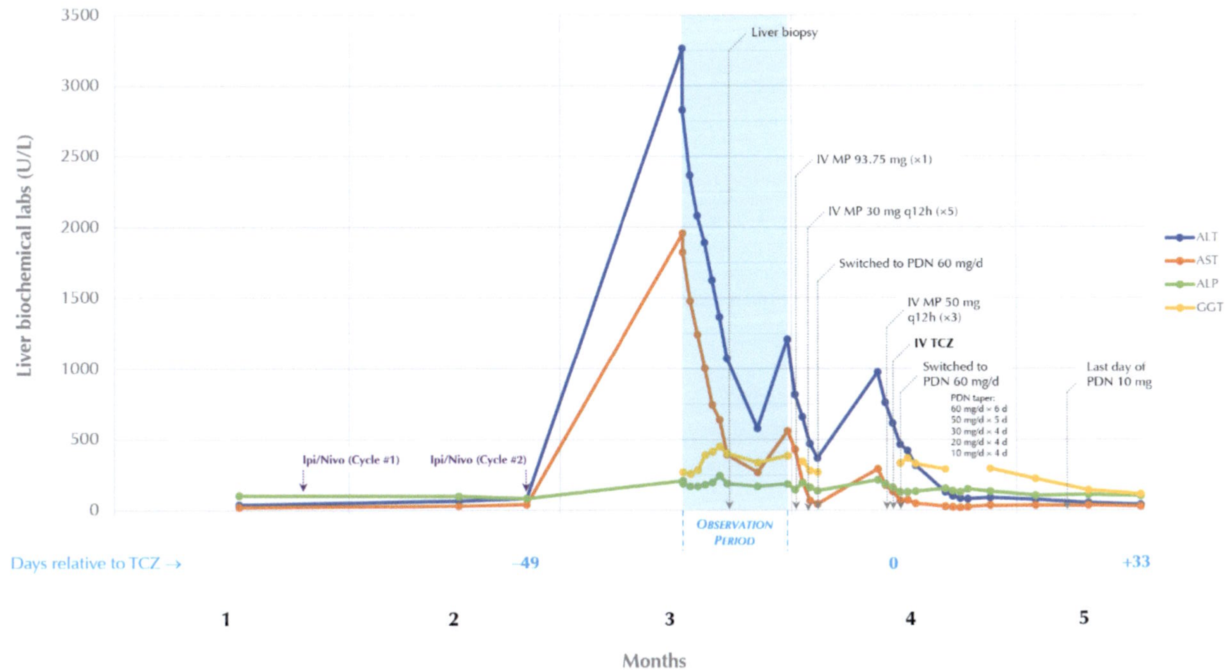

Fig. 35.1 Chronological trends of liver biochemical labs during the clinical course and with respect to management phases. This patient exhibited three distinct behaviors that have been observed with immune-mediated hepatotoxicity. In the first phase, observation alone without immunosuppression revealed that the liver was capable of spontaneous improvement, during which the patient was spared of steroid use, and significant improvement in ALT and AST occurred. When further natural improvement was not possible, this prompted the utilization of steroids to induce remission; this second phase is most familiar to clinicians as the mainstay of management for this toxicity. Despite initial response to intravenous steroids, oral steroids were not adequate, as evidenced by the resurgent ALT and AST levels, which represents the third phase. This third phase is the first cue to escalate the immunosuppression regimen. Because tocilizumab allows for decoupling of steroids, tocilizumab was administered followed by an accelerated steroid taper to compress the steroid exposure. Abbreviations: ALT, alanine aminotransferase; AST, aspartate aminotransferase; ALP, alkaline phosphatase; GGT, gammaglutamyl transferase; Ipi, ipilimumab; Nivo, nivolumab; d, day; IV, intravenous; MP, methylprednisolone; PRN, prednisone; TCZ, tocilizumab

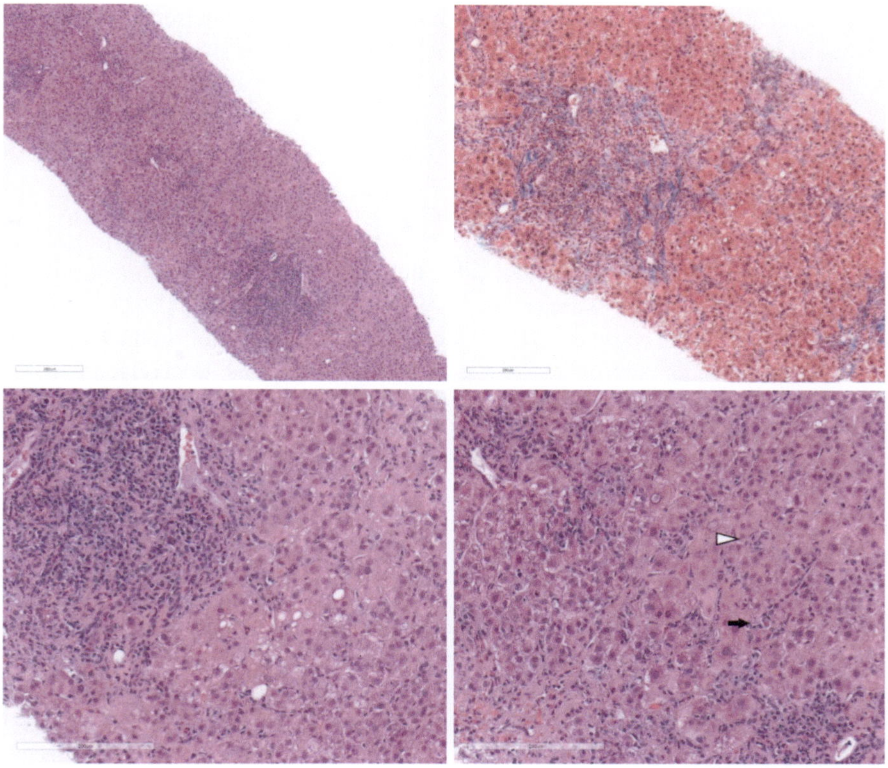

Fig. 35.2 Liver biopsy histologic evaluation (H&E stain). Predominantly hepatitic pattern of injury (left top panel) consisting of moderate portal and lobular mononuclear inflammation with interface activity (left hand, lower panel), zone 3 necrosis, hepatocyte dropout necrosis (arrow head, right lower panel), occasional acidophilic bodies (arrow, right lower panel), mixed micro- and macrovesicular steatosis involving less than 5% of hepatocytes, mild iron deposition in Kupffer cells (not shown), and septal and peri-sinusoidal fibrosis (score 3 of 4, Trichrome stain, right upper panel). These histological features are compatible with a drug reaction, including from immunotherapy

He was admitted to the hospital again for re-induction with IV steroids to determine whether his IMH would respond any further to steroids (Fig. 35.1). After receiving IV MP 100 mg/day, he again suffered from hyperglycemia. Given this trend, a diagnosis of steroid-refractory IMH was made. After discussion about different strategies for adjunctive therapies or rescue treatments, IV tocilizumab (TCZ) was selected as a steroid-sparing strategy to treat the IMH. IV TCZ 800 mg was given once, followed by a rapid steroid taper of prednisone across 23 days (Fig. 35.1). As such, it was not necessary to introduce mycophenolate mofetil, azathioprine, or tacrolimus, which would have otherwise required concurrent steroids with a gradual taper, prolonging duration of steroids longer than was needed compared to the TCZ strategy. The patient achieved steroid-free biochemical remission 33 days after the administration of TCZ, with ALT 39 U/L, AST 28 U/L, and ALP of 101 U/L

(Fig. 35.1; Table 35.1). Even 154 days after receiving TCZ, he remained in biochemical remission (Table 35.1). He was referred to radiation oncology in an effort to delay the re-initiation of systemic therapy given his prior IMH.

Summary of the Case

This is a case with a history of clear cell carcinoma treated with nephrectomy and combination ICI with ipilimumab and nivolumab, who developed CTCAE grade 4 IMH after his second cycle of ICI. He received a short course of prednisolone but showed evidence of steroid resistance and steroid induced hyperglycemia. He achieved steroid-free biochemical remission after TCZ. Summary of the timeline events is shown in Fig. 35.3.

Discussion

IMH is a heterogeneous entity both phenotypically and in its biochemical behavior. Clinical observations have supported the notion that about 33–50% of IMH cases resolve on their own without immunosuppression, whereas spontaneous improvement is the expectation in general cases of drug-induced liver injury [1–4]. The other proportion of patients require steroids to temper the immune response in the liver. The kinetics of transaminase improvement is also suggested to be similar whether the patient is treated with steroids or no steroids [5–8].

Upon first identification of acute abnormal liver biochemical tests and establishing CTCAE grade of the liver injury, the next 7 days is an opportunity to perform standard-of-care liver disease work-up including evaluation for acute viral hepatitis infection. Liver biochemical tests should be closely monitored (such as 2–3 times per week) for the next 7–14 days with the intent for the patient to undergo a diagnostic liver biopsy to confirm the diagnosis of IMH, particularly in those with CTACE grade 3–4 liver injury, and in select cases of grade 2 liver injury who do not improve. This offers the patient a steroid-free observation phase to determine whether steroids are warranted, and once histology confirms IMH, steroids can be initiated with confidence if the liver enzymes have not satisfactorily improved after 7–14 days (Fig. 35.2).

If IV systemic corticosteroids are initiated (at an induction dose of 60 mg/day or no greater than 1 mg/kg/day, even for high-grade IMH), response in liver enzyme levels should be apparent after 3 days, at which point transition to oral steroids, at its induction dose of 60 mg/day, is appropriate [9–12]. Clinicians should be aware that initial steroid-responsiveness is not a guarantee that the therapeutic effects of

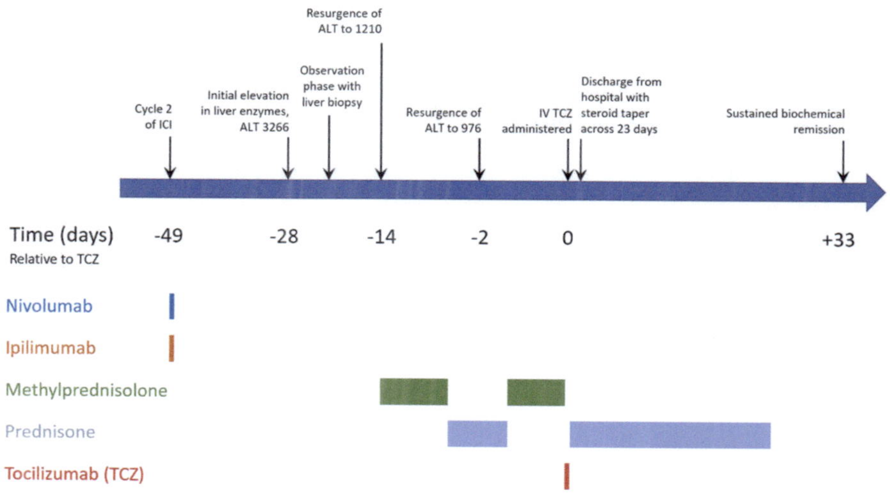

Fig. 35.3 Schematic of milestones in the clinical course of the patient's IMCH episode with respect to the day of tocilizumab administration. The patient developed IMCH after the second cycle of combination ICI treatment, with latency to first identification of CTCAE grade 4 liver enzyme elevations after 21 days, although the actual onset of IMH would have occurred prior to 21 days except for the absence of frequent routine tracking of liver enzymes. A 2-week course of observation without steroids were possible until steroids were deemed necessary to suppress the liver inflammation at the sign of the first acute resurgent ALT level. Despite induction IV steroids followed by oral prednisone without taper, liver enzymes exhibited resurgence nearly another 2 weeks later, which then prompted administration of IV tocilizumab after a very brief course of IV pulse steroids. The steroid taper thereafter was less than 1 month while liver enzymes approached biochemical remission. This strategy limited the systemic steroid exposure to less than 40 days for a steroid-refractory CTCAE grade 4 episode of IMH. *ALT* alanine aminotransferase, *TCZ* tocilizumab

steroids will be sustained, and not uncommonly, patients can exhibit a type of IMH that becomes steroid-dependent or even steroid-resistant.

Clinical observations suggest that 36% of IMH cases are overall steroid-responsive, but 29% may be steroid-refractory, with the remaining 35% of intermediate steroid-response [13]. Therefore, at the first sign of loss of optimal steroid response, the clinician should be prepared to escalate treatment with adjunctive therapies or rescue treatments.

This patient exhibited three behaviors of IMH during the same episode: (1) natural improvement of liver enzymes; (2) ongoing toxicity necessitating steroids; (3) development of steroid-resistance prompting escalation to TCZ (Fig. 35.1). Steroids were implemented only when necessary (*i.e.*, at the first sign of resurgence during the observation period) (Figs. 35.1 and 35.3). Prompt identification of steroid-resistance allowed for escalation to early TCZ treatment, obviating the need to add daily adjuncts like mycophenolate mofetil or azathioprine. The utilization of a steroid-sparing strategy with TCZ ultimately rescued a case of relapsed/

steroid-refractory IMH, which in turn enabled a shorter steroid tapering schedule, mitigating the associated adverse events from systemic steroids.

Society guidelines have been endorsing routine use of high-dose systemic corticosteroids to treat immune checkpoint IMH, with an additional steroid taper across 4–6 weeks after induction [14]. Observations reveal that many IMH cases do not require steroids given their self-resolving nature [13, 15]. Emerging experience showcases TCZ as a steroid-sparing strategy for IMH for refractory cases, a method still being studied but one that has shown early success [16–27]. In this case, the patient was managed using a systematic step-up approach from no immunosuppression to a steroid-sparing strategy based on the evolving behavior of his single IMH episode.

Conclusion

The understanding of treatment strategies for different phenotypes of IMH continues to evolve, with increasing evidence for the utilization of steroid sparing agents such as TCZ. We describe a systematic "step-up" approach to reduce overall systemic steroid exposure with early utilization of TCZ to ultimately manage IMH. In patients with steroid-dependent IMH, steroid-resistant IMH, or scenarios that may contraindicate prolonged steroid use, TCZ may ultimately serve an important role to rescue these patients in order to achieve steroid-free biochemical remission.

References

1. Miller ED, Abu-Sbeih H, Styskel B, Nogueras Gonzalez GM, Blechacz B, Naing A, et al. Clinical characteristics and adverse impact of hepatotoxicity due to immune checkpoint inhibitors. Am J Gastroenterol. 2020;115(2):251–61. https://doi.org/10.14309/ajg.0000000000000398.
2. De Martin E, et al. Characterization of liver injury induced by cancer immunotherapy using immune checkpoint inhibitors. J Hepatol. 2018;68(6):1181–90.
3. Gauci ML, et al. Immune-related hepatitis with immunotherapy: are corticosteroids always needed? J Hepatol. 2018;69(2):548–50.
4. Wang LS, Miller ED, Zhang HC. Moderate dose steroid treatment for immune checkpoint inhibitor-mediated hepatotoxicity (Su327). Digestive Disease Week 2021; virtual. Online 2021.
5. Postow MA, et al. Nivolumab and ipilimumab versus ipilimumab in untreated melanoma. N Engl J Med. 2015;372(21):2006–17.
6. Wang LS, et al. Moderate dose steroid treatment for immune checkpoint inhibitor-mediated hepatotoxicity (Su327). Digestive Disease Week 2021, virtual, 2021.
7. Johncilla M, et al. Ipilimumab-associated hepatitis: clinicopathologic characterization in a series of 11 cases. Am J Surg Pathol. 2015;39(8):1075–84.
8. Abu-Sbeih H, Styskel B, Blechacz B, Chalasani NP, Miller ED. Clinically significant hepatotoxicity due to immune checkpoint inhibitors is rare but leads to treatment discontinuation in a high proportion. Oral abstracts (abstracts 1–299). Hepatology, vol. 68; 2018. p. 25A–26A. https://doi.org/10.1002/hep.30256.

9. Li M, et al. Effect of corticosteroid dosing on outcomes in high-grade immune checkpoint inhibitor hepatitis. Hepatology. 2022;75(3):531–40.
10. Cheung V, Gupta T, Payne M, Middleton MR, Collier JD, Simmons A, et al. Immunotherapy-related hepatitis: real-world experience from a tertiary centre. Frontline Gastroenterol. 2019;10(4):364–71. https://doi.org/10.1136/flgastro-2018-101146.
11. Wang LS, et al.. Moderate dose steroid treatment for immune checkpoint inhibitor-mediated hepatotoxicity (Su327). Digestive Disease Week 2021. Virtual.
12. Pan JJ, Razumilava N. Corticosteroids for high-grade immune checkpoint inhibitor-mediated hepatitis: is less more? Hepatology. 2022;75(3):508–10.
13. Li M, et al. Predictors and outcomes of steroid-refractory ICI hepatitis in melanoma patients. In: AASLD the liver meeting digital experience 2020, hepatotoxicity lectures, Nov 2020. https://www.natap.org/2020/AASLD/AASLD_31.html.
14. Mack CL, Adams D, Assis DN, et al. Diagnosis and management of autoimmune hepatitis in adults and children: 2019 practice guidance and guidelines from the American Association for the Study of Liver Diseases. Hepatology. 2020;72(2):671–722. https://doi.org/10.1002/hep.31065.
15. Ziogas DC, Gkoufa A, Cholongitas E, Diamantopoulos P, Anastasopoulou A, Ascierto PA, Gogas H. When steroids are not enough in immune-related hepatitis: current clinical challenges discussed on the basis of a case report. J Immunother Cancer. 2020;8(2):e001322. https://doi.org/10.1136/jitc-2020-001322. PMID: 33144335; PMCID: PMC7607607.
16. Campochiaro C, et al. Tocilizumab for the treatment of immune-related adverse events: a systematic literature review and a multicentre case series. Eur J Intern Med. 2021;93:87–94. https://doi.org/10.1016/j.ejim.2021.07.016.
17. Lyles L, Farmer R, Abcugergi M. A potential new use for tocilizumab: refractory checkpoint inhibitor hepatitis. ACG Case Rep J. 2023;10(9):e01162. https://doi.org/10.14309/crj.0000000000001162. PMID: 37753105; PMCID: PMC10519460.
18. Moi L, et al. Personalized cytokine-directed therapy with tocilizumab for refractory immune checkpoint inhibitor-related cholangiohepatitis. J Thorac Oncol. 2021;16(2):318–26.
19. Reddy CA, et al. Nivolumab-induced large-duct cholangiopathy treated with ursodeoxycholic acid and tocilizumab. Immunotherapy. 2019;11(18):1527–31.
20. Stroud CR, et al. Tocilizumab for the management of immune mediated adverse events secondary to PD-1 blockade. J Oncol Pharm Pract. 2019;25(3):551–7.
21. Zhang HC, Eyada M, Taggart M, Miller E, Negrao M, Varghese S, Wang L. S2724 clinical presentation, treatment strategies, and chronic sequelae of immune checkpoint inhibitor-mediated cholangiopathy: a case study. Am J Gastroenterol. 2021;116:S1140. https://doi.org/10.14309/01.ajg.0000784428.93302.00.
22. Zhang HC, Taggart M, Miller E, Fossella F, Wang L. S2723 Extrahepatic biliary sequelae in immune checkpoint inhibitormediated cholangiohepatitis: urgent unmet need for early effective treatment. Am J Gastroenterol. 2021;116:S1139. https://doi.org/10.14309/01.ajg.0000784424.97540.d9.
23. Zhang, HC, Miller, ED, Wang, L. S2913 tocilizumab as an effective steroid-sparing agent for the treatment of recurrent and steroid-dependent immune checkpoint inhibitor-mediated hepatotoxicity: a case study and insight into pathophysiology. The American Journal of Gastroenterology 2022;117(10S):p e1896–e1897. https://doi.org/10.14309/01.ajg.0000868292.46390.96.
24. Zhang, HC, Miller, ED, Wang, L. S2977 Early Use of Tocilizumab as an Effective Steroid-Sparing Strategy for the Treatment of Immune Checkpoint Inhibitor-Mediated Cholangiopathy: Building Foundations for Personalized Management. The American Journal of Gastroenterology 2022;117(10S):p e1931. https://doi.org/10.14309/01.ajg.0000868548.94001.bc.
25. Zhang HC, Eyada M, Miller ED, Wang LS. Tocilizumab as an alternative treatment strategy for immunotherapy-mediated hepatobiliary toxicity: addressing an urgent unmet need. [Abstract; Poster] AASLD The Liver Meeting. Virtual, 2021.

26. Zhang HC, Wang LS, Miller E. Hepatobiliary and pancreatic adverse events. In: Naing A, Hajjar J, editors. Immunotherapy. Advances in experimental medicine and biology, vol. 1342. Cham: Springer; 2021. https://doi.org/10.1007/978-3-030-79308-1_13.
27. Zhang HC, Wang LS, Miller E. Hepatology (liver and bile duct). In: Wang Y, editor. Managing immunotherapy related organ toxicities. Cham: Springer; 2022. https://doi.org/10.1007/978-3-031-00241-0_7.

Chapter 36
Use of Immune Checkpoint Inhibitors Prior to and After Liver Transplantation

Alexander Philipp, Daniel Rössler, Helga Török, Christian Lange, and Enrico De Toni

Abbreviations

5-FU	5-Fluorouracil
AFP	Alpha-fetoprotein
BCLC	Barcelona Classification of Liver Cancer
CT	Computer tomography
Gem	Gemcitabine
HCC	Hepatocellular carcinoma
HDR	High dose rate
ICI	Immune checkpoint inhibitor
LT	Liver transplantation
MRI	Magnetic resonance imaging
Ox	Oxaliplatin
PD-L1	Programmed cell death ligand 1
PET-CT	Positron emission tomography and computed tomography
rIFNα2b	Recombinant alpha-2b interferon
TACE	Transarterial chemoembolization
VATS	Video-assisted thoracic surgery

A. Philipp (✉) · D. Rössler · H. Török · C. Lange · E. De Toni
Department of Medicine II, University Hospital, LMU Munich, Munich, Germany
e-mail: alexander.philipp@med.uni-muenchen.de; daniel.roessler@med.uni-muenchen.de; helga.toeroek@med.uni-muenchen.de; christian.lange@med.uni-muenchen.de; enrico.detoni@med.uni-muenchen.de

Y. Wang (ed.), *Challenging Cases in Immunotherapy Related Organ Toxicities*,
https://doi.org/10.1007/978-3-031-83533-9_36

Clinical Presentation

Case 1

This is a Caucasian male in his 30s with a history of liver transplantation for fibrolamellar carcinoma 18 years ago. He presented to our institution with a diagnosis of recurrent, metastatic fibrolamellar carcinoma, a rare variety of hepatocellular carcinoma (HCC) without established standard treatment. Previously, various surgical and local treatment approaches had been attempted, until widespread extrahepatic progression requiring systemic treatment occurred. An initial attempt with gemcitabine and oxaliplatin had to be halted due to intolerance to treatment and was followed by seven cycles of combined 5-Fluorouracil (5-FU) and interferon treatment. Despite this second-line treatment, tumor burden continued to progression with metastases to the lungs detected on a PET-CT scan. After thorough consultations involving various medical specialties and a comprehensive discussion with the patient and his family regarding the potential risks associated with immune checkpoint inhibitor (ICI) treatment in the post-transplant setting, the decision was made to start a salvage treatment with atezolizumab and bevacizumab. The initial immunosuppressive maintenance regimen he had been on (everolimus and mycophenolate) was eventually tapered down gradually. Following 3 months of treatment, a PET-CT scan indicated a notable reduction in tumor activity suggesting a favorable response (Fig. 36.1). Remarkably, throughout the treatment there were no observable signs of organ rejection. Therefore, treatment with atezolizumab and bevacizumab was extended for another 6 months. However, the patient subsequently lost his response with widespread disease progression and clinical decline, and eventually passed away 10 months after initiation of treatment. His transplanted liver remained to be in quiescent stable condition without rejection during the cancer treatment course.

Case Summary

In this case report a liver transplant recipient was treated successfully with ICI for HCC recurrence as last resort after failure of extensive prior therapies. Despite tapering of the immunosuppressive regimen no signs of liver transplant rejection occurred during a treatment duration of approximately 6 months although patient eventually deceased due to loss of response. Timeline events are summarized in Fig. 36.2.

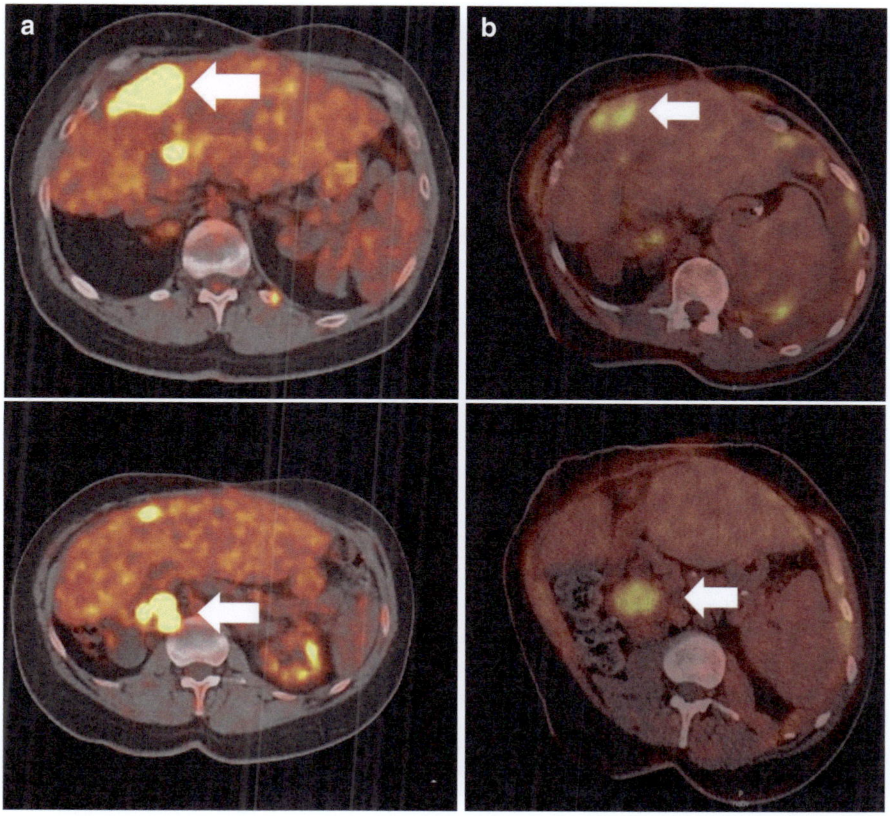

Fig. 36.1 Exemplary [18F] fluorodeoxyglucose positron emission tomography/computed tomography scans (**a**) before and (**b**) at cycle 3 of treatment with atezolizumab/bevacizumab. Arrows indicate representative lesions with decreasing metabolic activity

Case 2

This is a Caucasian male in his 50s with history of alcoholic liver cirrhosis who presented at our institution with locally advanced HCC confirmed on imaging and histology. Staging CT and MRI revealed multifocal HCC with at least two lesions larger than 3 cm and several other suspicious lesions. Thus, the Milan Criteria were not fulfilled. Nevertheless, no macrovascular invasion or extrahepatic spread was detected, classifying the tumor as Barcelona Classification of Liver Cancer (BCLC) stage B and leaving the window for a transplantation *out of Milan* open. Case discussion in the multidisciplinary Tumor Board concluded that the tumors were not amenable for local ablation and recommended transarterial chemoembolization (TACE) or screening for the DEMAND study, which examines the combination of TACE and systemic therapy with atezolizumab and bevacizumab, the latter being the standard of care for advanced HCC at the time.

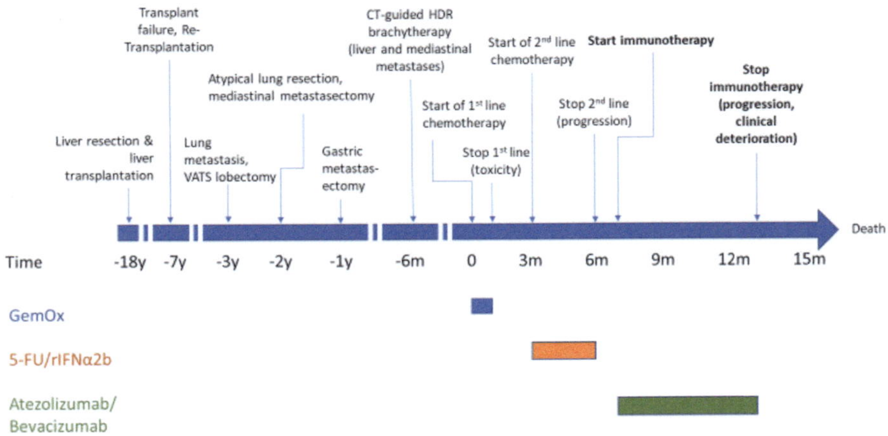

Fig. 36.2 Timeline of the patient's treatment course for Case 1

After the patient was successfully enrolled in the DEMAND trial, he was treated upfront with two cycles of TACE followed by treatment with atezolizumab and bevacizumab starting 3 days after the first TACE.

The first follow up assessment after approximately 6 weeks of treatment showed the sum of tumor diameters reduced by approximately 20% and complete devascularization of the lesions. Under continued cancer treatment all tumor lesions stayed stable and devascularized over the course of 1 year (total 18 cycles). The elevated tumor marker Alpha-fetoprotein (AFP) also decreased gradually and reached normal values after 5 months of therapy.

After multidisciplinary case discussion evaluation for liver transplantation was recommended. Patient received liver transplantation successfully after a washout phase of 3 months after the end of atezolizumab and bevacizumab. The transplanted liver remained within normal function and cancer free after transplantation for total of 16 months follow up. Histological workup of the explanted liver showed three necrotic lesions without vital tumor cells, and one lesions with a moderately differentiated HCC with 0.8 cm in size.

Case Summary

This patient received ICI therapy for locally advanced HCC which was not amenable for locoregional therapy but showed no signs of macrovascular invasion or extrahepatic spread. After 1 year of ICI treatment sustained tumor disease control could be established opening the opportunity for liver transplantation. ICI therapy was halted, and the patient underwent successful liver transplantation. After a follow-up of approximately 18 months the patient is still without evidence of disease,

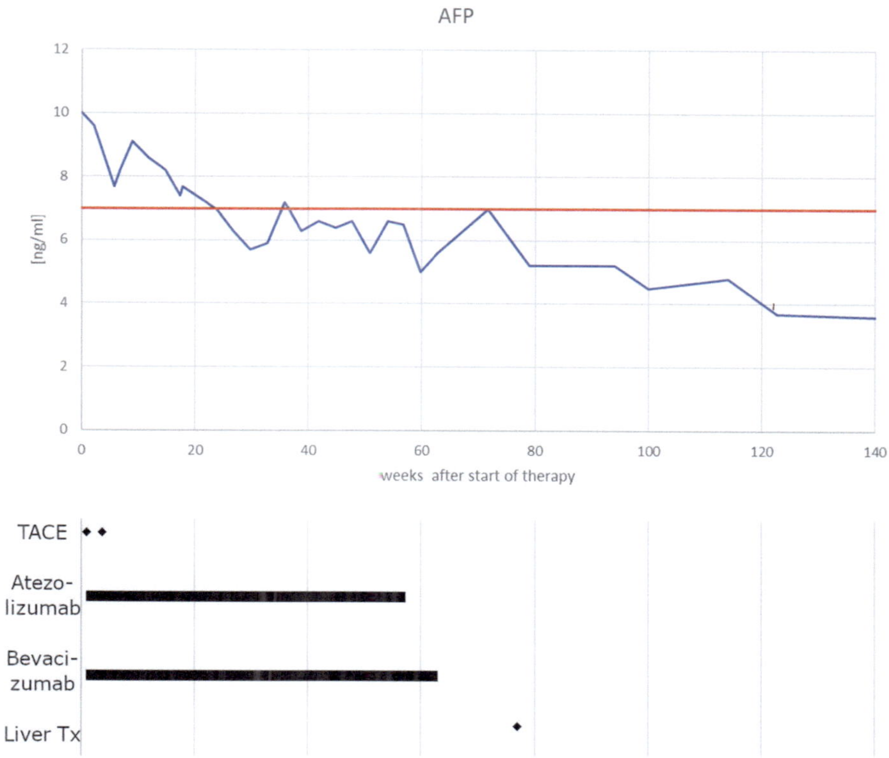

Fig. 36.3 Timeline and course of alpha-fetoprotein (AFP) after start of therapy with transarterial chemoembolization (TACE) followed by atezolizumab and bevacizumab. *Liver Tx: liver transplantation*

and no signs of transplant rejection have occurred. Timeline events are summarized in Fig. 36.3.

Discussion

The advent of immune checkpoint inhibitors (ICI) has radically affected response rates and clinical outcome across different tumor entities. However, the potential use of ICI in the setting of organ transplantation is still object of controversial debate owing to the concern that immune activation following exposure to ICI might cause organ rejection.

This is especially relevant to the case of liver transplant recipients because, despite optimized selection criteria, liver transplant recipients with a history of HCC remain at risk of HCC recurrence. This increasingly leads to the dilemma of whether ICI, recently established as standard of care for systemic treatment of HCC [1], could be an option in the post-transplant setting.

As patients with a history of organ transplantation are generally excluded from oncological trials, the evidence on the use of ICI in the transplant setting is still primarily based on case reports. The available data suggest nevertheless that acute organ failure as a result of organ rejection is not inevitable. A recent review of 33 studies including 57 patients reported a liver rejection rate of approximately 29% [2]. The time interval between ICI initiation and liver transplantation appears to influence the risk of rejection, as a longer time since transplantation seems to favor response. Additionally, there is anecdotic evidence showing negative programmed cell death ligand 1 (PD-L1) staining in patients who did not experience rejection upon treatment with ICI.

Effective clinical response and tumor control have been reported in post-transplant patients despite concomitant immunosuppression. However, it is important to recognize that the effect of ICI may be weakened by immunosuppression and that extrapolating data from non-liver-transplant patients to this group may not accurately reflect the true clinical benefit of ICI therapy. Consequently, due to the challenges in assessing the risk-benefit ratio of ICI therapy in this context, these agents should be considered a last-resort option only after the failure of other treatments and following thorough discussions with the patient.

ICI are also being increasingly used in intermediate stage HCC in combination with locoregional treatments [3]. This might lead to "stage-migration" or "downstaging" opening the opportunity of liver transplantation in selected cases. In case 2 presented above, the patient was treated with TACE and immune checkpoint inhibitors in a context of a study, an aggressive treatment resulting in a long-lasting response, eventually allowing the patient to undergo liver transplantation.

Acute organ rejection and failure in patients treated with ICI has been described. In a review of 9 studies [4] representing 27 patients, 4 cases of severe rejection were reported with 2 successful re-transplantations. Remarkably, Tabrizian and colleagues [5] recorded no instances of significant allograft rejection, tumor recurrence, or mortality in nine consecutive patients treated with ICI prior to transplantation, despite of the fact that most patients had received nivolumab merely 4 weeks before transplantation. It appears therefore reasonable to suggest that patients who have achieved tumor control should not be excluded from the transplantation list solely based on having received prior immune checkpoint inhibitor (ICI) treatment. Future investigations have to address optimal patient selection, minimum washout period between ICI treatment and transplantation as well as long-term safety and oncologic outcomes [4].

Conclusion

As an exception to the typical cases presented in this book, these two clinical cases illustrate instances in which ICI treatment did *not* result into organ rejection, the special kind of toxicity feared in the transplantation setting. Thus, ICI might be used under some circumstances in the context of transplantation, pre-transplant as well as post-transplant. However, dependable markers of toxicity are lacking, and ICI should not be offered as first-line treatment in the post-transplant setting. Thus, further research is essential. Until then, ICI therapy in the transplant setting must be cautiously evaluated on a case-by-case basis and comprehensive patient education regarding the potential risks is mandatory.

References

1. Singal AG, Llovet JM, Yarchoan M, Mehta N, Heimbach JK, Dawson LA, et al. AASLD practice guidance on prevention, diagnosis, and treatment of hepatocellular carcinoma. Hepatology. 2023;78(6):1922–65. https://doi.org/10.1097/hep.0000000000000466.
2. Wassmer C-H, El Hajji S, Papazarkadas X, Compagnon P, Tabrizian P, Lacotte S, et al. Immunotherapy and liver transplantation: a narrative review of basic and clinical data. Cancers (Basel). 2023;15:4574. https://doi.org/10.3390/cancers15184574.
3. Ben KN, Seidensticker M, Ricke J, Mayerle J, Oehrle B, Rössler D, et al. Atezolizumab and bevacizumab with transarterial chemoembolization in hepatocellular carcinoma: the DEMAND trial protocol. Futur Oncol. 2022;18:1423–35. https://doi.org/10.2217/fon-2021-1261.
4. Claasen MPAW, Sneiders D, Rakké YS, Adam R, Bhoori S, Cillo U, et al. European Society of Organ Transplantation (ESOT) consensus report on downstaging, bridging and immunotherapy in liver transplantation for hepatocellular carcinoma. Transpl Int. 2023;36:1–15. https://doi.org/10.3389/ti.2023.11648.
5. Tabrizian P, Florman SS, Schwartz ME. PD-1 inhibitor as bridge therapy to liver transplantation? Am J Transplant. 2021;21:1979–80. https://doi.org/10.1111/ajt.16448.

Part VII
Nephrology

Chapter 37
Acute Tubulointerstitial Nephritis Post Immune Checkpoint Inhibitor Therapy

Ala Abudayyeh, Jean Tayar, and Amanda Tchakarov

Abbreviations

AKI	Acute kidney injury
ATIN	Acute tubulointerstitial nephritis
ATN	Acute tubular necrosis
Cr	Creatinine
HPF	High power field
ICI	Immune checkpoint inhibitor
PD-L1	Programmed death ligand 1
RBC	Red blood cell
TNF	Tumor necrosis factor
UA	Urine analysis
UPCR	Urine protein:creatinine ratio
WBC	White blood cell

A. Abudayyeh (✉)
Section of Nephrology, Division of Internal Medicine, The University of Texas MD Anderson Cancer Center, Houston, TX, USA
e-mail: aabudayyeh@mdanderson.org

J. Tayar
Section of Rheumatology and Clinical Immunology, Department of General Internal Medicine, The University of Texas MD Anderson Cancer Center, Houston, TX, USA
e-mail: JHTayar@mdanderson.org

A. Tchakarov
Department of Pathology and Laboratory Medicine, University of Texas Health Science Center McGovern Medical School, Houston, TX, USA
e-mail: Amanda.S.Tchakarov@uth.tmc.edu

Y. Wang (ed.), *Challenging Cases in Immunotherapy Related Organ Toxicities*,
https://doi.org/10.1007/978-3-031-83533-9_37

Clinical Presentation

This is a Caucasian female in 60s diagnosed with stage IIIB triple negative, invasive ductal carcinoma of the breast (2.8 cm mass; multicentric). She was initially treated with four cycles of neoadjuvant dose dense Adriamycin/Cytoxan followed by an immune check point inhibitor (ICI) atezolizumab (anti-PD-L1 monoclonal antibody). Three months after starting her ICI she was admitted with fevers and acute kidney injury with a serum creatinine (Cr) level of 4.03 mg/dL (baseline Cr 0.70 mg/dL) which peaked to 7.47 mg/dL (Fig. 37.1). Her white blood cell (WBC) count was 19 K/uL, urinalysis (UA) had 36 red blood cells (RBC) per high power field (HPF), >182 WBC/HPF and UPCR 3.16 g. She also had severe hyperkalemia and dialysis was initiated. Renal biopsy revealed intense acute tubulointerstitial nephritis (ATIN) with neutrophils, lymphocytic tubulitis and focal tubular microabscesses (Fig. 37.2). Tubular epithelial injury consistent with acute tubular necrosis (ATN) secondary to ATIN was also present.

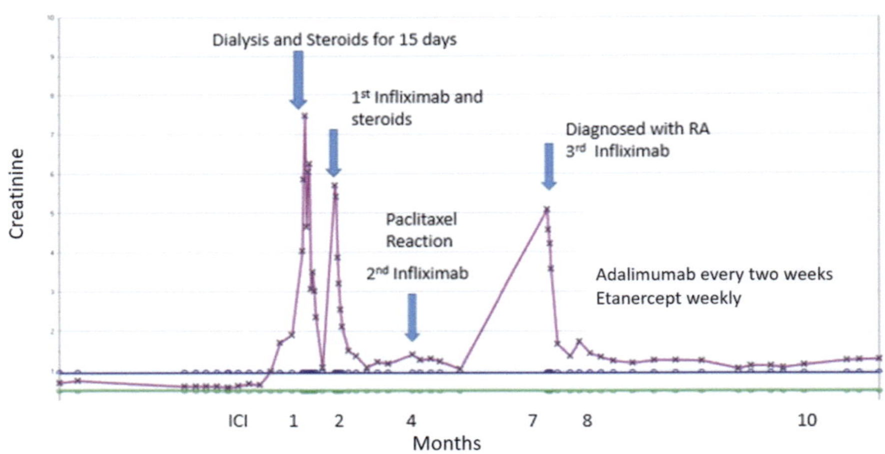

Fig. 37.1 Creatinine trend over time in months from ICI exposure and interventions associated with AKI

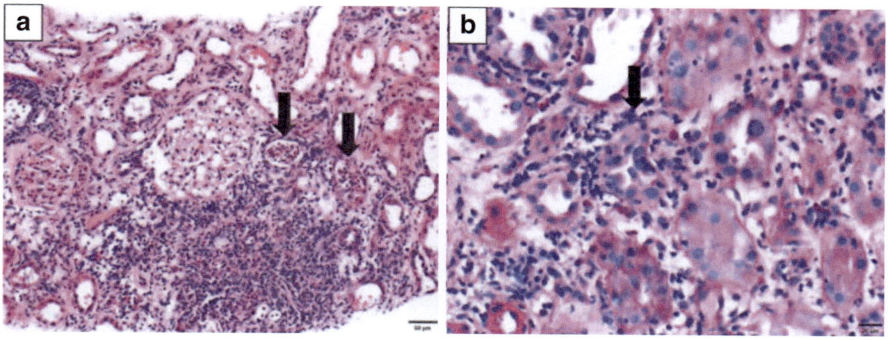

Fig. 37.2 Renal pathology associated with initial AKI after ICI exposure. (**a**) **(H&E stain)** tubulointerstitial inflammation with lymphocytes, neutrophils, and tubular microabscesses (arrows). (**b**) **(PAS stain)** lymphocytic tubulitis (arrow)

Differential Diagnosis

Patient's presentation with acute kidney injury with fever could have been attributed to acute tubular necrosis due to a systemic infection, however an initial workup there were no indications of infections. An increased cytokine syndrome associated with ICI exposure there is can explain her fever and AKI. Another leading diagnosis in setting of many WBC in the urine is acute interstitial nephritis. A glomerulonephritis is not likely since the patient had no proteinuria or hematuria noted. Based on the kidney biopsy with severe immune infiltrate, patient was diagnosed ATIN induced by ICI exposure.

Treatment and Outcome

Due to the severity of her renal injury she was initiated on high dose corticosteroids intravenous solumedrol which she initially responded well to; however during her steroid tapering period, she had a flare of her acute kidney injury with her Cr rising back to 5.9 mg/dL that warranted reinstating high dose of corticosteroids (prednisone) with the addition of a tumor necrosis factor alpha (TNF-alpha) inhibitor, infliximab at 5 mg/kg . This approach resulted in the remission of her AKI with improved Cr to baseline of 1.0 mg/dL (Fig. 37.1). One month later she had a milder flare of her renal disease with her Cr increasing to 1.4 m g/dL coinciding with a reaction to a paclitaxel infusion; nonetheless another dose of infliximab was given along with 7 days of prednisone with again a great response. Three months later the patient had a third flare of severe AKI associated with polyarthritis with a Cr of 5.09 mg/dL (Fig. 37.2). She was retreated with a third dose of infliximab and short dose of steroids with resolution of her AKI, Cr improving down to 1.2 mg/dL. Due to the recurrent episodes of pyuria and arthritis she was maintained on TNF-alpha blockade (adalimumab or etanercept) for 6 months and then weaned off with continued complete remission of her arthritis and nephritis. Three years as the last follow up since her first presentation with AKI, her urine analysis showed no WBC and her Cr was at 0.8 mg/dL.

Case Summary

This is a female patient in her 60s with a challenging disease course of multiple relapses of ATIN even after more than 6 months of ICI exposure. The patient was effectively managed with TNF-alpha blockade for over 6 months period with limited steroid exposure resulting in a maintained complete remission of her renal disease now 3 years later. In addition, she had a complete tumor response to her cancer therapy (Fig. 37.3).

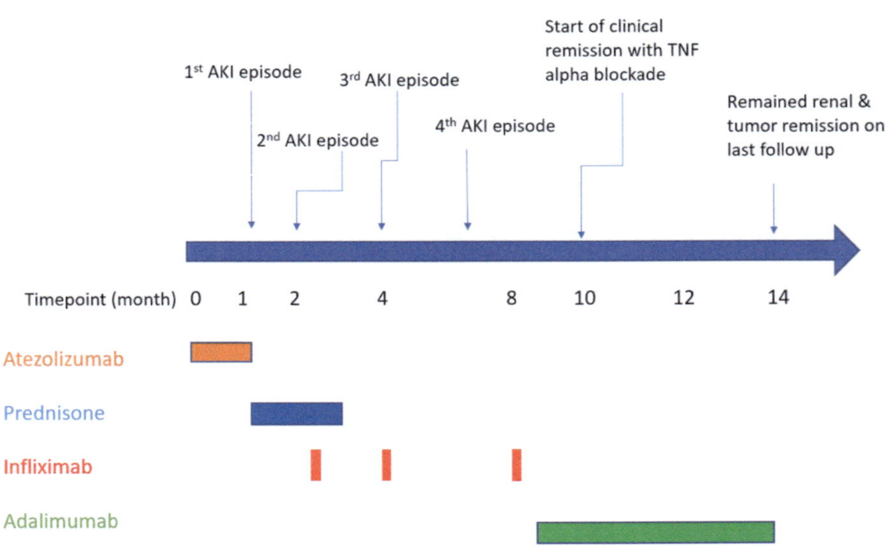

Fig. 37.3 Summary of timeline events (timepoint of 0 is ICI initiation)

Discussion

Acute kidney injury related to ICI has been noted to be as high as 17.0%, among which only 3.0–4.2% attributed to ICI therapy [1, 2] . In rare occasions, multiple relapses and refractory disease course that required prolonged immunosuppressive treatment even after ICI treatment cessation has been reported. These issues are even more evident since not all patients with ATIN have complete recovery kidney function to baseline (<50%) [3]. In addition, authors reported that relapse of ATIN is a challenge and associated with worse kidney prognosis than patients who experienced no relapse [4]. Re-challenge of ICI after ATIN even with continued steroid use has been noted to occur in 23% of the patients AKI. In the setting of ATIN some studies demonstrated that decreasing steroid treatment to 3 weeks was equally effective compared to the standard 4–6 weeks of steroid therapy in treating ICI-induced ATIN [5, 6]. In a recent retrospective study evaluating 35 kidney biopsies of confirmed ATIN pathologically we concluded that low levels of interstitial fibrosis in kidney tissue are associated with renal response to treatment for ICI-induced AIN, and the renal response and use of concurrent ICIs are associated with better OS in these patients. These findings further support the importance of early diagnosis and treatment of ATIN, while continuing concurrent ICI therapy [7].

Interest in steroid-sparing agents in the field of irAEs has grown over the past few years with proposed algorithms to use cytokine targeting agents and CD-20 inhibitors like rituximab extrapolated from autoimmune disease treatment and tissue based findings of irAE's [8]. Similarly, in ICI induced ATIN we have demonstrated a durable 80% response to treatment with infliximab without prolonged steroid exposure in cases of relapsed ICI-ATIN [6]. It has been reported that elevated urinary levels of tumor necrosis factor alpha and interleukin-9 were independently predictive of drug-induced ATIN and therefore may be involved in the pathogenesis of ICI-ATIN [9, 10]. Furthermore, nanostring analysis in a small ICI nephritis cohort of 14 patients showed a significant gene expression of IFN-y and TNF-alpha in kidney tissue in ICI-ATIN cases compared to non ICI induced AIN [11]. In a prospective of cohort of 24 patients of ICI induced nephritis samples of urine and kidney tissue had an elevated TNF-alpha levels using mass cytometry systems compared to other causes of AKI [12]. Therefore, in cases of ICI-ATIN, with cytokine elevation, biologic treatment has theoretical benefit which was validated by our case series and the current presented case [6]. This data further supports the utility of TNF-alpha blockade in ICI induced ATIN [13]. Future prospective studies in the use of TNF-alpha blockade to treat ICI induced ATIN would be of importance to further clarify the role of TNF-alpha and its treatment in ICI related renal adverse events.

References

1. Seethapathy H, Zhao S, Chute DF, et al. The incidence, causes, and risk factors of acute kidney injury in patients receiving immune checkpoint inhibitors. Clin J Am Soc Nephrol. 2019;14(12):1692–700. https://doi.org/10.2215/CJN.00990119.
2. Meraz-Muñoz A, Amir E, Ng P, et al. Acute kidney injury associated with immune checkpoint inhibitor therapy: incidence, risk factors and outcomes. J Immunother Cancer. 2020;8(1):e000467. https://doi.org/10.1136/jitc-2019-000467.
3. Cortazar FB, Kibbelaar ZA, Glezerman IG, et al. Clinical features and outcomes of immune checkpoint inhibitor-associated AKI: a multicenter study. J Am Soc Nephrol. 2020;31(2):435–46. https://doi.org/10.1681/ASN.2019070676. [Published Online First: 2020/01/02].
4. Caravaca-Fontán F, Shabaka A, Sánchez-Álamo B, et al. Recurrent acute interstitial nephritis: what lies beneath. Clin Kidney J. 2021;14(1):197–204. https://doi.org/10.1093/ckj/sfaa018. [Published Online First: 2020/03/11].
5. Lee MD, Seethapathy H, Strohbehn IA, et al. Rapid corticosteroid taper versus standard of care for immune checkpoint inhibitor induced nephritis: a single-center retrospective cohort study. J Immunother Cancer. 2021;9(4):e002292. https://doi.org/10.1136/jitc-2020-002292.
6. Lin JS, Mamlouk O, Selamet U, et al. Infliximab for the treatment of patients with checkpoint inhibitor-associated acute tubular interstitial nephritis. Onco Targets Ther. 2021;10(1):1877415. https://doi.org/10.1080/2162402X.2021.1877415.
7. Abudayyeh A, Suo L, Lin H, et al. Pathologic predictors of response to treatment of immune checkpoint inhibitor-induced kidney injury. Cancers (Basel). 2022;14(21):5267. https://doi.org/10.3390/cancers14215267.
8. Martins F, Sykiotis GP, Maillard M, et al. New therapeutic perspectives to manage refractory immune checkpoint-related toxicities. Lancet Oncol. 2019;20(1):e54–64. https://doi.org/10.1016/S1470-2045(18)30828-3.
9. Moledina DG, Wilson FP, Pober JS, et al. Urine TNF-α and IL-9 for clinical diagnosis of acute interstitial nephritis. JCI Insight. 2019;4(10):e127456. https://doi.org/10.1172/jci.insight.127456. [Published Online First: 2019/05/16].
10. Ernandez T, Mayadas TN. Immunoregulatory role of TNFalpha in inflammatory kidney diseases. Kidney Int. 2009;76(3):262–76. https://doi.org/10.1038/ki.2009.142. [Published Online First: 2009/05/13].
11. Lin J, Tchakarov A, Abdel-Wahab N, et al. 808 tertiary lymphoid structure gene signature detected in immune checkpoint inhibitor-associated renal immune related adverse event. J Immunother Cancer. 2021;9(Suppl 2):A845. https://doi.org/10.1136/jitc-2021-SITC2021.808.
12. Farooqui N, Zaidi M, Vaughan L, et al. Cytokines and immune cell phenotype in acute kidney injury associated with immune checkpoint inhibitors. Kidney Int Rep. 2023;8(3):628–41. https://doi.org/10.1016/j.ekir.2022.11.020.
13. Mamlouk O, Lin JS, Abdelrahim M, et al. Checkpoint inhibitor-related renal vasculitis and use of rituximab. J Immunother Cancer. 2020;8(2):e000750. https://doi.org/10.1136/jitc-2020-000750. [Published Online First: 2020/07/29].

Chapter 38
Vasculitis Post Immune Checkpoint Inhibitors Therapy

Sehrish Qureshi, Naszrin Arani, Maria Suarez-Almazor, Amanda Tchakarov, Mehmet Altan, and Ala Abudayyeh

Abbreviations

AKI	Acute kidney injury
anti-PR3 ANCA	Anti-neutrophil cytoplasmic antibodies-proteinase 3
ICI	Immune checkpoint inhibitor
PD-1	Programmed cell death protein-1

S. Qureshi · N. Arani
Division of Internal Medicine, Department of General Internal Medicine, The University of Texas MD Anderson Cancer Center, Houston, TX, USA
e-mail: SQureshi1@mdanderson.org; NArani@mdanderson.org

M. Suarez-Almazor
Department of Health Services Research and Section of Rheumatology and Clinical Immunology, The University of Texas MD Anderson Cancer Center, Houston, TX, USA
e-mail: msalmazor@mdanderson.org

A. Tchakarov
Department of Pathology and Laboratory Medicine, University of Texas Health Science Center McGovern Medical School, Houston, TX, USA
e-mail: Amanda.S.Tchakarov@uth.tmc.edu

M. Altan
Department of Thoracic/Head and Neck Medical Oncology, The University of Texas MD Anderson Cancer Center, Houston, TX, USA
e-mail: MAltan@mdanderson.org

A. Abudayyeh (✉)
Section of Nephrology, Division of Internal Medicine, The University of Texas MD Anderson Cancer Center, Houston, TX, USA
e-mail: aabudayyeh@mdanderson.org

Y. Wang (ed.), *Challenging Cases in Immunotherapy Related Organ Toxicities*,
https://doi.org/10.1007/978-3-031-83533-9_38

Clinical Presentation

This is a female in 50s with stage IIIA, T2a N2 M0 adenocarcinoma of the right lower lung status-post lobectomy and 4 cycles of chemotherapy with cisplatin and vinorelbine, completed 7 months post-surgery. She also has a past medical history of intermittent thyroiditis status-post total thyroidectomy. Restaging PET CT 9 years later showed FDG-avid soft tissue involvement in the right hilum and biopsy, confirming recurrent metastatic adenocarcinoma. Patient received definitive, concurrent chemoradiation followed by consolidative durvalumab, anti-PD-1 therapy as standard of care. Within 1 month she developed oral blisters, high fevers, hemoptysis, and a productive cough along with acute kidney insufficiency (AKI, creatinine 0.8–3.5 mg/dL) with hematuria and proteinuria of 2 g. She also developed possible splinter hemorrhages on her hands, leading to suspicion of endocarditis.

Evaluations and Diagnosis

Transesophageal echocardiogram showed a small (<1 mm) echogenic lesion attached to the atrial surface of the mitral valve. Blood cultures remained negative on multiple tests. The patient was diagnosed with culture-negative infectious endocarditis and treated with cefazolin at a dose of 1 g intravenously every 12 h (reflecting renal adjustment for kidney injury), which she continued for 6 weeks.

She had positive anti-neutrophil cytoplasmic antibodies-proteinase 3 (anti-PR3 ANCA) with proteinuria and hematuria, with same ANCA positivity even prior to ICI exposure was noted to be positive in serum samples collected prior to ICI exposure. Subsequently, kidney biopsy was performed, which revealed acute pauci-immune segmental necrotizing (50% of viable glomeruli) and crescentic (36% of viable glomeruli) glomerulonephritis, consistent with anti-PR3 ANCA–associated glomerulonephritis and/or systemic vasculitis (Fig. 38.1).

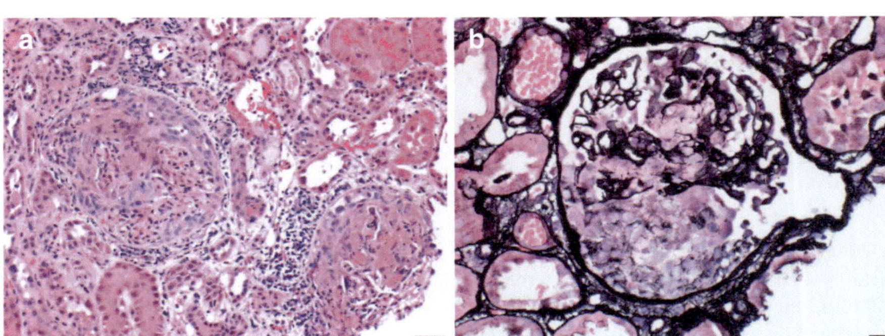

Fig. 38.1 **(a)** **(H&E stain)** Renal biopsy tissue showing crescentic and necrotizing glomeruli. **(b)** **(Silver stain)** Renal biopsy tissue showing a glomerulus with segmental necrosis and glomerular basement membrane disruption [1]

Differential Diagnosis

In setting of acute kidney injury (AKI) post ICI exposure, the more likely etiology would be acute interstitial nephritis. However, in the setting of the patient having proteinuria, hematuria, and positive anti-PR3 ANCA this is more consistent with autoimmune induction and vasculitis. Patient had splinter hemorrhages, fevers, oral ulcers, hemoptysis, and indications of endocarditis but with negative blood cultures which is also consistent with ANCA related vasculitis.

Treatment

The patient was aggressively treated with pulsed methylprednisolone at a dose of 500 mg for 3 days and plasmapheresis for 4 days. Durvalumab was permanently discontinued. She was treated with one dose (1 g) of rituximab, followed by a second dose 2 weeks after the first dose (Fig. 38.2). Her baseline serum creatinine level of 0.56 mg/dL peaked at 3.22 mg/dL and improved to 1.0 mg/dL after treatment with rituximab. A subsequent maintenance dose of rituximab (500 mg) was given at 8 months from the induction dose.

The patient's renal disease subsequently went into almost complete remission; on 3-year follow-up her creatinine was 0.98 mg/dL with bland urine, and ANCA was negative (Fig. 38.2a, b). Her skin changes, lung wheezing, and suspected endocarditis had also resolved (Fig. 38.3), and the cancer remained in remission at 2 years after discontinuing ICIs at the last follow up.

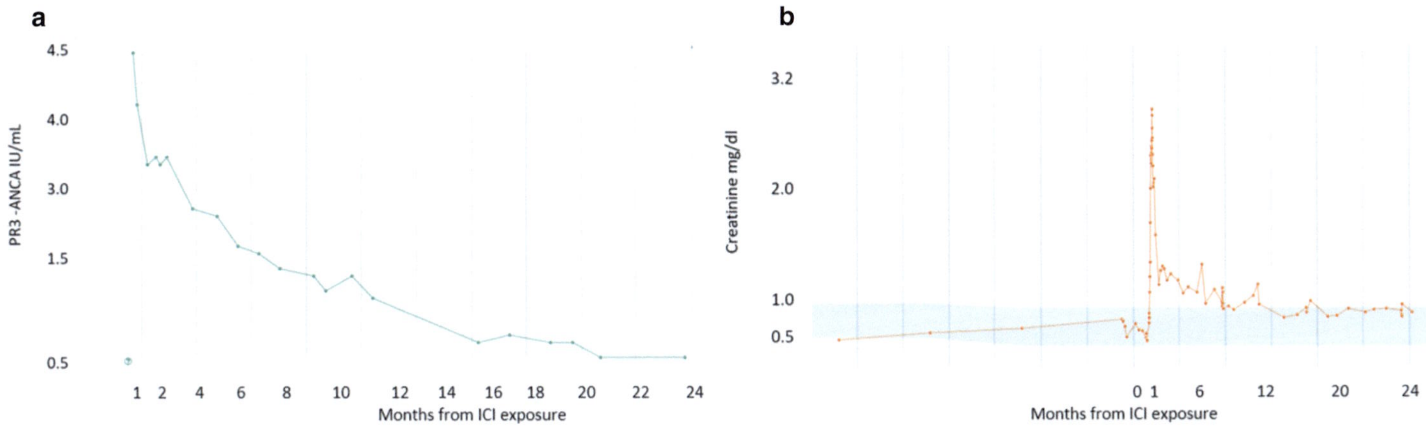

Fig. 38.2 (**a**) Proteinase 3 antibody after treatment with pulse steroids, plasmapheresis, and rituximab. (**b**) Creatinine trend after treatment with pulse steroids, plasmapheresis, and rituximab

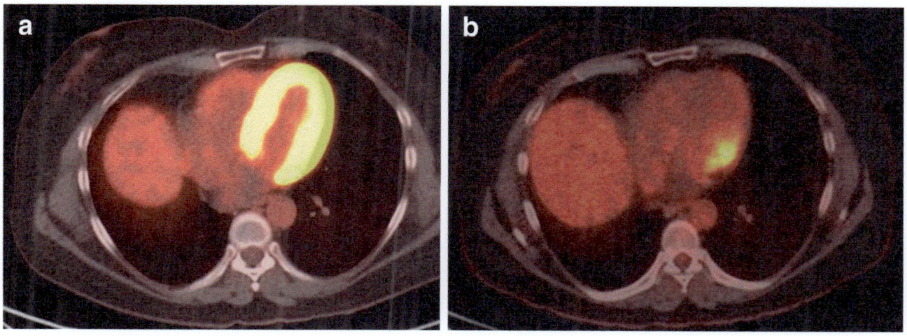

Fig. 38.3 Cardiac positron emission tomography/computed tomography images obtained (**a**) during initial hospitalization, showing FDG activity surrounding the myocardium, and (**b**) 4 months after hospitalization, showing improvement of FDG activity surrounding the myocardium [1]

Case Summary

This is a case with positive anti-PR3 ANCA vasculitis with multiorgan involvement who was successfully treated with steroids, rituximab and plasmapheresis with continued both renal remission and tumor response. Both anti-PR3 ANCA and creatinine continued to decline overtime with no relapse in her disease. Summary of the timeline events is shown in Fig. 38.4.

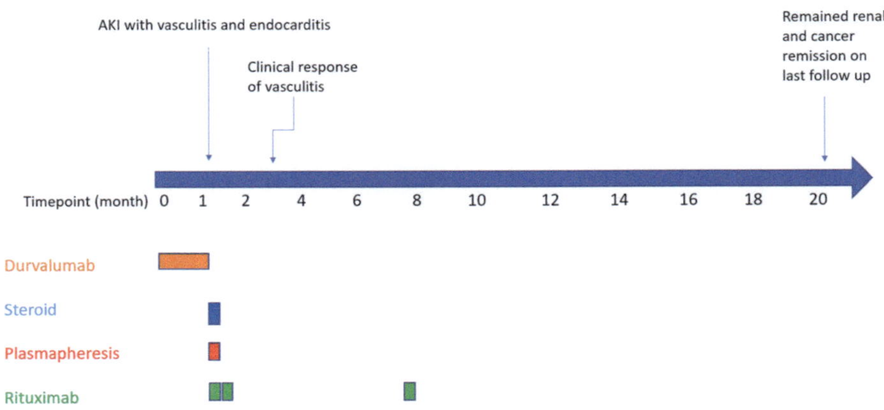

Fig. 38.4 Summary of timeline events (timepoint of 0 is ICI initiation)

Discussion

This case displays the challenges with autoimmune reactivation or induction after ICI therapy [1]. It is evident in this case that the patient had an underlying positive anti-PR3 ANCA that was not manifesting into vasculitis but after exposure to ICI there was a pronounced activation with multiorgan involvement. Current guidelines indicate the use of steroids only for immune related events of the kidney; however, as evident in this case, an autoimmune induction necessitated the use of plasmapheresis and rituximab to both remove and halt the anti-PR3 ANCA activity related organ injury. In a small cohort of five patients diagnosed with ICI-induced renal vasculitis, treatment with rituximab resulted in partial to complete renal recovery and no renal relapses [2]. Although glomerulonephritis after ICI exposure is rare (<3%), it can complicate cancer treatment and therefore affect survival. In a recent meta-analysis of de novo glomerular diseases after ICI exposure, pauci-immune glomerulonephritis and renal vasculitis accounted for 27% of glomerular disease cases, followed by minimal change disease (20%) and C3 glomerulonephritis (11%), and 41% of the patients had concomitant acute tubulointerstitial nephritis [3]. The median time to glomerular disease diagnosis after starting ICI therapy was 93 days (interquartile range 44–212 days); 98% of patients received corticosteroids, and 31% had complete recovery and 42% had partial recovery from acute kidney injury. Approximately 19% of the patients underwent dialysis, and of these, approximately one-third died (Fig. 38.5).

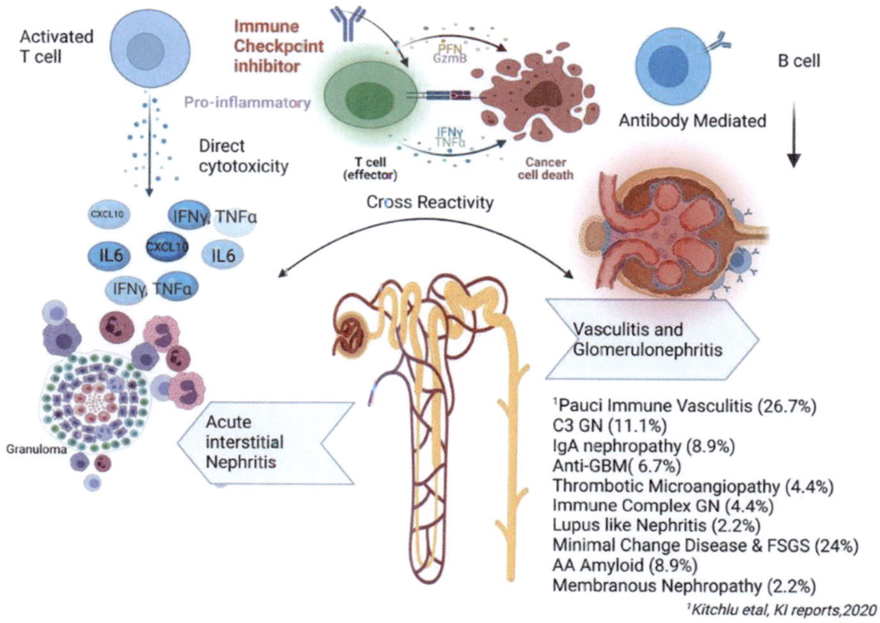

Fig. 38.5 Overview of ICI induced renal injury

References

1. Qureshi S, Arani N, Parvathareddy V, et al. Case report: immune checkpoint inhibitor-induced multiorgan vasculitis successfully treated with rituximab. Front Nephrol. 2023;3:1168614. https://doi.org/10.3389/fneph.2023.1168614.
2. Mamlouk O, Lin JS, Abdelrahim M, et al. Checkpoint inhibitor-related renal vasculitis and use of rituximab. J Immunother Cancer. 2020;8(2):e000750. https://doi.org/10.1136/jitc-2020-000750. [published Online First: 2020/07/29].
3. Kitchlu A, Jhaveri KD, Wadhwani S, et al. A systematic review of immune checkpoint inhibitor-associated glomerular disease. Kidney Int Rep. 2021;6(1):66–77. https://doi.org/10.1016/j.ekir.2020.10.002.

Chapter 39
Membranous Nephropathy Post Immune Checkpoint Inhibitors

Ala Abudayyeh, Adi Diab, and Amanda Tchakarov

Abbreviations

ANA	Antinuclear antibody
Anti-PLA2R	Phospholipase A2 antibody
CTLA-4	Cytotoxic T-lymphocyte-associated protein 4
DsDNA	Anti-double stranded DNA
GN	Glomerulonephritis
ICI	Immune checkpoint inhibitors
irAE	Immune related adverse event
MN	Membranous nephropathy
PD-1/PD-L1	Programmed cell death protein-1/ligand 1

A. Abudayyeh (✉)
Section of Nephrology, Division of Internal Medicine, The University of Texas MD Anderson Cancer Center, Houston, TX, USA
e-mail: aabudayyeh@mdanderson.org

A. Diab
Department of Melanoma Medical Oncology, The University of Texas MD Anderson Cancer Center, Houston, TX, USA
e-mail: ADiab@mdanderson.org

A. Tchakarov
Department of Pathology and Laboratory Medicine, University of Texas Health Science Center McGovern Medical School, Houston, TX, USA
e-mail: Amanda.S.Tchakarov@uth.tmc.edu

Y. Wang (ed.), *Challenging Cases in Immunotherapy Related Organ Toxicities*,
https://doi.org/10.1007/978-3-031-83533-9_39

Clinical Presentation

This is a male in 60s has a history of prostate cancer, melanoma and chronic kidney disease e.g. primary membranous nephropathy (GN) diagnosed 50 years ago and off immunosuppression 8 years ago. In addition, he also has hypertension, diabetes, with no proteinuria and creatinine at baseline of 1.4 mg/dL.

About 1 year ago, patient presented with proteinuria (urine protein was 2.2 g) with no clinical symptoms. Patient underwent secondary workup for his proteinuria which included antinuclear antibody (ANA), anti-double stranded DNA (DsDNA), complements, serum protein electrophoresis, and urine protein electrophoresis which were all negative. He therefore was referred for a kidney biopsy which showed membranous nephropathy with negative Phospholipase A2 antibody (which is usually found to be associated with primary membranous nephropathy, Fig. 39.1). In setting of his likely secondary membranous nephropathy with the typical leading cause would be cancer, he underwent extensive cancer workup including a CT of his chest and abdomen, which identified a large mass in the lung with adrenal and brain metastatic disease. He was started on ipilimumab and nivolumab and achieved significant cancer response after 4 infusions along with progression of proteinuria to the level of 6 g and colitis.

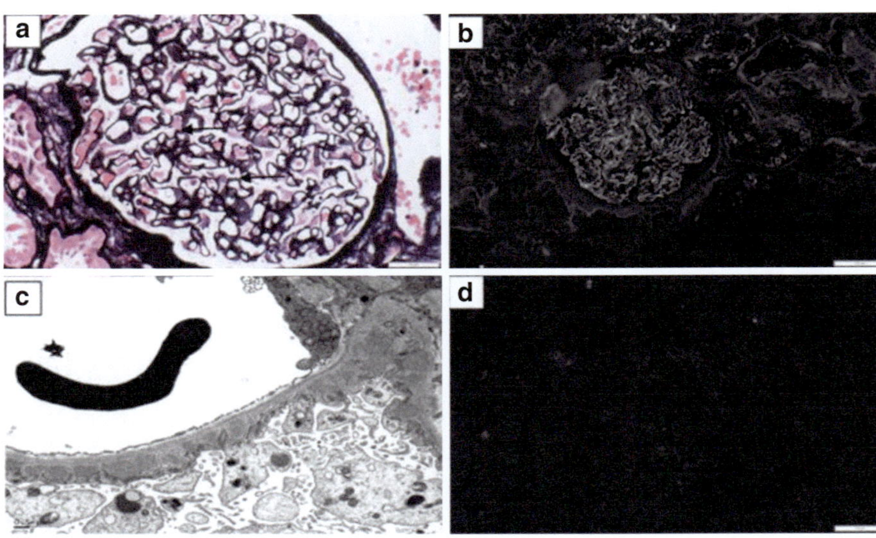

Fig. 39.1 (**a**) (Silver stain) segmental small glomerular basement membrane spikes (arrows), (**b**) (IgG immunofluorescence) global granular capillary and mesangial deposits, (**c**) (electron microscopy) subepithelial electron-dense deposits, (**d**) (PLA2r immunofluorescence) negative within glomerular deposits

Treatment

He started budesonide at 9 mg/day with quick resolution of diarrhea. Once off steroids, urine protein increased to 15 g and creatinine to 2.0 mg/dL. Since there was a concern of further kidney function decline, the patient was started on a 3-week prednisone taper and intravenous rituximab 1 g for one dose. Within 3 weeks, urine protein was improved to 3 g. At 2 years from starting ICI he has maintained both cancer and kidney remission with proteinuria <1 g and creatinine of 1.3 mg/dL on single agent nivolumab for 19 cycles.

Case Summary

We presented a patient with history of autoimmune disease of the kidney which was reactivated after cancer diagnosis and exacerbated with immune checkpoint inhibitor (ICI) treatment. Patient's reactivation of membranous nephropathy was due to a secondary cause which was the dual ICI therapy for his metastatic melanoma. Rituximab achieved excellent response and resolution of proteinuria after one cycle which was maintained on ICI for over 2 years with no exacerbation of his membranous nephropathy. Summary of the timeline events is shown in Fig. 39.2.

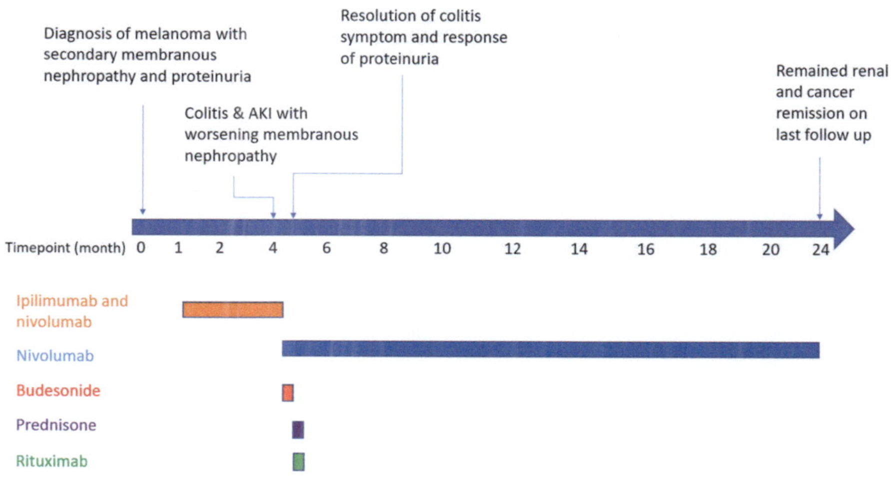

Fig. 39.2 Summary of timeline events (timepoint of 0 is cancer diagnosis)

Discussion

More than one third of patients with pre-existing rheumatic or autoimmune disease have experienced flares of their prior disorders in association with treatment after Immune checkpoint inhibitors. More commonly reported with anti–PD-1/PD-L1 agents than with CTLA-4 blockade (62% vs. 36%), de novo irAEs were more common among patients treated with CTLA-4 blockade (42% vs. 26%) [1, 2]. Adverse events were more likely to correlate with a partial or complete tumor response [3]. In a large retrospective cohort by Toi et al., in a multivariate analysis the presence of pre-existing antibodies were independently associated with irAEs (odds ratio, 3.25; 95%CI, 1.59–6.65; P = 0.001) [4].

Rituximab has been shown to be beneficial in treating ICI induced autoimmune diseases of kidney [5–7]. Rituximab, a monoclonal anti-CD20 antibody, disrupts pathogenic B-lymphocyte interaction with cytotoxic T lymphocytes, reduces chemokine production, and limits endothelial injury which, to-date, has not been shown to inhibit the anti-neoplastic effects of ICI therapy [8, 9]. In our center experience, we favor rituximab opposed to other cytotoxic therapies which are the typical first line treatments for glomerulonephritis (GN) in cases of GN and vasculitis in cancer patients to avoid T cell inhibition that are activated for the cancer care of the patient. We also recommend with minimal treatment duration of rituximab after achieving remission of the GN or vasculitis induced by ICI since B cells are classically known to further the activation and proliferation of the T-cells through antigen presentation [10]. A biopsy tailored approach to treatment is recommended as displayed in our institutionally approved ICI induced nephritis algorithm [11].

References

1. Ibis B, Aliazis K, Cao C, et al. Immune-related adverse effects of checkpoint immunotherapy and implications for the treatment of patients with cancer and autoimmune diseases. Front Immunol. 2023;14:1197364. https://doi.org/10.3389/fimmu.2023.1197364.
2. Abdel-Wahab N, Shah M, Lopez-Olivo MA, et al. Use of immune checkpoint inhibitors in the treatment of patients with cancer and preexisting autoimmune disease: a systematic review. Ann Intern Med. 2018;168(2):121–30. https://doi.org/10.7326/M17-2073.
3. Abdel-Wahab N, Shah M, Lopez-Olivo MA, et al. Use of immune checkpoint inhibitors in the treatment of patients with cancer and preexisting autoimmune disease. Ann Intern Med. 2018;169(2):133–4. https://doi.org/10.7326/L18-0209.
4. Toi Y, Sugawara S, Sugisaka J, et al. Profiling preexisting antibodies in patients treated with anti-PD-1 therapy for advanced non-small cell lung cancer. JAMA Oncol. 2019;5(3):376–83. https://doi.org/10.1001/jamaoncol.2018.5860.
5. Mamlouk O, Lin JS, Abdelrahim M, et al. Checkpoint inhibitor-related renal vasculitis and use of rituximab. J Immunother Cancer. 2020;8(2):e000750. https://doi.org/10.1136/jitc-2020-000750. [published Online First: 2020/07/29].
6. Kitchlu A, Jhaveri KD, Wadhwani S, et al. A systematic review of immune checkpoint inhibitor-associated glomerular disease. Kidney Int Rep. 2021;6(1):66–77. https://doi.org/10.1016/j.ekir.2020.10.002.

7. Lin JS, Wang DY, Mamlouk O, et al. Immune checkpoint inhibitor associated reactivation of primary membranous nephropathy responsive to rituximab. J Immunother Cancer. 2020;8(2):e001287. https://doi.org/10.1136/jitc-2020-001287. [published Online First: 2020/10/07].
8. Néel A, Bucchia M, Néel M, et al. Dampening of CD8+ T cell response by B cell depletion therapy in antineutrophil cytoplasmic antibody-associated vasculitis. Arthritis Rheumatol. 2019;71(4):641–50. https://doi.org/10.1002/art.40766. [published Online First: 2019/03/08].
9. Damsky W, Jilaveanu L, Turner N, et al. B cell depletion or absence does not impede anti-tumor activity of PD-1 inhibitors. J Immunother Cancer. 2019;7(1):153. https://doi.org/10.1186/s40425-019-0613-1. [published Online First: 2019/06/14].
10. LeBien TW, Tedder TF. B lymphocytes: how they develop and function. Blood. 2008;112(5):1570–80. https://doi.org/10.1182/blood-2008-02-078071.
11. Abudayyeh A. Evalutaion and management of suspected immune-mediated nephritis. 2023. https://www.mdanderson.org/content/dam/mdanderson/documents/for-physicians/algorithms/clinical-management/clin-management-nephritis-web-algorithm.pdf.

Part VIII
Neurology

Chapter 40
Encephalitis/Meningoencephalitis Post Immune Checkpoint Inhibitor Therapy

Sudhakar Tummala

Abbreviations

CSF	Cerebrospinal fluid
EEG	Electroencephalogram
FLAIR	MRI sequence—fluid attenuated inversion recovery
GAD 65 Ab	Anti-glutamic acid decarboxylase antibody
IVIG	Intravenous immunoglobulin
LP	Lumbar puncture
MOCA	Montreal cognitive assessment
MP	Methylprednisolone
NFLC	Neurofilament light chain
TPO Ab	Thyroid peroxidase antibody

Case #1 Presentation

A Caucasian female patient in 40s with past medical history of hypertension, hypothyroidism, stage III C melanoma of the L ankle (initial diagnosis 4 years prior) that was treated with local excision. Melanoma recurred in the ankle with positive sentinel lymph node 6 months prior to current presentation. Patient underwent local excision followed by local adjuvant radiation. Adjuvant Nivolumab was started at 240 mg iv q 2 weeks. After 8 doses, cluster of new neurological complaints have evolved over 10 days. This included personality changes, panicky spells, confusion,

S. Tummala (✉)
Division of Cancer Medicine, Department of Neuro-Oncology, The University of Texas MD Anderson Cancer Center, Houston, TX, USA
e-mail: stummala@mdanderson.org

Y. Wang (ed.), *Challenging Cases in Immunotherapy Related Organ Toxicities*,
https://doi.org/10.1007/978-3-031-83533-9_40

and memory difficulty. Patient's confusion is mainly categorized as anterograde amnesia with difficulty in new memories and recalling recent events, with good recall of distant events. Patient had visual, and auditory hallucinations. Patient also exhibited changes in personality with hypomania like behavior and affect. Patient mentions deja vu like sensations and lack of insight in familiarity of faces or events. Patient appeared confused doing daily tasks. No repetitive behaviors or involuntary movements were described. No balance difficulty or bladder or bower disturbance reported. Other relevant complaints on initial evaluation were blood pressure lability in systolic BP ranging between 170 s and 110 s.

Initial neurological examination showed MOCA 27/30 (−3 for memory recall). Cranial nerve, motor examination was normal with no dysmetria or any abnormal movements. Other organ dysfunction at time of neurological presentation was thyroid—TSH increased to 80 μunit/mL (normal range: 0.27–4.20) from normal value done few weeks prior to neurological symptoms. Remaining Pituitary endocrine evaluation was normal. Patient was diagnosed with ICI thyroiditis with positive TPO Ab at 654 IU/mL (0–35 IU/mL). Neurological differential diagnosis includes Hashimoto encephalopathy (HE)/steroid responsive encephalopathy associated with autoimmune thyroiditis (SREAT). Patient baseline levothyroxine dose was optimized. Brain MRI on admission with and without contrast in comparison to 6 months prior normal study showed new T2 FLAIR hyperintensity within the mesial temporal lobes, hippocampi, and insula, right greater than left (Fig. 40.1a). Initial EEG done at the admission to the hospital was normal. CSF revealed wbc −6 (92% lymphocytes), protein 50, "0" oligoclonal bands. There were absent malignant cells and moderately increased numbers of small lymphoid cells on cytology. Serum GAD 65 was 4.02 nmol/L (normal range ≤0.02 nmol/L), CSF GAD65 Ab titer was 2.22 nmol/L (normal range <0.02). Intrathecal synthesis (IS) was 2 (>1 suggests intrathecal synthesis). Follow up GAD65 at 1 year was 1.73.

Patient was subsequently diagnosed with limbic encephalitis based on the clinical, laboratory and radiological evidence, treated initially with intravenous Methylprednisolone (MP) 1 g × 5 days. This was subsequently followed by prednisone 1 mg/kg/day with reduction by 10 mg/weekly.

Follow Up

Patient had neuropsychological evaluation at 2 months follow up. Moderate impairments in visual learning and memory consistent with her neuroradiologic abnormalities (right > left) were noted. Other domains of cognitive function assessed including orientation, verbal learning and memory, attention, processing speed, expressive and receptive language, visuospatial function, and executive function were within the low average to superior range.

Three months after initial neurological evaluation, while on 30 mg of prednisone, patient was readmitting for memory lapses, confusion, and increased anxiety. Work up showed stable MRI findings (Fig. 40.1b). EEG showed periodic complexes

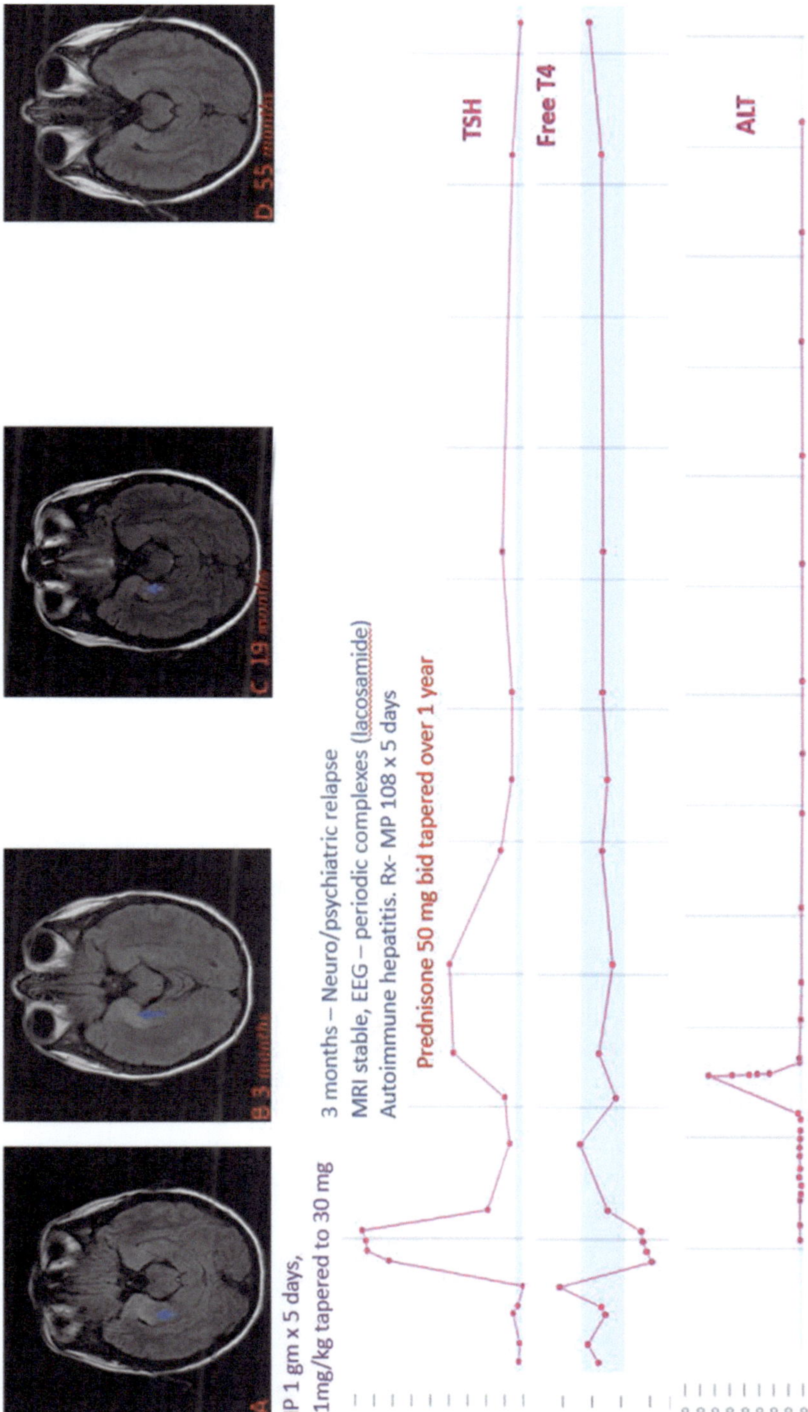

Fig. 40.1 Treatment summary and other organ toxicities are shown. Likely a milder recrudescence of CNS inflammation at time of autoimmune hepatitis. Blue arrows point the limbic encephalitis related temporal lobe FLAIR signal changes

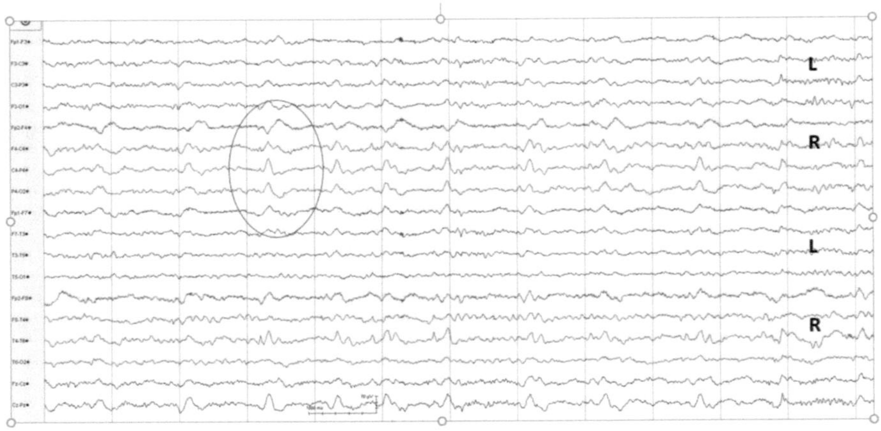

Fig. 40.2 EEG shows periodic complexes (blue circle). Differential diagnosis includes viral encephalitis and it is good practice to add acyclovir until viral cultures are available

(Fig. 40.2), that were not present at initial diagnosis. These are present, right more than left, at approximate at 1–1.5 s on the right and inconsistent with much lower amplitude at 5–7 s on the left temporal regions (BIPD—bilateral independent periodic discharges). These are suggestive of cortical irritability (epileptiform). Patient was also noted to have liver function abnormalities with ALT elevation to 1281 U/L (≤33) and diagnosed with autoimmune hepatitis. Treated with MP −1.5 mg/kg/day. With very rapid improvement of liver enzymes and improvement of neuropsychiatry symptoms. Patient was started on antiepileptic lacosamide given the presence of periodic complexes on EEG and to help with neuropsychiatric symptoms (anxiety, mood stabilization). There was also concern for episodic tingling and episodic confusion, which was thought to be related to anxiety or temporal lobe seizure manifestations. Patient was transitioned to oral prednisone at 100 mg/day and tapered slowly over the next 1 year, in gradual decrements at 5 mg and 2.5 mg/every 2 weeks. EEG at 1 year was normal. MRI at 19 months was normal (Fig. 40.1c).

Throughout her course patient psychiatric issues required medications (trial of escitalopram that was switched to sertraline, clonazepam, and olanzapine as needed) and psychotherapy.

Last clinic follow up and last MRI at 55 months (Fig. 40.1d) resolution of prior seen temporal findings and negative metastasis. Patient was maintaining good functioning status and cancer was in remission. Patient's limbic encephalitis clinical course is summarized in Fig. 40.3.

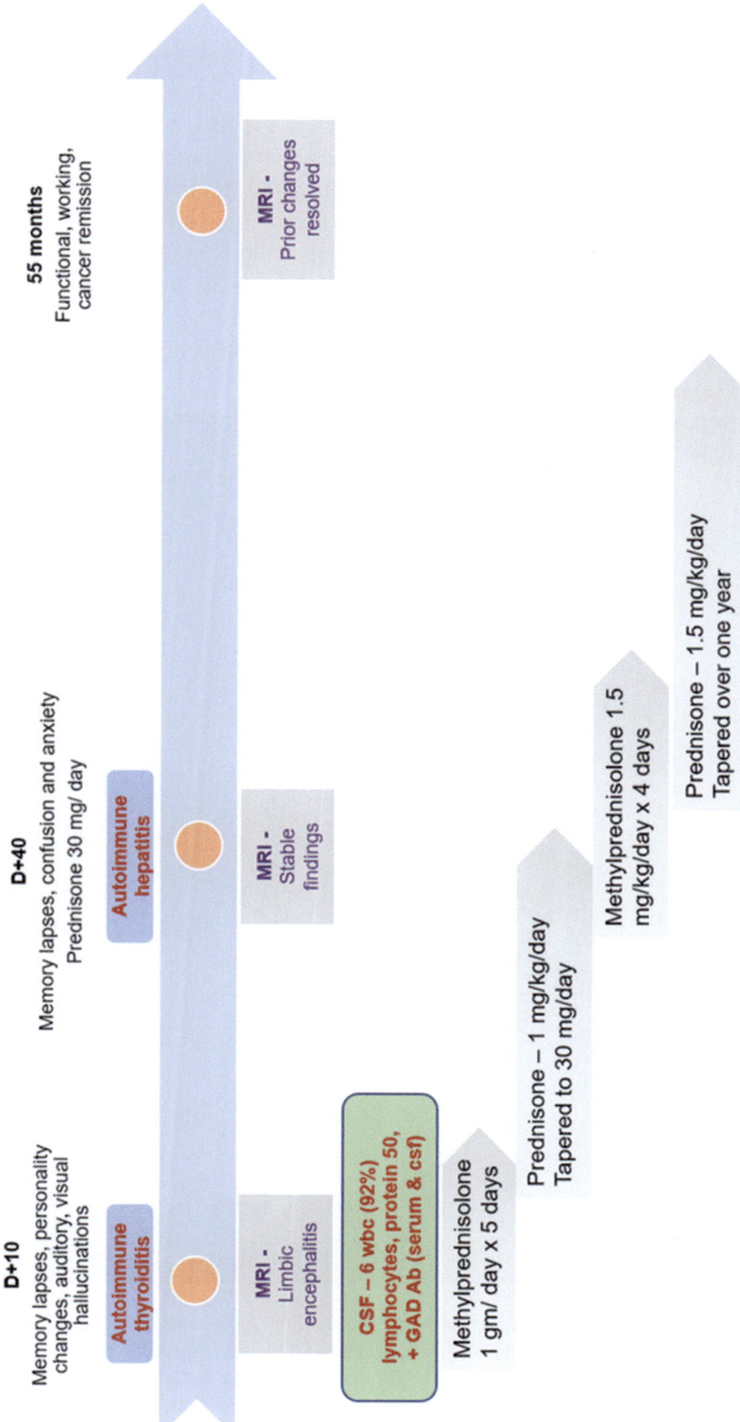

Fig. 40.3 Clinical and treatment summary. Timepoint of 0 is hospital admission

Case #2 Presentation

A Caucasian female in 60s with stage IV lung adenocarcinoma—KRAS G12D—PD-L1 TPS 5% with bone and brain metastasis, at the time of cancer diagnosis. Patient was asymptomatic from the brain lesions. About 1 month after the diagnosis, patient underwent gamma knife to the 11 small metastatic brain lesions, without any complications. Patient was subsequently started on frontline nivolumab and ipilimumab induction as part of lone star trial regimen. Follow up MRI 3 months later showed good response of brain lesions except left thalamic lesion with radiation treatment effects (blue arrow Fig. 40.4). However, follow up brain MRI another 2 months later revealed asymptomatic new small metastasis and resolution of the

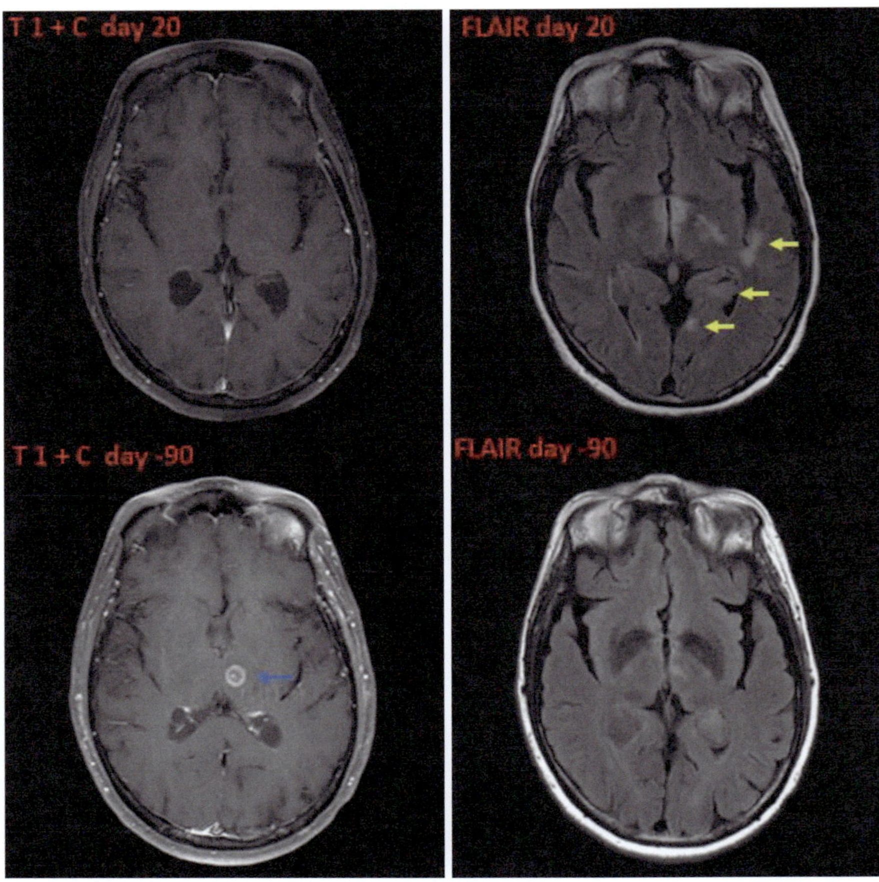

Fig. 40.4 Brain MRI. T1 post contrast 3 months after gamma knife showed radiation treatment effects of prior treated left thalamic metastasis (blue arrow). This has resolved over time as seen on the image day 20. Yellow arrows show new FLAIR signal changes in the temporal lobes, hypothalamic and other regions in keeping with encephalitis. Timepoint of 0 is hospital admission for mental status changes

left thalamic treatment effects. Patient developed fatigue and diarrhea which lead to temporary holding of immune checkpoint inhibitor therapy after first cycle, then was admitted to the hospital 1 week later for 5 days history of mental status changes. Confusion, speech difficulty, visual hallucinations were the main symptoms. No headache was reported. On initial neurology consultation, patient was only oriented to self only, perseverates, followed simple commands only and had right central facial palsy. No meningeal signs were noted. Patient had accompanying electrolyte abnormalities, e.g. sodium of 120 mEq/Lt on admission with labs consistent with Syndrome of Inappropriate Antidiuretic Hormone Secretion (SIADH) (Table 40.1). MRI of the brain on admission showed subacute FLAIR signals with subtle diffusion changes involving multiple regions of brain especially temporal lobes and hypothalamus. There was interval resolution of the prior seen new small metastasis before the initiation of ICI therapy. Repeat MRI on day 12 and 20 showed more FLAIR hyperintensities throughout the brain parenchyma including para-hippocampal, bilateral temporal lobes, occipital frontal regions, and left striatum. PET scan showed stable lung carcinoma with resolution of prior know adrenal gland metastasis and more apparent lymph diffuse nodes. Figure 40.5 summarizes the timeline for this patient. Patient had developed DVT & PE further complicating the hospital course, limiting use of IVIG. Discharged to rehab facility with overall stability but no clear neurological improvements with limited interaction and dense

Table 40.1 Lab values

	D + 8 (LP#1)	D + 19 (LP#2)	D + 22	D + 26 (LP#3)	D + 33	D + 38
CSF WBC (0–5)	68	46		43		
CSF lymphocytes	96%	98%		98%		
CSF protein (mg/dL)	66	50		37		
CSF oligoclonal bands (<2)	1	1		2		
CSF paraneoplastic panel	Negative × 1					
CSF cytology	Polymorphous lymphocytes and infrequent plasma cells. Lymphocytes are predominantly small to medium-sized with occasional large cells and monocytes. No malignant cells × 3					
Serum paraneoplastic panel	Negative					
Sodium (mEq/L)	120	133	134	139	138	140
Plasma neurofilament light chain (NFLC ≤28.0 pg/mL)					111	182
EEG	Diffuse slowing		Diffuse slowing			

Serum and CSF immunology antibody panels were negative. CSF inflammation persisted despite plasma exchange, high dose steroids. Tacrolimus added after third spinal tap on D + 26. SIADH can be seen in encephalitis that was corrected with fluid restriction, salt tabs and Ure-Na

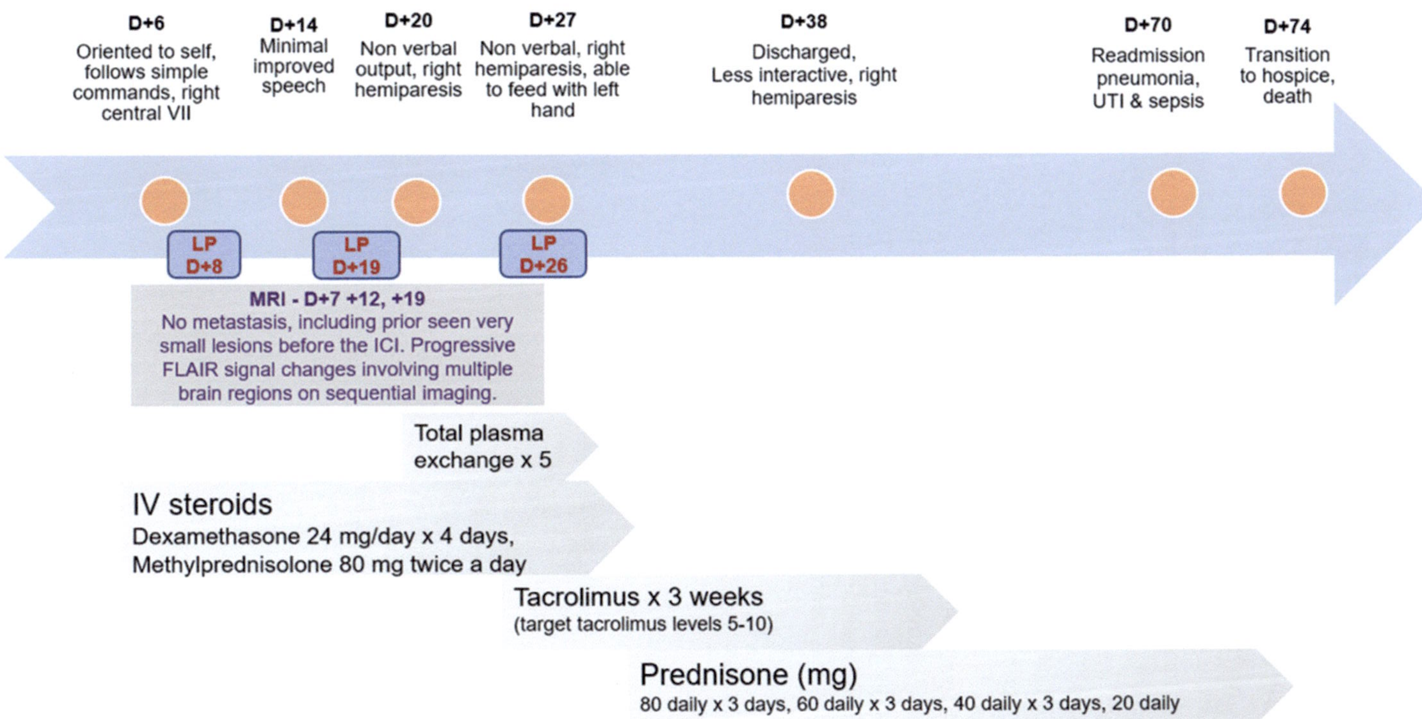

Fig. 40.5 Persistent CNS inflammation seen, despite multiple immunosuppressive/immunomodulation interventions. Patient can be at high risk for infections

right hemiparesis. Patient was readmitted 32 days later with pneumonia and urinary tract infections. No further neurological work up was done as family elected comfort care. EEG done on readmission showed toxic metabolic encephalopathy features.

Summary of Cases 1 and 2 Immune check point inhibitors encephalitis can present with focal limbic encephalitis predominantly involving temporal lobes (case 1) or extra-limbic encephalitis (case 2). GAD 65 (anti-glutamic acid decarboxylase) Ab identified in case 1, is generally associated with good outcomes. Presence of antibody and intrathecal synthesis rate >1 increases the sensitivity of diagnosing GAD 65 encephalitis, as the antibody can be present in cancer and diabetic patients. Case 2 highlights progressive disease despite aggressive multimodal immunosuppression. Recognition that ICI encephalitis can be associated with poor outcomes would help providers inform, engage and guide family members, from the beginning, along with consideration for multi-modal immunosuppressive therapy.

Discussion

ICI encephalitis can present with neuropsychiatric disturbance similar to autoimmune encephalitis in non-cancer patients [1–3]. Acute or subacute onset of working memory deficits, seizures, and psychiatric symptoms are suggestive of limbic system involvement. MRI can reveal medial temporal abnormalities, with FLAIR sequences being more sensitive. EEG an important mandatory needed test could show epileptic activity from the involved temporal lobes. Extra-limbic encephalitis could involve other regions of the brain. Monophasic with or without milder recrudescence or persistent progressive patterns can be seen. CSF pleocytosis is generally present, however can be normal if lumbar puncture is performed after initiation of high dose steroids. Differential diagnosis especially viral encephalitis should be rapidly excluded, and patient's should receive acyclovir initially. Hyponatremia can be seen with autoimmune encephalitis. Rapid initiation of high dose steroids is recommended. Multi modal approach could be considered in steroid refractory status with addition of other B & T cell suppressive agents like rituximab, cyclophosphamide, tacrolimus. Florid initial presentation with status epilepticus, significant MRI findings and marked CSF pleocytosis could warrant multimodal immune suppressive/modulation from the beginning with plasma exchange and high dose steroids followed by rituximab or cyclophosphamide. IVIG can also be considered. Variable relapses can occur, and patients need close clinical follow ups. There should be low index of suspicion for seizures. Temporal lobe seizures symptoms can have varied autonomic (vomiting, flushing, goosebumps), motor (automatisms, behavioral arrest), sensory (smell, illusions, peculiar taste, Alice in wonderland syndrome), emotional (anxiety, laughter, crying spells, intense happiness), cognitive (Déjà vu, jamais vu, forced thinking, memory disturbance) symptoms. Routine EEG or continuous EEG can be helpful in the seizure diagnosis. There should be low threshold for antiseizure medication which helps both the seizures/ seizure aura and the accompanying psychiatric symptoms. Autoimmune antibodies can be positive in serum and their presence in CSF increases the sensitivity. Patients with GAD Ab or other cell surface antibody (NMDA Ab, CASPR-2 Ab) have better outcomes compared to antineuronal antibodies (Hu-Ab, Ri-Ab, Ma-Ab). Lack of antibodies does not preclude the diagnosis of autoimmune encephalitis, as repertoire of testing methodology and identification of novel antibodies continues to expand. Antibodies can be present for much longer duration despite resolution of neuroinflammation. Other potential biomarkers like NFLC (neurofilament light chain) which is not specific but sensitive of neuronal stress can guide immunosuppressive therapy. Concomitant inflammation of other organ systems can occur and treatment of which is urgent to minimize toxic metabolic encephalopathy. Psychiatric consultation is recommended to manage accompanying psychiatric symptoms, which can be varied (anxiety, depression, compulsions, psychosis, visual and or auditory hallucinations, personality changes, behavioral changes aggressiveness). Other neurological manifestations of autoimmune encephalitis include movement disorders (chorea, myoclonus, orofacial dyskinesias, tremors), sleep disorders, cerebellar ataxia, autonomic instability, needs prompt assessment and treatment. Neuropsychiatric evaluation is highly recommended and will help in guiding further cognitive rehabilitation, job placement as needed. ICI encephalitis can also occur in patients with known brain metastasis, and vigilance is recommended. Other ICI CNS complications could include meningitis, meningoencephalitis, mid brain dysfunction, cerebellar dysfunction, transverse myelitis, brain and spinal cord demyelinating disorders [2].

References

1. Velasco R, Villagrán M, Jové M, Simó M, Vilariño N, Alemany M, Palmero R, Martínez-Villacampa MM, Nadal E, Bruna J. Encephalitis induced by immune checkpoint inhibitors: a systematic review. JAMA Neurol. 2021;78(7):864–73.
2. Vogrig A, Muñiz-Castrillo S, Joubert B, Picard G, Rogemond V, Marchal C, Chiappa AM, Chanson E, Skowron F, Leblanc A, Ducray F, Honnorat J. Central nervous system complications associated with immune checkpoint inhibitors. J Neurol Neurosurg Psychiatry. 2020;91(7):772–8.
3. Müller-Jensen L, Zierold S, Versluis JM, Boehmerle W, Huehnchen P, Endres M, Mohr R, Compter A, Blank CU, Hagenacker T, Meier F, Reinhardt L, Gesierich A, Salzmann M, Hassel JC, Ugurel S, Zimmer L, Banks P, Spain L, Soon JA, Enokida T, Tahara M, Kähler KC, Seggewiss-Bernhardt R, Harvey C, Long GV, Schöberl F, von Baumgarten L, Hundsberger T, Schlaak M, French LE, Knauss S, Heinzerling LM. Characteristics of immune checkpoint inhibitor-induced encephalitis and comparison with HSV-1 and anti-LGI1 encephalitis: a retrospective multicentre cohort study. Eur J Cancer. 2022;175:224–35.

Chapter 41
Neuromuscular Complications Post Immune Checkpoint Inhibitor Therapy

Sudhakar Tummala

Abbreviations

Ab	Antibody
BP	Blood pressure
CTCAE	Common terminology criteria for adverse events
EMG/NCS	Electromyogram/nerve conduction studies
FVC	Forced vital capacity
ICI	Immune checkpoint inhibitors
LVEF	Left ventricular ejection fraction
NIF	Negative inspiratory force
N-irAE	Neurological immune related adverse events
PNS-irAEs	Peripheral nervous system immune related adverse events
SFEMG	Single fiber electromyogram

Case Presentation

This is a female patient in 70s with history of hypertension on no medications, stage IB melanoma of the right forearm about 10 years ago, s/p wide lesion excision with negative margins. Recently diagnosed with in-transit recurrence at the medial aspect of the right upper arm and planned to receive two cycles of neoadjuvant single agent nivolumab. Approximately 15 days after first dose (480 mg), patient started developing blurred vision, dropping of eyes, double vision, muscle weakness, shortness of breath and dyspnea, that evolved over few days in acute fashion. Up until 1 week

S. Tummala (✉)
Division of Cancer Medicine, Department of Neuro-Oncology, The University of Texas MD Anderson Cancer Center, Houston, TX, USA
e-mail: stummala@mdanderson.org

Y. Wang (ed.), *Challenging Cases in Immunotherapy Related Organ Toxicities*,
https://doi.org/10.1007/978-3-031-83533-9_41

prior she was playing golf. Patient reports of trouble getting up from seated position such as bathroom commode and was apprehensive to eat solid foods for fear of choking. Patient was also noted to have high blood pressure (Systolic BP 190–196, Diastolic BP 91–96), that was easily controlled with blood pressure medications.

Initial neurological examination, at the time of hospital admission revealed normal cognitive functions. Cranial examination showed bilateral ptosis which did not improve with icepack test (see below). Patient was only able to count only up to 10 following single breath (see below). Extraocular eye movements were intact. She does endorse double vision following 60 s of sustained upward gaze, that was corrected by closing one eye (binocular diplopia- suggestive of neuromuscular weakness). No obvious neck ptosis noted. Muscle strength revealed proximal shoulder girdle and pelvic girdle muscles 4/5 MRC grade. Distal muscles showed full strength 5/5. Deep tendon reflexes are present.

Evaluation

On admission, forced vital capacity is 990 ml (15 mL/kg, see below), with NIF at −40. Admitting CK-4247 (26–192 μ/mL), troponin T-320 (<19 ng/mL). Troponin I-97 (53 pg/mL), ALT—270 (≤33 u/L), AST—355 (≤32 u/L). Aldolase—115.6 (7.7 units/L), Myoglobin—2439 (90 μg/L). Myasthenia panel is summarized in Table 41.1.

Patient had urgent cardiac catheterization and underwent myocardial biopsy (Table 41.2). Initial cardiac echo showed LVEF of 29%. Chest X-ray did not show congestive heart failure.

Table 41.1 Myasthenia panel

ACh receptor (muscle) binding Ab (ref ≤0.02)	0.99 nmol/L (admission) → 0.15 nmol/L (day 60)
P/Q-type calcium channel Ab (ref ≤0.02)	0.00 nmol/L
Myositis Ab	Negative

Table 41.2 Imaging evaluation and biopsy

Cardiac transthoracic echocardiogram	Admission LV is dilated using volumetric criteria Left ventricular systolic function is severely reduced LVEF—29%	Day 10 LV is dilated. Left ventricular systolic function is severely reduced LVEF—30% to 35%	Day 36 LV is dilated using volumetric criteria There is moderate segmental LV systolic dysfunction LVEF—35%	Day 60 LV is dilated using volumetric criteria LVEF—39%	Day 180 Left ventricular systolic function is moderately reduced. There is normal left ventricular wall thickness. There is moderate global hypokinesis of the left ventricle LVEF—37%
Cardiac cath	Diffusely reduced LV wall motion; mildly elevated L and R filling pressures. Mean PA = 23 mmHg. Mean PCW = 18 mmHg. Thermodilution Cardiac Outputs = 5.50 L/min. Thermodilution Cardiac Index = 3.03 L/min/m^2. Fick CO = 3.43 L/min. Fick CI = 1.89 L/min/m^2				
Cardiac Bx (right ventricle myocardium)	Lymphohistiocytic myocarditis (negative CD21, more CD 68 positive histiocytes than CD3 positive T-Lymphocytes and reversed CD4:CD8 ratio (1:5) IHC showed weakly positive PD-L1 staining at the inflamed areas in both infiltrating cells and in myocytes				
Brain MRI	No metastasis. No leptomeningeal disease. Chronic microvascular changes				

Diagnosis and Treatment Course

Patient was diagnosed with 3 M's (Myocarditis, Myositis, Myasthenia) and admitted to intensive care unit. Patient has started immediately on methylprednisolone 500 mg on day 1 and increased to 1 g day 2 after first plasma exchange given there is no decline in respiratory function (high dose steroids could potentially precipitate myasthenia crisis in idiopathic myasthenic patient). Plasma exchange was continued along with high dose steroids.

Patient was able to advance to small frequent regular food after clearance by Speech evaluation.

Patient received supplemental nasal cannula during daytime and continuous NIV-ST (non-invasive ventilation-spontaneous timed) at night without requirement for intubation and ventilation support.

Patient had good initial response to high-dose steroids and plasma exchange, with improvement of ptosis, muscle strength. Patient also started on pyridostigmine 30 mg twice a day slowly increased to 3 times a day. CK, myoglobin, aldolase have normalized over the subsequent days. However, by around day 10 there is worsening of ptosis, and subjective feeling of weakness with significant fatigue component. There was accompanying decreased vital capacity varying between 500 and 800 mL based on her effort. Patient was started on IVIG, followed by rituximab. With gradual improvement of her fatigue, improved respiratory dynamics (forced vital capacity improving to 1000–1200 mL) and completion of 2 doses of rituximab, patient transferred to inpatient rehabilitation. Steroids have been tapered prior to the transfer. In the inpatient rehab unit, patient showed declining muscle endurance, fatigue, that coincided with slight elevation of myoglobin and aldolase (recrudescence of labs), with again declining vital capacity to 800–900 mL range (Fig. 41.1).

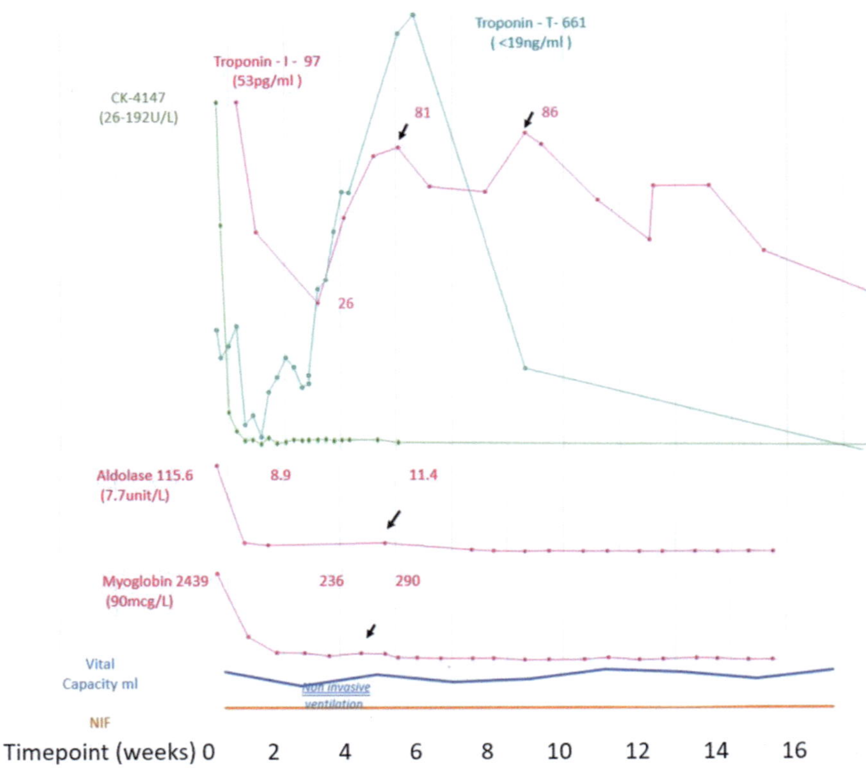

Fig. 41.1 Lab trends. Timepoint of 0 is the onset of neuromuscular toxicity

IVIG maintenance therapy has been continued along with addition of abatacept (abatacept binds to the costimulatory molecules CD80 and CD86 on antigen-presenting cells (APC), thereby blocking interaction with CD28 on T cells). Non-invasive ventilation has been started. During this prolonged hospital stay, patient had localized small bowel intestinal perforation treated conservatively with intravenous antibiotics, and total parenteral nutrition. Patient stabilized from neuromuscular standpoint, and eventually discharged on day 72. In the outpatient setting, she continues to show improving muscular strength, moving from walker to being able to ambulate independently. Vital capacity at the time of discharge was consistently seen in the range of 1000–1100 mL. Patient tolerating oral feeds at the time of discharge. Towards the later part of her admission, at the time of discharge, and at outpatient follow-up's, patient's eyelid ptosis has completely resolved without steroids or pyridostigmine. IVIG maintenance infusions were continued at 1 g/kg every 3 weeks × 3 followed by increased time intervals to every 4 weeks. CK, aldolase and myoglobin continue to be normal in the outpatient setting. Cardiac left ventricular ejection fraction stabilized at 37%.

Case Summary

This is a case with melanoma underwent surgery and nivolumab therapy, developed myocarditis, myositis, and myasthenia that required hospital admission. Patient responded to steroids, TPE, IVIG, rituximab, abatacept and ultimately achieved remission for both toxicities and cancer until the last follow up 8 months later. Summary of the events is depicted in Fig. 41.2.

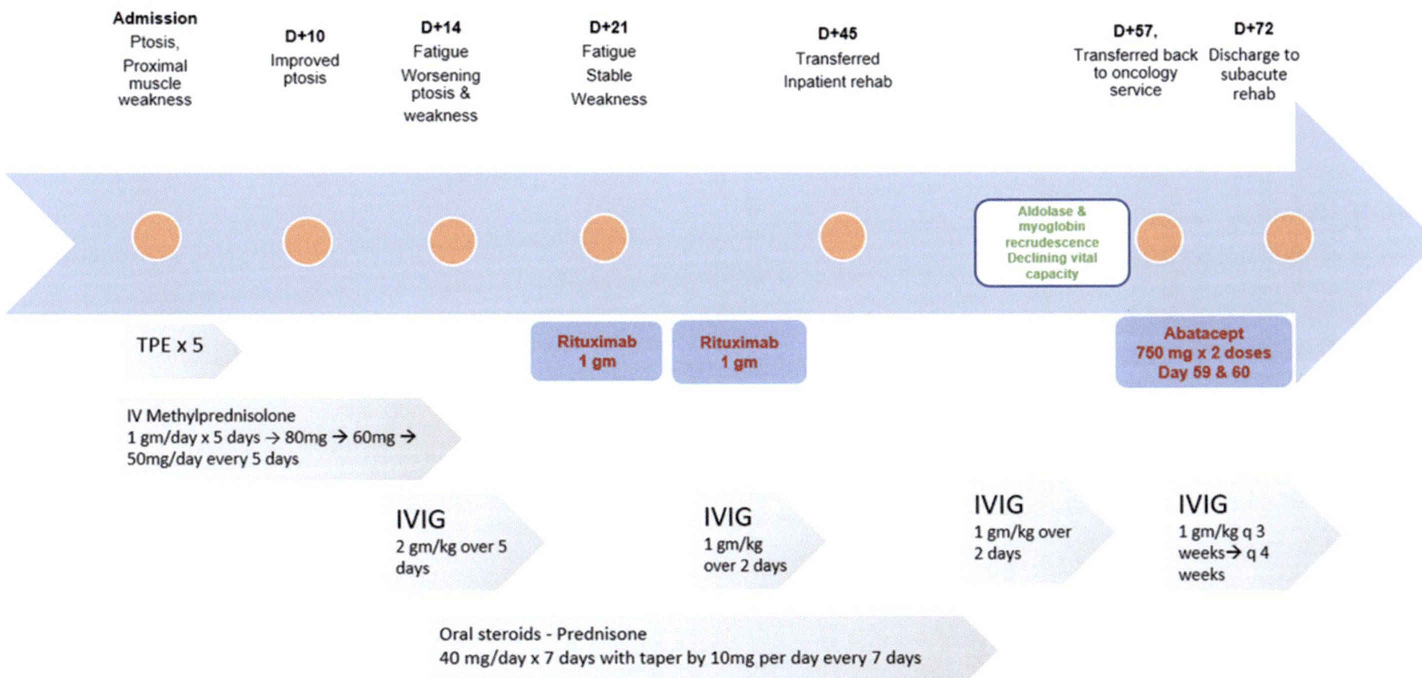

Fig. 41.2 Patient treatment summary

Discussion

ICI neurological side effects (N-irAE) can involve peripheral nervous system (PNS-irAEs), with weakness as the primary component that frequently need neurology evaluation. It is recommended to hold ICI therapy, as individual patients' clinical trajectory can vary significantly. Neuromuscular weakness needs prompt workup for nerve, muscle, and neuromuscular junction dysfunction as a package when indicated given the concern of multiple sites involvement. These include evaluation for inflammatory demyelinating or axonal cranial/peripheral polyneuropathy, myositis, and myasthenia gravis [1]. Fluctuating weakness (eyelid ptosis, binocular diplopia, bulbar muscle weakness, limb muscle weakness), positive myasthenia antibody titers, and supportive findings from neurophysiological testing (decrement seen on repetitive nerve stimulation, abnormalities seen on single-fiber EMG if available) are suggestive of myasthenia gravis. Most common myasthenia antibody seen is anti-acetylcholine receptor antibody, while MUSK antibody or LR P4 antibody are very rare. Post neuromuscular junction disorder Lambert-Eaton myasthenic syndrome with positive anti voltage-gated calcium channel antibody is very rarely reported. This is seen in the context of small cell lung cancer and accompanied by autonomic symptoms (dry mouth, eyes blurred vision), and diminished deep tendon reflexes in comparison to myasthenia gravis. Fixed muscle weakness (cranial nerves with negative icepack test, bulbar muscles, limb muscles), EMG findings of irritable myopathy, elevated CK, aldolase, myoglobin, positive myositis antibody, and much rare HMGCR or anti-cN-1 antibody are suggestive of myositis [2]. Work-up for myocarditis include troponin I, cardiac MRI, echocardiogram, with patient's being monitored on telemetry for any new cardiac arrhythmias. Because of the peculiar facial and ocular involvement (ptosis), myositis can mimic myasthenia gravis at the initial clinical evaluation, and the negative icepack test, elevated muscle enzymes (CK, aldolase, myoglobin) favor myositis. Skeletal and cardiac muscle biopsies could be considered depending on the patient clinical status, and local expertise. Necrotizing myopathy is the most common findings seen on muscle biopsies, with endomysial inflammation (CD63+ macrophages, CD8+/PD-L1+ T-cells). Work-up for myositis, myocarditis, and myasthenia are detailed in Fig. 41.3.

ICI related neuropathy adverse events can be varied. Clinical presentation can be varied and include cranial neuropathies, radiculopathy, inflammatory neuropathies (Gilliam Barré syndrome variants), chronic inflammatory demyelinating polyneuropathy, vasculitis, radiculopathies, brachial plexopathy, isolated mononeuropathies like median (carpal tunnel) and phrenic neuropathies. Work-up includes lumbar puncture for cerebrospinal fluid analysis which can show cytoalbumin dissociation (high protein with no white cells). However frequently in ICI related adverse events there are increased white cells which could represent primed CD8+ T cells [3]. Patients could be screen for presence of ganglioside antibodies. Appropriate work-up should be done with MRI of the brain and spine for metastasis including leptomeningeal disease. If appropriate based on the clinical status, nerve biopsy could be considered. Treatment approaches include similar approaches with myositis and

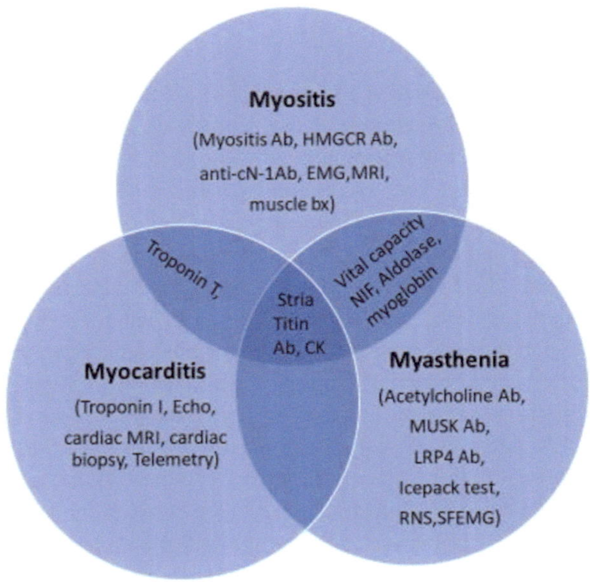

Fig. 41.3 3 M's (Myositis myocarditis and Myasthenia) proposed needed work up. Some of workup overlaps. Troponin I is very sensitive for myocarditis. Clinicians are recommended to include appropriate workup. Elevations in CK, Stria-Striational Antibody, Titin Ab can be seen in all three entities. EMG (electromyogram), RNS (repetitive nerve stimulation), SFEMG (single-fiber EMG)

myasthenia gravis. Clinical stratification (CTCAE grading) and early multimodal aggressive immunosuppressive and immunomodulating therapies could be considered for patients with greater weakness. Like myasthenia and myositis, bulbar and respiratory weakness should be considered as severe toxicity. Neck ptosis can be seen with myasthenia, myositis and neuropathy and generally suggestive of higher-grade toxicity.

For ICI related neuromuscular weakness, patient's need prompt evaluation for bulbar weakness and respiratory muscle weakness at admission, and frequently during the hospital stay. Speech therapy consultation, and as needed alternative feeding via gastric tube feeds or total parenteral nutrition need to be addressed promptly given the patients are at high risk for aspiration. Respiratory muscle weakness including the diaphragm needs close attention by daily and frequent pulmonary functions assessment by forced vital capacity (FVC) and negative inspiratory force (NIF) [4, 5].

Patients with myositis and myasthenia with accompanying myocarditis overlap syndrome can be associated high mortality rate. Prompt recognition, evaluation and treatment for cardiac arrhythmia, and early multimodal immunosuppressive/immunomodulatory therapy is recommended. Rapid initiation of high dose steroids, total plasma exchange or intravenous immunoglobulins, is recommended followed by other agents like rituximab and abatacept. This approach limits steroid exposure.

Patient can be re-challenged after improvement of the neurological symptoms [1]. Higher CTCAE grades [6, 7], with residual neurological sequelae, needs multidisciplinary team approach, with greater collaboration between oncology and neurology teams, balancing the risks, and a very careful close patient follow-up [6]. Similarly, patients with underlying autoimmunity prior to the initiation of immune checkpoint inhibitors (known myasthenia gravis, chronic inflammatory demyelinating polyneuropathy), when stable at lower maintenance therapies, can likely be started on checkpoint inhibitors with close clinical follow-up.

Conclusion

ICI related neuromuscular complications need prompt recognition and treatment. Patients with unique combination of 3 M's (myositis, myasthenia and myocarditis) need close clinical and laboratory follow up. One entity may be predominant than the others in the presentation. Earlier aggressive multimodal approach is needed early in the disease course. Prompt recognition of clinical and laboratory recrudescence would lead to addition of more immunosuppressive/immunomodulatory agents.

Specific considerations in managing patients with neuromuscular weakness.

1. Daily CK, aldolase, myoglobin, and Troponin I are recommended twice a week to recognize recrudescence early.
2. Liver tests ALT, AST could be elevated from muscle disease. Aldolase can be elevated in fasciitis.
3. Clinical diagnosis is needed when antibody testing is negative.
4. Rheumatological adverse events related to checkpoint inhibitors, like polymyalgia rheumatica, inflammatory arthritis, fasciitis, can mimic neuromuscular weakness.
5. Ice pack test is performed by applying ice over eyelids for approximate 2–5 min, depending on tolerability and the eyelid elevation is re-measured after that. If there is improvement of 2 mm or more, and are improvement in extraocular eye movements, it's considered a positive test. Test is considered sensitive and specific for myasthenia gravis, while it has no effect on ptosis from other causes (myositis). The reported sensitivity is up to 80%.
6. Single breath count test is performed by asking patients to take a deep breath and count as far as possible in their normal voice at an approximate rate of 2 counts per second. Normal is 50 and less than 15 correlates with reduced vital capacity.
7. Forced vital capacity (FVC), less than 15 mL/kg (normal is >25 mL/kg) in patients with neuromuscular weakness, should prompt urgent intensive care referral for careful watch and possible endotracheal intubation in anticipation of progressive respiratory weakness leading to hypercarbia. Supine and sitting vital capacity should be measured. Decreased FVC in supine position by 15–20% could represent diaphragm weakness. Negative inspiratory force (NIF) normal is −80 to −100 and respiratory support indicated for −20 to 0.
8. Lumbar puncture for CSF analysis should be done in patients for inflammatory cranial/peripheral neuropathies. Leptomeningeal disease should be ruled out

along with regular indices like protein, glucose, cell count with differential, infectious panel, oligoclonal bands, paraneoplastic panel.

9. Appropriate neuroimaging (MRI of the brain, spine, with and without contrast) is recommended for evaluation of metastasis, especially for neuropathies.
10. NIV (non-invasive ventilation)—can aid patients with neuromuscular weakness affecting ventilation. Nocturnal use in sleep could help with improving sleep apnea and resting muscles [1, 3].
11. Pyridostigmine side effects including increased secretions. Recommendation are for needed dose adjustments or holding.
12. In patients with facial and cranial muscle weakness and high CK it is reasonable to start high doses steroids. There is a higher incidence of myocarditis and mortality in these patients. Rapid initiation of high dose of steroids in idiopathic myasthenia gravis not related to checkpoint inhibitors can precipitate myasthenic crisis needing intubation. However, this is not seen in ICI related myositis and myasthenia overlap with or without myocarditis.

References

1. Rossi S, Gelsomino F, Rinaldi R, Muccioli L, Comito F, Di Federico A, De Giglio A, Lamberti G, Andrini E, Mollica V, D'Angelo R, Baccari F, Zenesini C, Madia P, Raschi E, Cortelli P, Ardizzoni A, Guarino M. Peripheral nervous system adverse events associated with immune checkpoint inhibitors. J Neurol. 2023;270(6):2975–86.
2. Garibaldi M, Calabrò F, Merlonghi G, Pugliese S, Ceccanti M, Cristiano L, Tartaglione T, Petrucci A. Immune checkpoint inhibitors (ICIs)-related ocular myositis. Neuromuscul Disord. 2020;30(5):420–3.
3. Rubio-Perez C, Planas-Rigol E, Trincado JL, Bonfill-Teixidor E, Arias A, Marchese D, Moutinho C, Serna G, Pedrosa L, Iurlaro R, Martínez-Ricarte F, Escudero L, Cordero E, Cicuendez M, Ruiz S, Parra G, Nuciforo P, Gonzalez J, Pineda E, Sahuquillo J, Tabernero J, Heyn H, Seoane J. Immune cell profiling of the cerebrospinal fluid enables the characterization of the brain metastasis microenvironment. Nat Commun. 2021;12(1):1503.
4. Patel N, Howard IM, Baydur A. Respiratory considerations in patients with neuromuscular disorders. Muscle Nerve. 2023;68(2):122–41.
5. Carlucci A, Fusar PB. getting it right in restrictive lung disease. J Clin Med. 2023;12(10):3353.
6. Hundsberger T, Schreiner B, Roth P. Immune checkpoint inhibitors induced side effects of the peripheral nervous system. Curr Opin Neurol. 2023;36(5):427–31.
7. Jordan B, Benesova K, Hassel JC, Wick W, Jordan K. How we identify and treat neuromuscular toxicity induced by immune checkpoint inhibitors. ESMO Open. 2021;6(6):100317.

Chapter 42
Hyperosmia Secondary to Immune Checkpoint Inhibitor Therapy

Jane M. Taylor, Marcus S. Dempster, Jung-Min Song, Lucy Boyce Kennedy, and Pauline Funchain

Abbreviations

AI	Adrenal insufficiency
ICI	Immune checkpoint inhibitor
irAE	Immune-related adverse event
T-VEC	Talimogene laherparepvec

Clinical Presentations

This is a female in her 60s with a history of uterine fibroids and endometriosis who presented to an oncology clinic for management of Stage IIIC malignant melanoma of the left heel. She underwent a wide local excision and a sentinel lymph node biopsy of the left groin. After local excision, she was started on adjuvant immune checkpoint inhibitor (ICI) nivolumab 480 mg every 28 days. During the first cycle of nivolumab, she experienced multiple adverse events, including fatigue,

J. M. Taylor · L. B. Kennedy
Taussig Cancer Institute, Cleveland Clinic Foundation, Cleveland, OH, USA
e-mail: taylorj41@ccf.org; kennedl5@ccf.org

M. S. Dempster
Department of Hematology and Medical Oncology, Roswell Park Comprehensive Cancer Center, Buffalo, NY, USA
e-mail: ma56010@roswellpark.org

J.-M. Song
Department of Hematology/Oncology, Metro Health, Cleveland, OH, USA
e-mail: JSong1@metrohealth.org

P. Funchain (✉)
Division of Oncology, Department of Medicine, Stanford Cancer Institute, Stanford University, Stanford, CA, USA
e-mail: funchap@stanford.edu

Y. Wang (ed.), *Challenging Cases in Immunotherapy Related Organ Toxicities*,
https://doi.org/10.1007/978-3-031-83533-9_42

intermittent flu-like symptoms, diffuse myalgia and arthralgia of multiple joints, mild nausea, and mild constipation. Due to development of immune-related hypothyroidism at the start of cycle 3, she was started on levothyroxine 75 μg daily. Additionally, the patient reported persistent cough, congestion, and rhinitis while receiving ICI.

Five months into the course of adjuvant nivolumab, the patient was diagnosed with unresectable in-transit metastases of the left foot, for which she received talimogene laherparepvec (T-VEC) to her left foot. She received four cycles of T-VEC in combination with nivolumab therapy. By the eighth cycle of nivolumab, the patient reported increased fatigue, ongoing myalgias and arthralgias, and increased nausea. As the cycles of therapy continued, the patient continued to experience subsequent adverse events including a new grade 1 pruritic rash, for which she was prescribed triamcinolone cream.

Extreme sensitivity to smell and worsening seasonal allergies were first noted on her cycle 13 visit. The patient reported that she began experiencing rhinorrhea, cough, esophageal burning, pleuritic pain, and wheezing when exposed to irritants like smoke, paint, aerosols, perfume, and dust. The patient acknowledged that her onset of hyperosmia was likely much earlier during her course of therapy, and notes it was, however, masked due to the timing of the pandemic and remaining at home more frequently. By cycle 16, the patient had new onset of severe arthralgia and treatment was ultimately held. Systemic steroids were not pursued. Persistent cough, congestion, and rhinitis that the patient experienced from the time of ICI initiation slowly improved after cessation of therapy. The patient continued to have a complete intolerance to smells with associated unpleasant systemic reactions. Her quality of life became very limited in order to minimize her exposures.

One month after the patient's last cycle of nivolumab, she experienced a systemic reaction to a common household cleaner, with associated bronchitis, neutrophilia, and leukocytosis (Fig. 42.1). She was seen in clinic around that time and laboratory tests revealed an elevated WBC of 19.9 k/uL and an absolute neutrophil count of 17.7 k/uL. She reported that she experienced rhinorrhea, cough, pleuritic pain, esophageal burning, a sensation of esophageal swelling, and wheezing during this exposure. The patient's hyperosmia subjectively worsened at that time. Following subsequent exposures to chemicals and other irritants, the patient continued to experience similar adverse symptoms. A steroid inhaler was not prescribed at that time.

The patient was evaluated by an allergy specialist early during the disease course. Evaluation revealed no history of nasal polyps or tumors and no known allergies, other than a prior, mild intolerance to perfume and mild seasonal allergies. Per the allergist's recommendations, she was started on olopatadine nasal spray and cetirizine 10 mg once daily. Treatment with this regimen was not associated with any improvement in the patient's hyperosmia or systemic symptoms following exposure to aerosols or other irritants. The patient's reactive symptoms are best managed by avoidance and by using an N-95 mask with a charcoal filter. When she has an exposure, she uses a saline nasal mist to flush away lingering unpleasant sensations. She continues to follow with allergy regularly; her symptoms of hyperosmia persist and

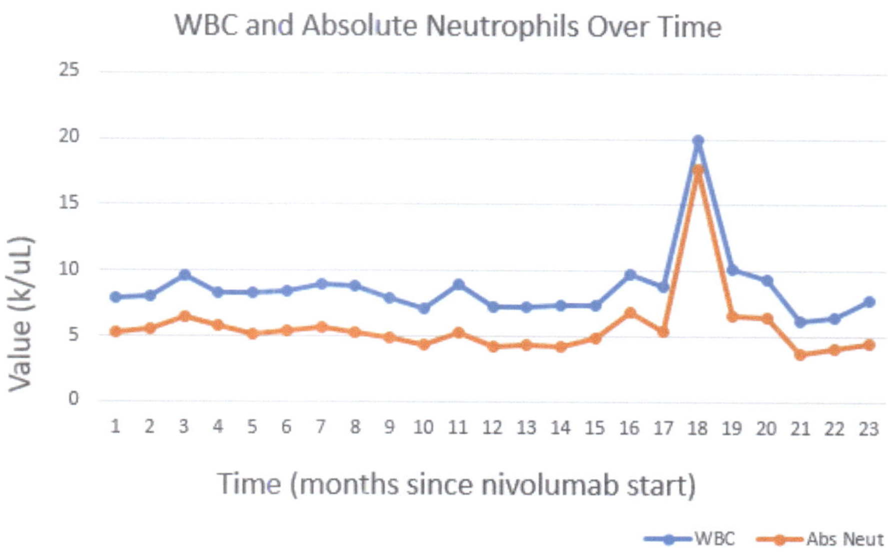

Fig. 42.1 Leukocytosis and neutrophilia after systemic reaction to a common household cleaner

her quality of life has remained limited at 60 months since initiation of ICI, the time of her last follow up (Fig. 42.2).

Differential Diagnoses

Hyperosmia is associated with some autoimmune disorders such as ICI related endocrine adverse event, e.g. adrenal dysfunction, which is less frequently reported. Common symptoms of adrenal insufficiency (AI) include fatigue, muscle ache, weakness, dizziness, nausea, and vomiting. The patient experienced temporary fatigue, muscle weakness and nausea concurrent with T-VEC injections and had no chronic symptoms consistent with AI.

There is an increasingly recognized association between dysosmia and respiratory infections, including with COVID-19. The patient reported chronic respiratory infection-like symptoms throughout the duration of her ICI, including persistent cough, congestion, and rhinitis. While the most reported form of dysosmia associated with viral infections is anosmia, hyperosmia has been reported as a less common and potential deregulatory olfactory episode [1].

Olfactory disturbances may also be associated with nasal cranial polyps and tumors. The patient's brain MRI at the time of diagnosis and prior to beginning ICI revealed no notable abnormalities. Other differentials for hyperosmia that were automatically excluded for this patient include pregnancy, epilepsy, multiple sclerosis, and idiopathic environmental intolerance.

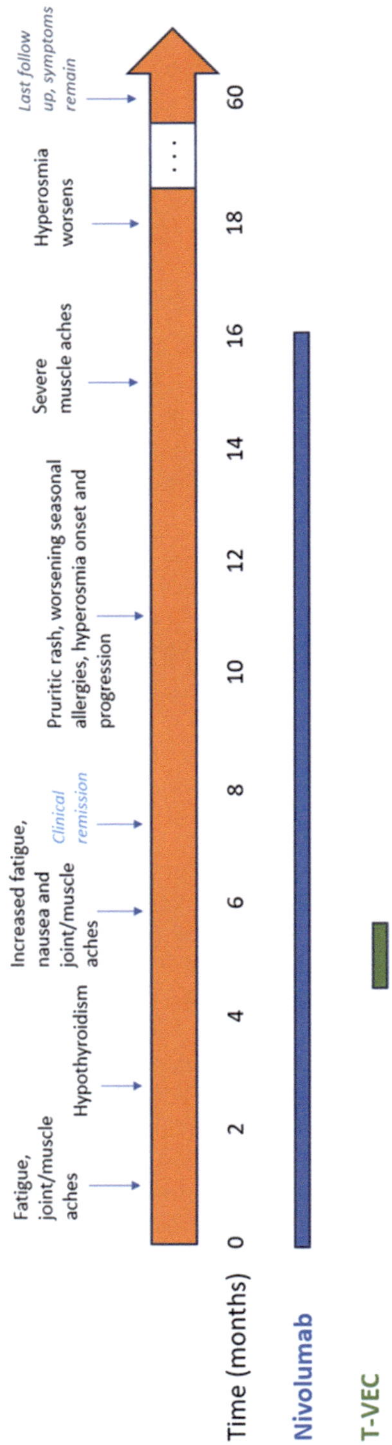

Fig. 42.2 Timeline of adverse events and onset of hyperosmia

Follow Up and Outcome

Three and a half years post cessation of ICI, the patient experiences persistent sensitivity to smell, with associated cough, sneezing, wheezing, mild dyspnea, pleuritic pain, and esophageal burning when exposed to synthetic and natural chemicals. Her symptoms vary depending on the type of exposure; she reports occasional palpitations, nausea, muscle pain, and joint pain. Following reactive episodes, she continues to use saline mist to flush away lingering sensations. She uses budesonide-formoterol inhaler preventatively and an albuterol inhaler as recovery after exposures, although notes minimal improvement in symptoms with this regimen, with resolution of acute symptoms spontaneously occurring in around a few hours. She continues to take cetirizine 10 mg daily and utilize preventive methods to minimize her sensitivity, primarily by avoidance and wearing an N-95 mask with an activated charcoal filter. She also continues levothyroxine 100 μg daily for immune-related hypothyroidism. The patient's quality of life is significantly impacted by the need to limit activities to minimize her exposures.

Case Summary

This case illustrates the acute onset of hyperosmia almost 1 year after the initiation of anti-PD-1 monotherapy. This patient remains in clinical remission without evidence of recurrent melanoma but continues to have persistent symptoms of hyperosmia. Her sensitivity to smell has not improved since cessation of ICI despite different treatments and continues to severely impact her quality of life.

Discussion

Hyperosmia as an adverse event attributed to ICI has not been reported. Hyperosmia is rare, may be difficult to ascertain a definitive etiology, and is associated with several disorders including Addison's disease, multiple sclerosis, psychiatric conditions, epilepsy, pregnancy, and nasal/cranial polyps and tumors [2, 3]. Neurologic side effects of ICI are among the least frequently reported immune-related adverse events (irAEs) [4]. Hyperosmia can be a symptom of autoimmune or endocrine disorders, and it is important to consider comprehensive inflammatory reactions from ICIs for involvement of further multidisciplinary management. While more rare than other adverse events, hyperosmia and associated symptoms can significantly impact quality of life and should be included as part of a general awareness of irAEs with neurologic and endocrine etiologies. The development of subjective hypersomnia from ICI highlights an association between immune surveillance and olfaction. This case of olfactory dysregulation demonstrates that the efficacy of ICIs is not without a myriad of unexpected presentations.

References

1. Di Stadio A, D'Ascanio L, De Luca P, Roccamatisi D, La Mantia I, Brenner MJ. Hyperosmia after COVID-19: hedonic perception or hypersensitivity? Eur Rev Med Pharmacol Sci. 2022;26(6):2196–200.
2. Haugh AM, Probasco JC, Johnson DB. Neurologic complications of immune checkpoint inhibitors. Expert Opin Drug Saf. 2020;19(4):479–88.
3. Cameron EL. Pregnancy and olfaction: a review. Front Psychol. 2014;5:67. Published 2014 Feb 6.
4. Norès JM, Biacabe B, Bonfils P. Olfactory disorders and general pathology. Analysis and review of the literature. Rev Med Interne. 2000;21(1):95–104.

Part IX
Ophthalmology

Chapter 43
Optic Neuritis Post Immune Checkpoint Inhibitor Therapy

May Ameri, Andrew Whyte, and Nagham Al-Zubidi

Abbreviations

CRP	C-reactive protein
CT	Computerized tomography
CTCAE	Common terminology criteria for adverse events
ESR	Erythrocyte sedimentation rate
HVF	Humphrey visual field
ICI	immune checkpoint inhibitor
IrAE	Immune related adverse events
LP	Lumber puncture
OCT	Optical computerized tomography
OD	Right eye
OS	Left eye
OU	Both eyes
PD1	Programmed cell death protein 1
PET	Positron emission tomography
RAPD	Relative afferent pupillary defect
RNFL	Retinal nerve fiber layer

M. Ameri
McGovern Medical School, University of Texas Health Science Center, Houston, TX, USA
e-mail: may.ali.a.alameri@uth.tmc.edu

A. Whyte
Department of Head and Neck Surgery, The University of Texas MD Anderson Cancer Center, Houston, TX, USA
e-mail: ATWhyte@mdanderson.org

N. Al-Zubidi (✉)
Department of Ophthalmology, McGovern Medical School, University of Texas Health Science Center, Houston, TX, USA

Department of Head and Neck Surgery, The University of Texas MD Anderson Cancer Center, Houston, TX, USA
e-mail: nsal@mdanderson.org

Y. Wang (ed.), *Challenging Cases in Immunotherapy Related Organ Toxicities*,
https://doi.org/10.1007/978-3-031-83533-9_43

WNL Within normal limits

Clinical Presentation

Patient is a Caucasian male in his 80s with history of stage IIA melanoma status post wide local excision and sentinel lymph node biopsy who presented a year later with recurrent melanoma of scalp. The recurrent lesion was excised at an outside hospital with a Positron emission tomography (PET) and computerized tomography (CT) scan that revealed disease spread to left parotid gland and lymph node and right neck lymph node. Biopsy of nodes were consistent with metastatic disease (Stage IV M1a). He was subsequently started on pembrolizumab, a Programmed cell death protein 1 (PD-1) inhibitor, and completed one cycle. The patient was seen by ophthalmology for baseline screening prior to treatment per protocol. Initially the patient had no visual complaints with a best corrected vision of 20/20 bilaterally (OU). Intraocular pressure (IOP) was within normal limit (WNL), color vision was WNL with pupil exam being normal without a relative afferent pupillary defect (RAPD). Slit lamp microscopy (SLM) was positive for 2+ nuclear sclerosis, dilated fundus examination was unremarkable.

Cycle 2 of pembrolizumab was delayed for 4 months due to severe colitis which required a course of steroid taper from 40 mg/day and two doses of infliximab. A restaging MRI brain showed a 3 mm enhancing nodule involving the right frontal lobe suspicious for metastasis and cycle 2 was reinstated.

Eleven days post cycle 2 pembrolizumab treatment he presented with new onset blurry vision of both eyes. The following day (day 12), his local ophthalmologist described bilateral optic nerve swelling and raised concerns for optic neuritis. Cycle 3 pembrolizumab was held and patient was given 5-day methylprednisolone dose pack (1000 mg/day) which improved his visions slightly after 2 days. Patient denied headaches, jaw pain, eye pain, temporal pain, no ocular discomfort with ocular motilities. The patient presented to neuro-ophthalmology clinic with continued symptoms of progressive bilateral blurry vision, most apparent on left and inferior gaze. The deterioration in VA was clinically significant with a best corrected vision 20/40 OD and 20/60 OS with decreased color vision (9/13) OU. Dilated fundus exam exhibited Friesen IV/V optic disc edema with peripapillary hemorrhage OU and cup-to-disc ratio of 0.0, which was confirmed on OCT RNFL and Humphrey Visual Field (HVF) testing (Figs. 43.1 and 43.2, respectively). Patient had grade 3 ocular toxicity based on Common Terminology Criteria for Adverse Events (CTCAE).

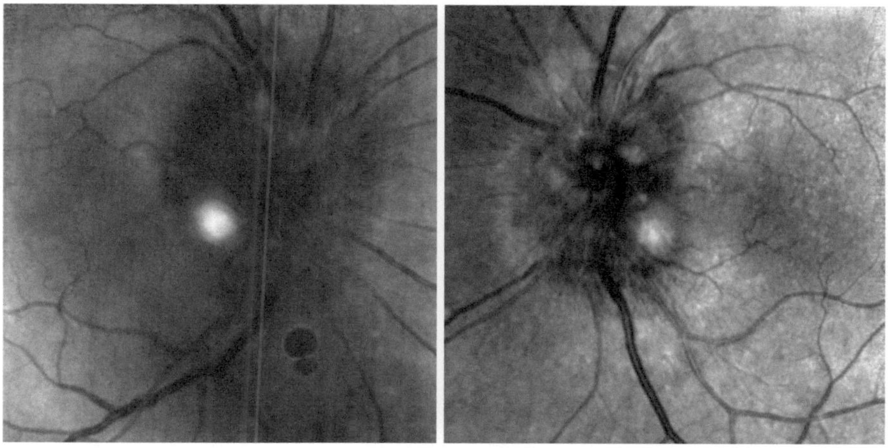

Fig. 43.1 Red free fundus photographs showing optic disc edema of right and left eyes

Differential Diagnosis

The challenges we face in our patient population when a patient exhibits new ocular symptoms and signs is whether it is the cancer itself (direct, metastatic, infectious or indirect paraneoplastic effect) vs. cancer treatment related conditions (e.g., radiation, chemotherapy, or immune related adverse events (irAE) from immune checkpoint inhibitors). Further work-up was considered including temporal artery biopsy and baseline Erythrocyte sedimentation rate (ESR) and C-reactive protein (CRP) rule out low-suspicion for Giant Cell Arteritis and lumber puncture (LP) for opening pressure and cytology; however, the patient denied lumbar puncture due to improvement on empiric therapy. The patient's repeat MRI with and without contrast confirmed 3 mm punctate enhancement within right anterior frontal lobe metastasis, unchanged from his early imaging prior to treatment, thus leptomeningeal metastasis causing ocular disturbance and optic nerve compression was ruled out. This signifies the difficulty in isolating and confirming the diagnosis of neuro-ophthalmic irAEs, given patient's high diagnostic burden—a more extensive workup that could lead to discomfort, harm, and increase healthcare costs in populations who already overburdened with testing—and the difficulty of a dechallenge-rechallenge protocol. There are two hypotheses for the difference in features of optic neuritis post-immune checkpoint inhibitor (ICI) therapy: one is that the pathogenesis is truly different to classic optic neuritis and the other is that previous reported causes have been mislabeling non arteritic anterior ischemic optic neuropathy as optic neuritis.

In our case, given the evidence of temporal relationship between the onset of symptom and the initiation of pembrolizumab, lack of systemic signs of infection, equal and bilateral presentation suggestive of systemic effect, exclusion of toxic and metabolic etiologies, and negative imaging and infectious or autoimmune process, it was determined that the most likely etiology of these new signs and symptoms

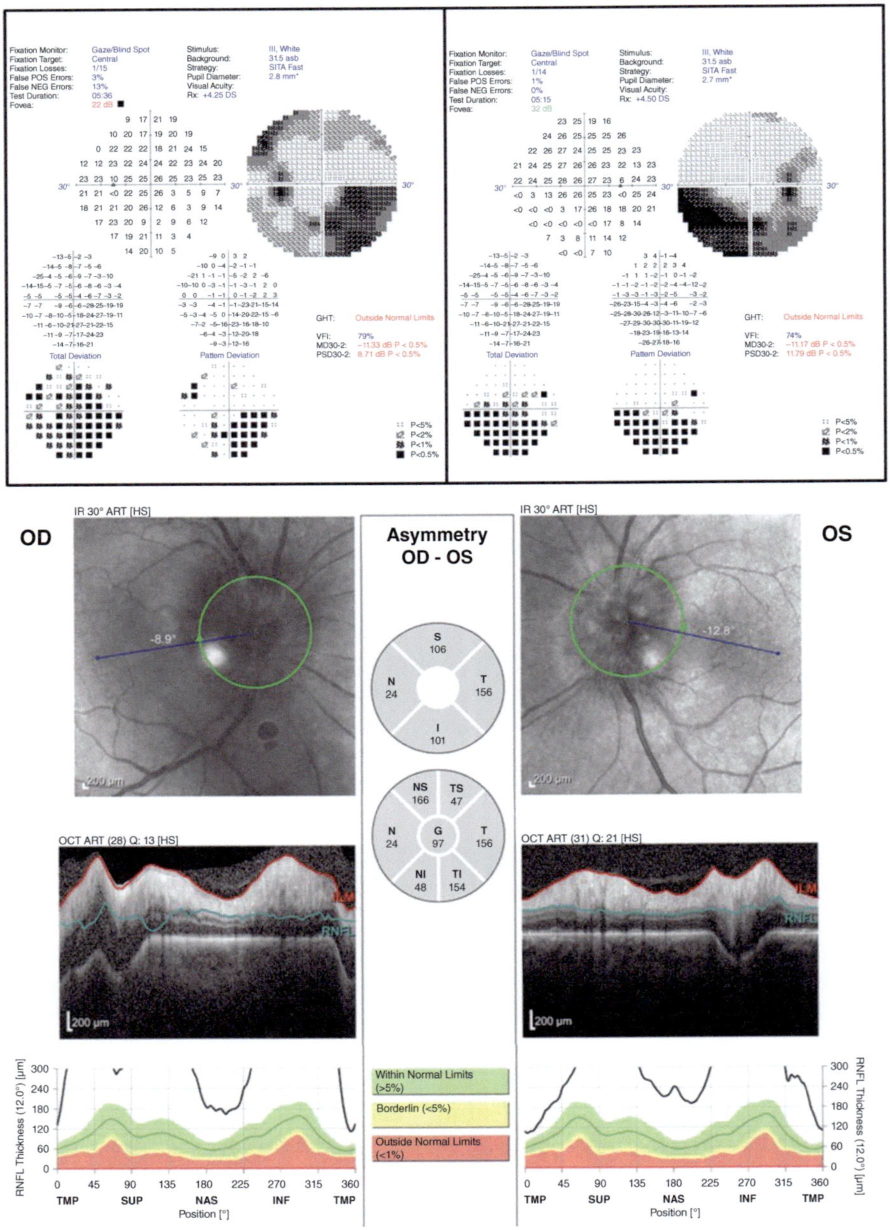

Fig. 43.2 HVF (top) showing partial outer inferior temporal and inferior nasal defect bilaterally and OCT RNFL scan (bottom) exhibiting grade V disc edema

were a toxic side effect of the immune checkpoint inhibitor therapy e.g. optic neuritis. We are bound by the ethics of non-maleficence; thus, re-challenging the patient with the suspected therapy would potentially cause harm and would be unethical unless the benefit outweighed the risk. Finally, we were unable to completely rule out other less plausible disease given the patient's wishes against more invasive testing for less likely causes and the clinical improvement. The criteria were then determined to have been met to the best possible degree (between probable and certain) in the given circumstances and the causal relationship of pembrolizumab was established and used to guide treatment.

Management and Outcome

Our patient was taken off pembrolizumab and started on 5 days of high-dose IV methylprednisolone 1 g/day followed by oral prednisone 60 mg/day with a 10 mg taper every 5 days conditional on response. On the first follow up 1 week later, the patient's vision remained stable, but his visual field had improved on HVF (Fig. 43.3). On dilated fundus exam the patient had improvement of the disc edema from the initial Friesen IV to grade II confirmed on OCT RNFL (Figs. 43.4 and 43.5).

Summary and Timeline

In summary, this was a patient with melanoma developed optic neuritis 11 days after second cycle of pembrolizumab treatment. Patient improved with intravenous steroid and withholding pembrolizumab, although vision did not return to baseline post treatment, patient's visual field and optic disc edema improved. The decision was made not to rechallenge with pembrolizumab. Patient is still undergoing

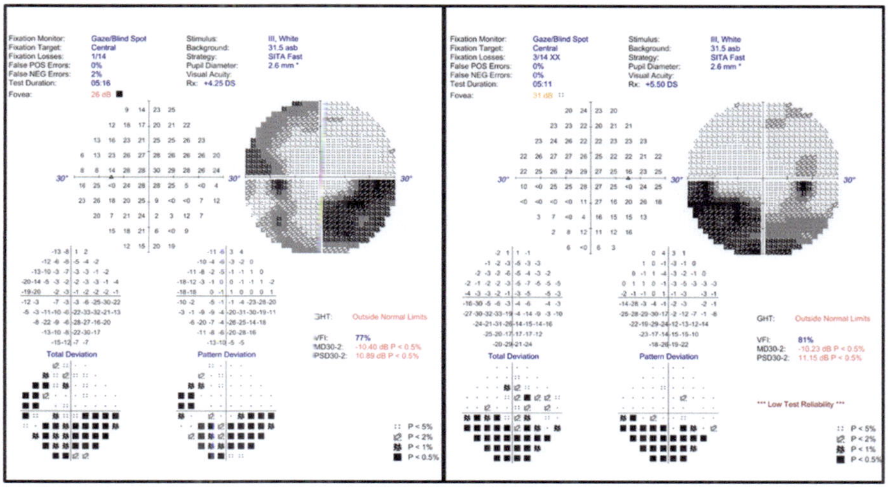

Fig. 43.3 HVF showing improvement in patient's visual field exam

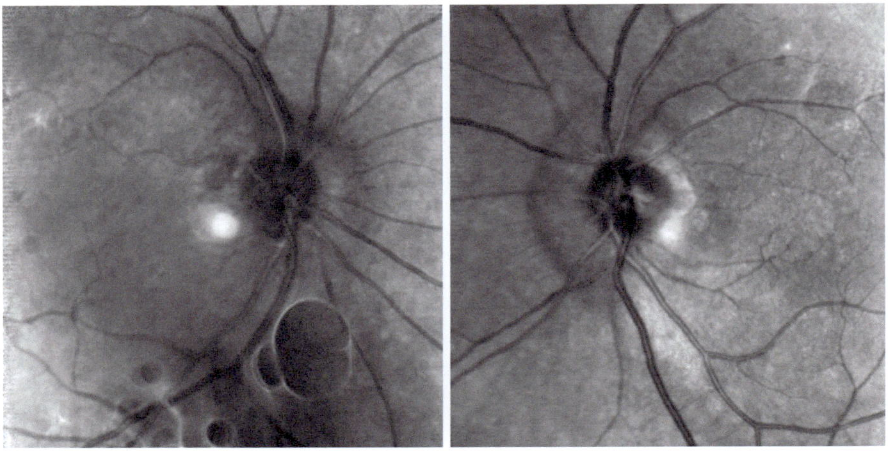

Fig. 43.4 Red free fundus photography showing improvement of the optic disc edema bilaterally

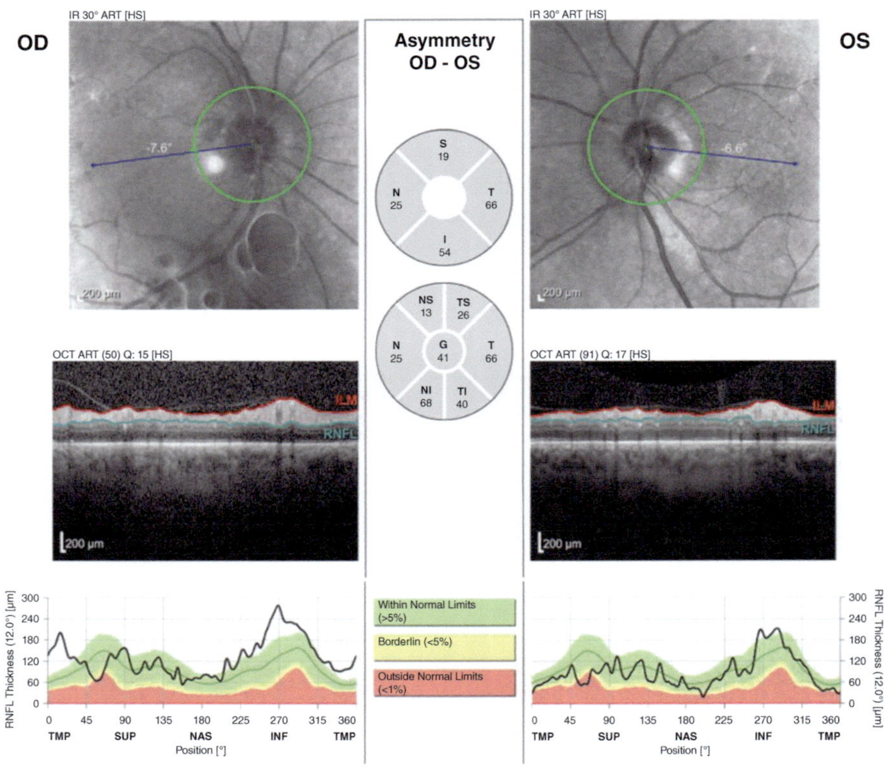

Fig. 43.5 OCT RNFL showing improvement of optic disc edema

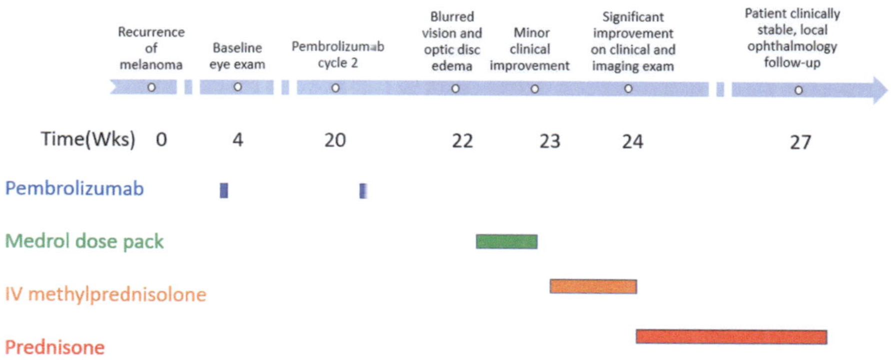

Fig. 43.6 Timeline of events (timepoint of 0 is melanoma recurrence)

different cancer treatment and was discharged to follow-up with local ophthalmologist. Figure 43.6 showed the summary of the timeline of all the events.

Discussion

Overall, the incidence of ICI-associated optic neuropathy is estimated to be 0.46% [1]. It is reported as either optic neuritis or non-arteritic anterior ischemic optic neuropathy. Optic neuritis makes up 12.8% of cases [2]. It may not always have all the classic clinical findings of pain, blurry vision, RAPD, decrease in visual acuity and color vision. According to one retrospective review, only 10% of patients reported painful vision loss and 67% had dyschromatopsia [2]. In a large case study, it was found that pembrolizumab and its ICI category (PD-1) are associated with 32% of neuro ophthalmic manifestations, such as uveitis and optic neuritis [2–4]. However, a systemic review of all reported case studies found that 60% of ICI associated optic neuritis were associated with ipilimumab [1]. There is no consensus on diagnosis and management of ocular irAEs. Recommendations are based on level V evidence and grade B level of recommendation (strong or moderate evidence for efficacy but with a limited clinical benefit, generally recommended) [5]. High dose intravenous (IV) corticosteroids followed by a slow prednisone taper is the mainstay for treatment for optic nerve disc edema. There is currently no evidence for using non-steroid immune modulating agents in the treatment of ICI-associated optic neuritis, however most patients (79.8%) experienced improvement or complete resolution of neuro-ophthalmic symptoms from cessation of ICI and immunosuppression with systemic corticosteroids.

References

1. Yu CW, Yau M, Mezey N, Joarder I, Micieli JA. Neuro-ophthalmic complications of immune checkpoint inhibitors: a systematic review. Eye Brain. 2020;12:139–67. https://doi.org/10.2147/EB.S277760.
2. Haanen JBAG, Carbonnel F, Robert C, Kerr KM, Peters S, Larkin J, et al. Management of toxicities from immunotherapy: ESMO clinical practice guidelines for diagnosis, treatment and follow-up. Ann Oncol. 2017;28(Suppl 4):iv119–42. https://doi.org/10.1093/annonc/mdx225.
3. Telfah M, Whittaker TJ, Doolittle GC. Vision loss with pembrolizumab treatment: a report of two cases. J Oncol Pharm Pract. 2019;25(6):1540–6. https://doi.org/10.1177/1078155219841683. Epub 2019 Apr 18. PMID: 30997872.
4. Makri OE, Dimitrakopoulos FI, Tsapardoni F, Tsekouras I, Argyriou AA, Kalofonos H, Georgakopoulos CD. Isolated optic neuritis after pembrolizumab administration for non-small-cell lung carcinoma. Int J Neurosci. 2022;132(7):643–8. https://doi.org/10.1080/00207454.2020.1831489. Epub 2020 Oct 14. PMID: 32998608.
5. Causality assessment of an adverse event following immunization (AEFI): user manual for the revised WHO classification (second edition). ISBN 978-92-4-151365-4.

Chapter 44
Uveitis Post Immune Checkpoint Inhibitor Therapy

Zachary DeZeeuw, Azadeh Razmandi, and Nagham Al-Zubidi

Abbreviations

BRAF	B-rapidly accelerated fibrosarcoma
CT	Computed tomography
CTCAE	Common terminology criteria for adverse events
IOP	Intraocular pressure
irAEs	Immune related adverse events
IV	Intravenous
MEK	Mitogen activated protein kinase
MRI	Magnetic resonance imaging
OCT	Optical coherence tomography
OD	Right eye
OU	Both eyes
PD-1	Programmed cell death protein 1
RAPD	Relative afferent pupillary defect
RNFL	Retinal nerve fiber layer

Z. DeZeeuw
Department of Ophthalmology, The University of Texas Medical Branch, Galveston, TX, USA
e-mail: zadezeeu@utmb.edu

A. Razmandi
Department of Head and Neck Surgery, The University of Texas MD Anderson Cancer Center, Houston, TX, USA
e-mail: arazmandi@mdanderson.org

N. Al-Zubidi (✉)
Department of Ophthalmology, McGovern Medical School, University of Texas Health Science Center, Houston, TX, USA

Department of Head and Neck Surgery, The University of Texas MD Anderson Cancer Center, Houston, TX, USA
e-mail: nsal@mdanderson.org

Y. Wang (ed.), *Challenging Cases in Immunotherapy Related Organ Toxicities*,
https://doi.org/10.1007/978-3-031-83533-9_44

SCM	Sternocleidomastoid muscle
SLM	Slit lamp microscopy
WNL	Within normal limits

Case Presentation

Patient is a Caucasian male in 60s with a history of stage IVC (cT4b, cN1b, cM1) anaplastic thyroid carcinoma status post total thyroidectomy at an outside hospital presented 1 month later to MD Anderson with swelling of the neck associated with shortness of breath and hoarseness. Patient underwent testing for the BRAF mutation and a CT of the soft tissue of the neck showed extensive residual and progressive mass in left thyroid bed (13.2 × 6.8 × 9.7 cm) with secondary severe tracheal stenosis, invasion of sternocleidomastoid muscle (SCM), bilateral strap muscles, and extension to the skin of anterior lower neck. He was also found to have multiple bilateral lung nodules up to 1.5 cm and pleural metastasis.

While awaiting BRAF status, he received one bridging dose of carboplatin/paclitaxel. BRAF testing was positive, and he was subsequently started on dabrafenib (BRAF-inhibitor), trametinib (MEK 1/2-inhibitor), pembrolizumab (PD-1 inhibitor). The patient was seen by ophthalmology for a baseline screening prior to treatment per protocol. Initially the patient had no visual complaint with a best corrected vision of 20/20 bilaterally (OU). Intraocular pressure (IOP) was within normal limit (WNL), with pupil exam being normal without a relative afferent pupillary defect (RAPD). Slit lamp microscopy (SLM) was positive for non-visually significant nuclear sclerosis, dilated fundus examination was unremarkable.

Two months post treatment he presented with a new onset of blurred vision worse at near and floaters. Ophthalmology exam showed best corrected vision of $20^{-1}/20^{-1}$ OU. SLM showed bilateral anterior uveitis +3 cells, flare of the right eye (OD) and 360-degree posterior synechiae of the iris OU (Fig. 44.1). Dilated fundus exam exhibited grade V optic disc edema OU and central serous retinopathy OU which was confirmed on Optical Coherence Tomography (OCT) of the retinal nerve fiber layer (RNFL) and OCT macula (Figs. 44.2 and 44.3, respectively). Patient had grade 3 anterior uveitis with grade 3 retinopathy based on Common Terminology Criteria for Adverse Events (CTCAE).

Magnetic resonance imaging (MRI) of the brain with and without contrast was unremarkable with no evidence of intracranial metastasis.

Differential Diagnosis

Given the evidence of temporal relationship between the onset of symptom and the initiation of chemotherapy, lack of systemic symptoms of infection, bilaterality of presentation suggestive of systemic effect, exclusion of toxic and metabolic etiologies, negative imaging and infectious or autoimmune process, it was determined

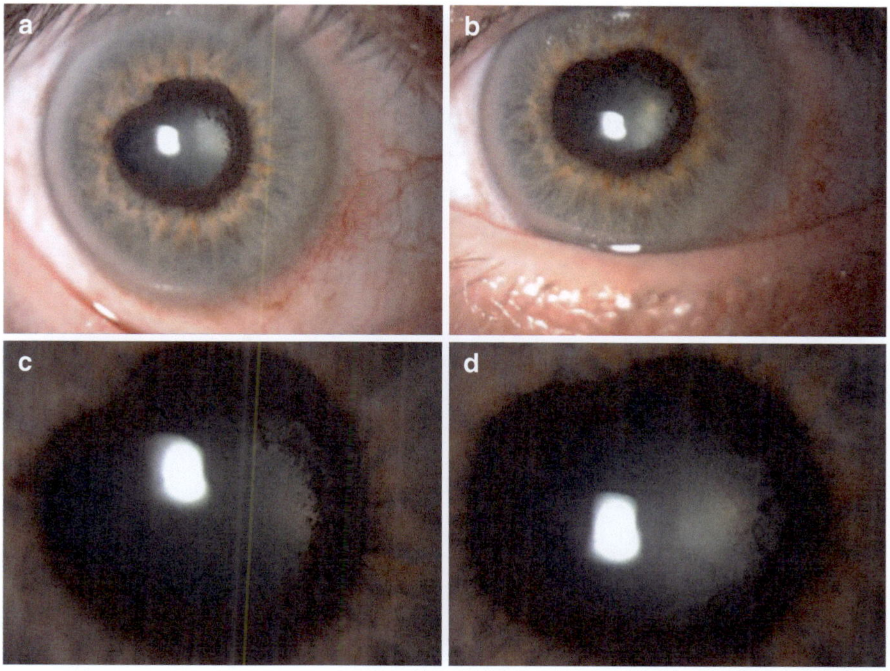

Fig. 44.1 Anterior segment photographs displaying irregular pupils OU with 360 posterior synechiae: (**a**) right eye, (**b**) left eye, (**c**) right eye zoomed in, (**d**) left eye zoomed in

that the most likely diagnosis of the patients' new signs and symptoms were a toxic side effect of the immune checkpoint inhibitor therapy resulting in a pan-uveitis and optic neuropathy. Further work-up was attempted, however the patient denied lumbar puncture due to improvement on empiric therapy, which highlights the challenge of balancing the treatment burden on the patient while still being diligent in doing what you can to acquire the appropriate diagnosis.

Using the Austin-Bradford-Hill criteria for causality, there is a plausible cause for the immune checkpoint inhibitors to cause uveitis and optic neuropathy as it has been reported in the literature. We are bound by the ethics of non-maleficence so re-challenging the patient with the suspected therapy would doing the patient harm and would be unethical unless the benefit outweighed the risk of rechallenge. There is a temporal relationship to when the suspected therapy and the onset of symptoms occurred. The Strength correlation cannot be tested for the same reasoning as discussed when addressing consistency. Specificity was evaluated using imaging and clinical judgement as only pembrolizumab has been associated with both uveitis and optic nerve involvement [1, 2]. Finally, the change in the risk factor was evaluated by stopping the presumed offending medication and witnessing the improvement in the patient. It is of note that treatment with systemic and topical therapies were also started at this time and as such would be a confounding effect on the observation of improvement of the patient's condition solely by removal of the

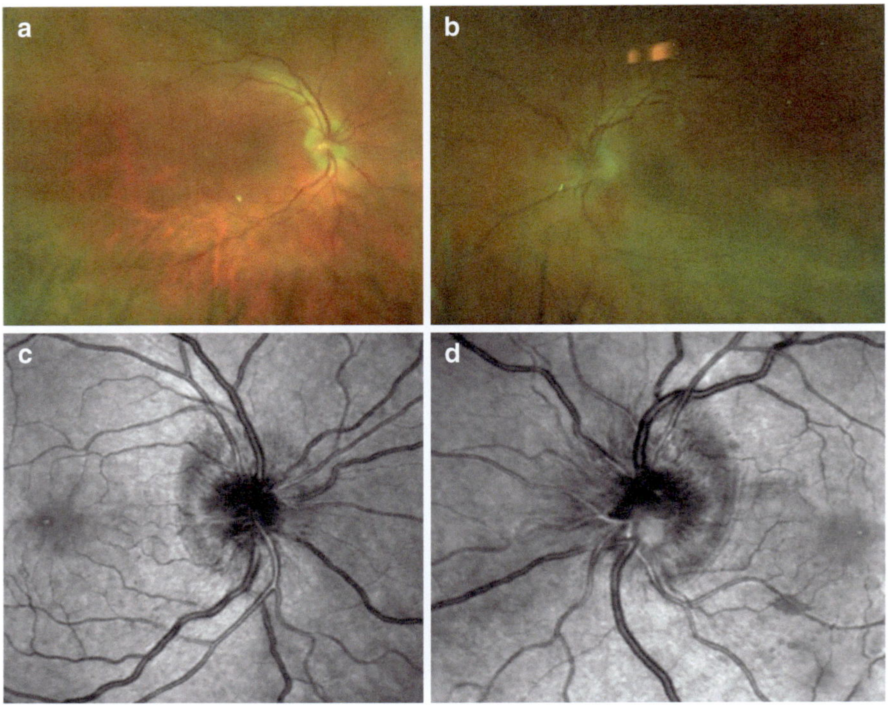

Fig. 44.2 Fundus photographs showing optic disc edema—(**a**) right eye, (**b**) left eye, (**c**) right eye, (**d**) left eye

offending agent. The criteria were then determined to have been met to the best possible degree in the given circumstances and the causal relationship of Pembrolizumab was established and used to guide treatment.

Management Options

There are no consensus statements on diagnosis and management of ocular immune related adverse events (irAEs). Recommendations are based on level V evidence (Studies without control group, case reports, expert opinions) and grade B level of recommendation (Strong or moderate evidence for efficacy but with a limited clinical benefit, generally recommended).

High dose intravenous (IV) corticosteroids followed by a slow prednisone taper is the mainstay for treatment for optic nerve disc edema. Therefore, our patient was taken off pembrolizumab and started on intravenous (IV) methylprednisolone 1000 mg for 3–5 days followed by oral prednisone 1 mg/kg/day then tapered gradually [3]. In addition to IV therapy, topical steroids and cycloplegics can be added to help control the anterior and intermediate uveitis. In our patient topical Difluprednate

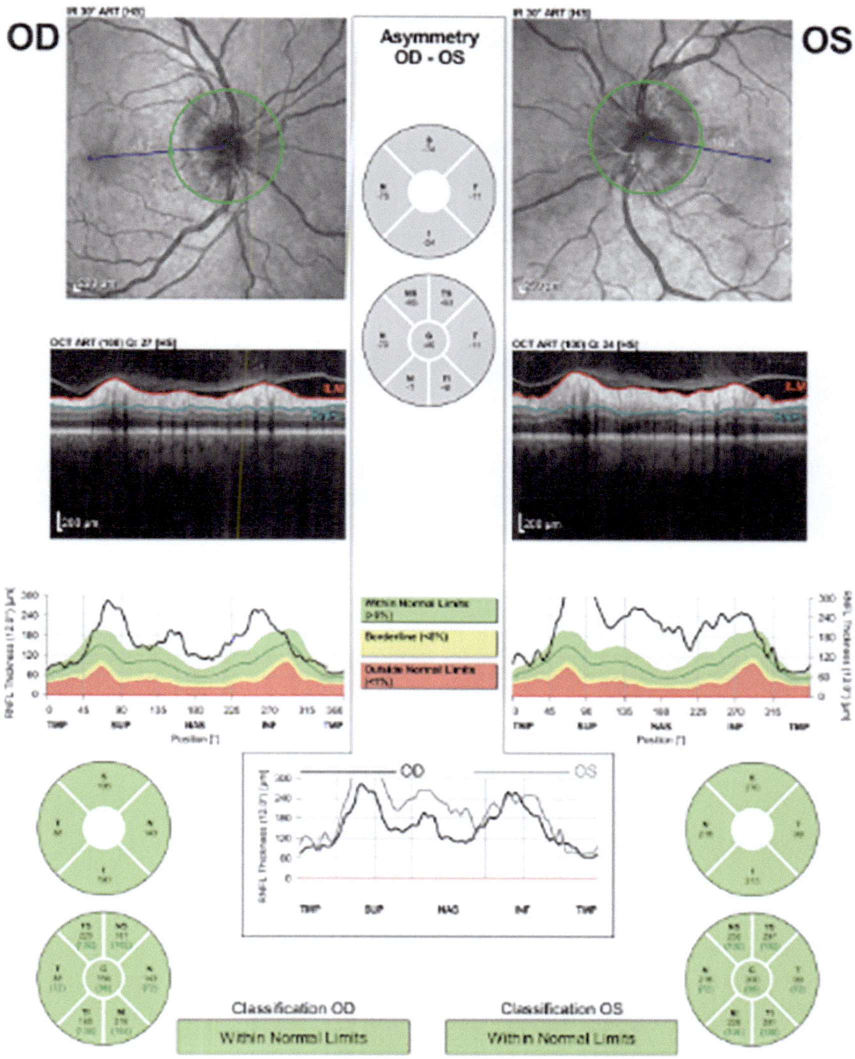

Fig. 44.3 OCT of the optic nerve and macula demonstrating optic disc edema and sub-foveal fluid

eye drop four times daily for 1 week then followed by weekly taper to three times daily for a week then twice daily for a week then once daily for a week. Atropine eye drops were added twice daily to help control the anterior and intermediate immune reaction.

Follow Up and Outcome

After the cessation of the pembrolizumab and the starting of topical and systemic therapies on his first follow up, his vision had improved to 20/25 and 20/20 OU. On SLM showed resolution of the anterior uveitis. Pupils remained fixed at 6 mm but there was improvement in the 360-degree posterior synechiae. On dilated fundus exam the patient had improvement of the disc edema from the initial grade IV to grade I and resolution of the subretinal fluid in the macula, confirmed on OCT RNFL and OCT macula (Figs. 44.4 and 44.5).

Summary and Timeline

In summary, this was a Caucasian male in his 60s with anaplastic thyroid carcinoma being treated at MD Anderson Cancer Center with dabrafenib, trametinib, and pembrolizumab leading to bilateral anterior uveitis, optic neuritis and central serous retinopathy after 2 months. Patient improved with intravenous steroid and withholding pembrolizumab, topical difluprednate, and topical atropine, with vision returned to baseline post treatment. The decision was made not to rechallenge with pembrolizumab. Patient is still undergoing cancer treatment with marked clinical and radiographic improvement showing resolution of metastatic pulmonary disease and near resolution of lower neck disease at 1 month follow up post uveitis (Fig. 44.6).

Discussion

The challenges we face in our patient population when a patient exhibits new ocular symptoms and signs is whether it is the cancer itself (direct, metastatic, infection or indirect paraneoplastic effect) vs. cancer treatment related conditions (e.g., radiation, chemotherapy, immune related adverse events from immune checkpoint inhibitors, such as irAEs).

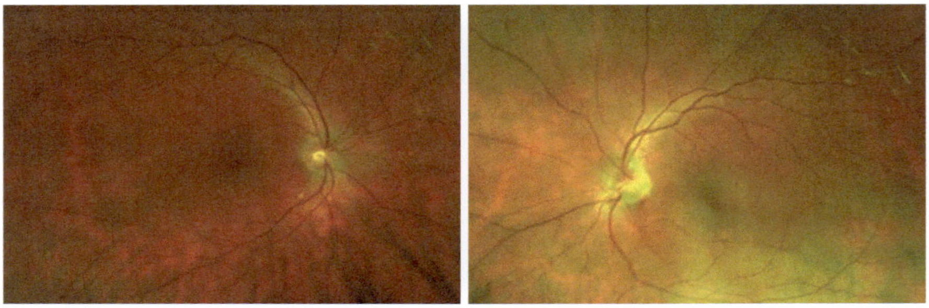

Fig. 44.4 Fundus photo showing improvement of the optic disc edema

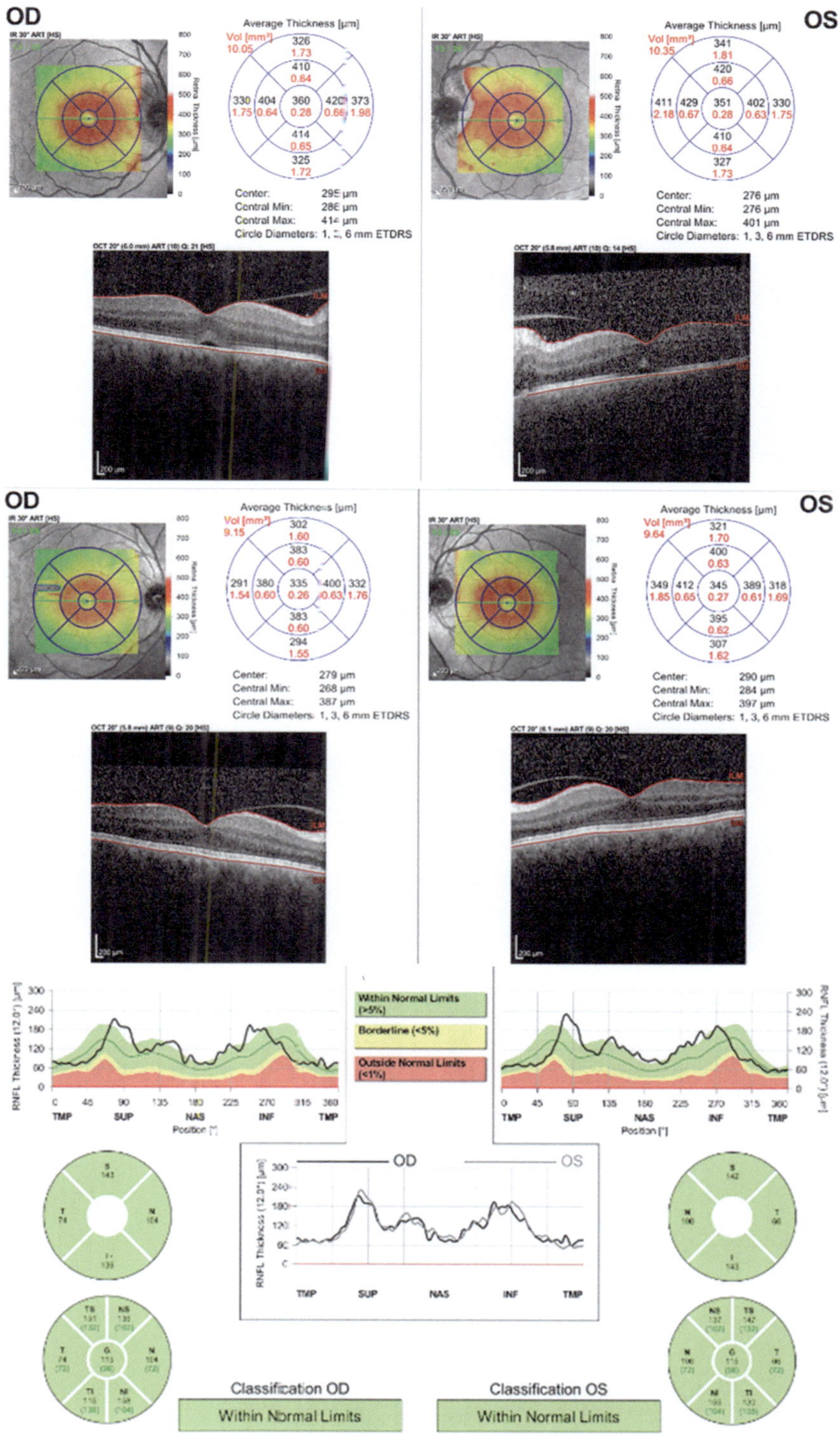

Fig. 44.5 OCT of the macula and RNFL showing improvement of the subretinal fluid and optic disc edema

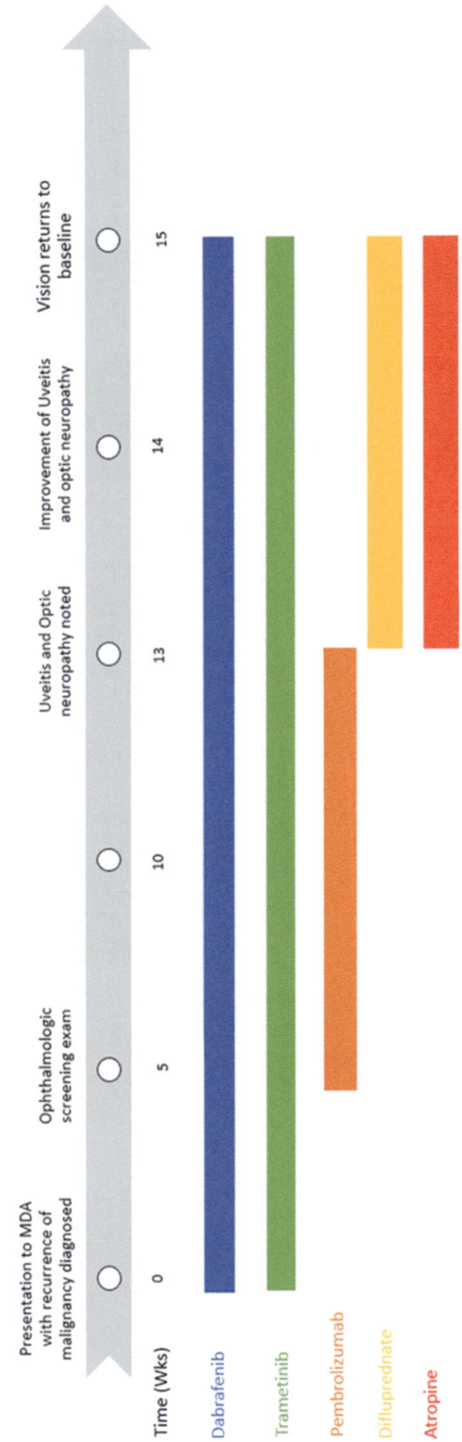

Fig. 44.6 Summary of patient's disease course with timeline of events (timepoint of 0 is cancer recurrence)

The three cancer treatment medications dabrafenib (BRAF-inhibitor), trametinib (MEK 1/2-inhibitor), pembrolizumab (PD-1 inhibitor) all can cause irAEs [4]. BRAF-inhibitors and MEK 1/2-inhibitors have been reported to be associated with central serous retinopathy and uveitis [5, 6]. PD-1 inhibitors have been reported to cause uveitis and optic neuritis [1, 2]. Given that this patient had a life threatening cancer and needed triplet therapy, after a multidisciplinary discussion between ophthalmology, oncology, endocrinology, it was determined to stop only one agent at a time as opposed to stopping all three. Pembrolizumab was held as being the only agent with a known association with optic neuritis. Under ideal circumstances the patient would undergo evaluation using the Bradford-hill criteria for causality [7].

While the severity of ocular involvement can widely vary, it is important that providers of all specialties that treat patients undergoing oncologic treatment be aware of the potential ocular side effects of such treatments. In this case the patient was able to return to his baseline vision without any apparent permanent deficits thanks to the timely recognition and action to manage these off target affects by his multi-disciplinary team of providers. The use of such a team led to not only the patient recovering from his vision but also the ability to remain on the majority of their treatment regimen, highlighting the balance between maintaining treatment of the patient's primary condition and management of the symptoms that might arise from that treatment.

References

1. Telfah M, Whittaker TJ, Doolittle GC. Vision loss with pembrolizumab treatment: a report of two cases. J Oncol Pharm Pract. 2019;25(6):1540–6. https://doi.org/10.1177/1078155219841683. Epub 2019 Apr 18. PMID: 30997872.
2. Makri OE, Dimitrakopoulos FI, Tsapardoni F, Tsekouras I, Argyriou AA, Kalofonos H, Georgakopoulos CD. Isolated optic neuritis after pembrolizumab administration for non-small-cell lung carcinoma. Int J Neurosci. 2022;132(7):643–8. https://doi.org/10.1080/00207454.2020.1831489. Epub 2020 Oct 14. PMID: 32998608.
3. Haanen JBAG, Carbonnel F, Robert C, Kerr KM, Peters S, Larkin J, et al. Management of toxicities from immunotherapy: ESMO clinical practice guidelines for diagnosis, treatment and follow-up. Ann Oncol. 2017;28(Suppl 4):iv119–42. https://doi.org/10.1093/annonc/mdx225.
4. Ramos-Casals M, Brahmer JR, Callahan MK, et al. Immune-related adverse events of checkpoint inhibitors. Nat Rev Dis Primers. 2020;6:38. https://doi.org/10.1038/s41572-020-0160-6.
5. Sarny S, Neumayer M, Kofler J, El-Shabrawi Y. Ocular toxicity due to Trametinib and Dabrafenib. BMC Ophthalmol. 2017;17(1):146. https://doi.org/10.1186/s12886-017-0541-0. PMID: 28818062; PMCID: PMC5561643.
6. Tarım B, Kılıç M. Ocular side effects of Trametinib and Dabrafenib: a case report. J Ophthalmic Inflamm Infect. 2023;13:17. https://doi.org/10.1186/s12348-023-00339-0.
7. Fedak KM, Bernal A, Capshaw ZA, Gross S. Applying the Bradford Hill criteria in the 21st century: how data integration has changed causal inference in molecular epidemiology. Emerg Themes Epidemiol. 2015;12:14. https://doi.org/10.1186/s12982-015-0037-4. PMID: 26425136; PMCID: PMC4589117.

Chapter 45
Autoimmune Retinopathy Secondary to Nivolumab

Phillip Saikaly, Charles Drescher, Sharel C. Ongchin, and Kelly G. Paulson

Abbreviations

ALT	Alanine aminotransferase
AST	Aspartate aminotransferase
dMMR	Mismatch repair deficient
FIGO	Federation Internationale de Gynecolgie et d'Obstetrique
IADL	Instrumental activity of daily living
iRAE	Immune related adverse event

P. Saikaly
Elson S Floyd College of Medicine, Washington State University, Spokane, WA, USA
e-mail: psaikaly@wsu.edu

C. Drescher
Departments of Gynecology-Oncology and Medical Oncology, Providence-Swedish Cancer Institute, Seattle, WA, USA

Fred Hutchinson Cancer Center, Seattle, WA, USA
e-mail: cdresche@fredhutch.org

S. C. Ongchin
Retina Consultants of Seattle, Seattle, WA, USA
e-mail: songchin@rcseattle.com

K. G. Paulson (✉)
Elson S Floyd College of Medicine, Washington State University, Spokane, WA, USA

Departments of Gynecology-Oncology and Medical Oncology, Providence-Swedish Cancer Institute, Seattle, WA, USA
e-mail: kelly.paulson@providence.org

Y. Wang (ed.), *Challenging Cases in Immunotherapy Related Organ Toxicities*,
https://doi.org/10.1007/978-3-031-83533-9_45

Clinical Presentation and Clinical Course

A female patient in her 50 s presented with abdominal pain and was found to have mismatch repair deficient (dMMR) FIGO stage IVB endometrial cancer. She received initial surgical debulking followed by carboplatin and paclitaxel chemotherapy. Given the poor response to chemotherapy, she then received second-line ipilimumab and nivolumab per clinical trial [1]. Initial dual checkpoint blockade was complicated by several iRAEs including grade 2 rash, grade 1 autoimmune hepatitis and grade 1 pneumonitis. These toxicities were readily managed with corticosteroids, which were tapered off successfully. Patient then returned to nivolumab monotherapy. Patient achieved complete remission radiographically. Hepatitis and pneumonitis remained quiescent.

25 months after nivolumab resumption patient developed slowly progressive visual findings including blurred vision, difficulty with night vision, and loss of peripheral vision. Soon she developed difficulties with IADLs such as driving. There was not redness or pain in either eye. On ophthalmologic evaluation, she was noted to have marked decline in visual acuity to 20/60 along with bilateral extensive retinal pigment degeneration involving the macula and peripheral retina. Confirmatory exam by retina specialist was significant for bilateral loss of the outer retinal layer with loss of both the ellipsoid layer and photoreceptors. Exam was further notable for macular edema along with a parafoveal ring of enhanced autofluorescence with normal autofluorescence within the ring and hypoautofluorescence mottling outside the ring (Fig. 45.1).

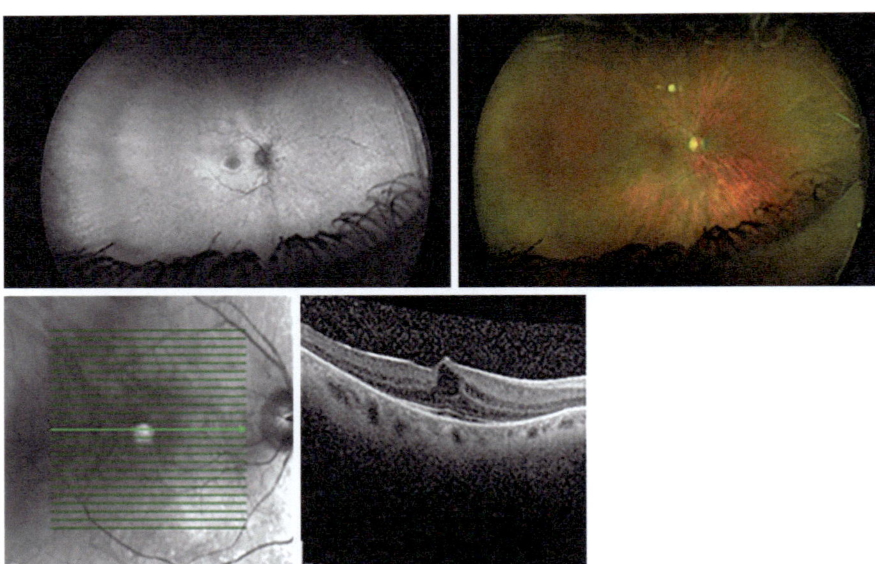

Fig. 45.1 Retinal Findings (right eye) at time of symptom peak are shown. Bilateral pigment degeneration and macular edema was observed along with a parafoveal ring of enhanced autofluorescence with normal autofluorescence within the ring and hypoautofluorescence outside the ring

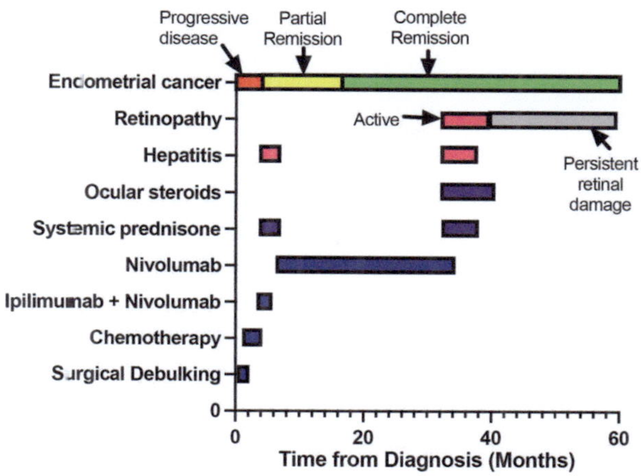

Fig. 45.2 Timeline. Timeline of events as described in the case report are shown, with 0 representing the time of diagnosis

Laboratory studies at the time of ocular findings were significant for recurrence of the autoimmune hepatitis with AST and ALT values between 3–5× upper limit of normal and a normal bilirubin. Laboratory studies were otherwise unremarkable. Anti-recoverin and anti-retinal antibody panel were negative. Cross-sectional imaging was again with no evidence of disease.

Systemic corticosteroids (prednisone starting at 1 mg/kg and tapering by 5-10 mg weekly) and topical corticosteroids were initiated and then tapered over a 3-month period (systemic) and 6-month period (topical), with taper speed dictated by patient's hepatitis (Fig. 45.2). With steroid treatment, vision rapidly improved although did not return to pre-treatment baseline. Repeat imaging studies showed no progression of photoreceptor loss and overall stability of hyperautofluorescent and hypoautofluorescent lesions in both eyes.

Clinical Outcome

4.5 years from ipilimumab/nivolumab initiation and 2 years from last nivolumab treatment, patient remained cancer remission. She has not had further flares in ocular symptoms and there has been no progression on retinal imaging. Some loss of visual acuity persisted (20/30) and patient has returned to most iADLs (still limited in night driving) until last follow up 2 weeks ago.

Summary of the Case

This is a case with advanced dMMR endometrial cancer received ipilimumab/nivolumab therapy followed by nivolumab maintenance. After approximately 2 years of maintenance she developed new clinically significant vision deficits and was found to have pronounced retinal findings. Systemic and ocular corticosteroid successfully improved the visual symptoms and halted the progression of the retinal condition.

Discussion

Ocular adverse events represent rare but increasingly recognized iRAEs from immune checkpoint blockade [2]. The most commonly reported ocular iRAEs are uveitis, followed by dry eye, conjunctival inflammation, and ocular myasthenia. Here we report a case of significant retinopathy induced by nivolumab with findings characteristic of autoimmune retinopathy [3]. The retinopathy can be distinguished from paraneoplastic cancer associated etiology by the lack of active cancer at time of development, rapid improvement on corticosteroids, and negative anti-recoverin antibodies [4]. Retinopathy improved with cessation of nivolumab and corticosteroids but did not fully resolve. Clinicians should be aware of this potential toxicity of immune checkpoint inhibition, which is not well characterized but has been reported in at least one other case with similar symptoms and imaging findings [5]. The delayed onset of the retinopathy in the nivolumab treatment course from presently reported case is also notable to reflect a wide window of iRAEs development that warrants vigilant surveillance and early recognition.

Conclusion

Autoimmune retinopathy is an iRAE that may be caused by immune checkpoint blockade. Early detection of this toxicity is critical as it has a potential for long term visual loss, which could be prevented by prompt treatment.

References

1. Mangat PK, Halabi S, Bruinooge SS, et al. Rationale and Design of the Targeted Agent and Profiling Utilization Registry (TAPUR) study. JCO Precis Oncologia. 2018;2018:00122. https://doi.org/10.1200/PO.18.00122.
2. Fang T, Maberley DA, Etminan M. Ocular adverse events with immune checkpoint inhibitors. J Curr Ophthalmol. 2019;31(3):319–22. https://doi.org/10.1016/j.joco.2019.05.002.
3. Grange L, Dalal M, Nussenblatt RB, Sen HN. Autoimmune retinopathy. Am J Ophthalmol. 2014;157(2):266–272.e1. https://doi.org/10.1016/j.ajo.2013.09.019.
4. Goldstein SM, Syed NA, Milam AH, Maguire AM, Lawton TJ, Nichols CW. Cancer-associated retinopathy. Arch Ophthalmol. 1999;117(12):1641–5. https://doi.org/10.1001/archopht.117.12.1641.
5. Ghoraba H, Or C, Karaca I, et al. Immunotherapy-induced retinopathy mimicking cancer associated retinopathy. Am J Ophthalmol Case Rep. 2022;26:101449. https://doi.org/10.1016/j.ajoc.2022.101449.

Part X
Pancreatology

Chapter 46
Pancreatitis Related to Immune Checkpoint Inhibitor Therapy

Sidra Naz, Sireesha Yedururi, Yinghong Wang, Suresh Chari, and Anusha S. Thomas

Abbreviations

CT	Computed tomography
ICI	Immune checkpoint inhibitor
irAEs	Immune related adverse events

Introduction

Immune checkpoint inhibitors (ICI) have revolutionized the treatment of various malignancies. However, these therapies are associated with immune-related adverse events (irAEs), which can significantly impact patient management. Pancreatic irAEs are rare and may have a varied spectrum of clinical presentation as is demonstrated in the case series to follow.

PATIENT 1: Asymptomatic Elevation of Lipase Following Nivolumab Plus Ipilimumab Immunotherapy in a Patient with Urothelial Carcinoma.

A Caucasian male in 60 s with recently diagnosed lung and intrathoracic nodal metastatic disease from previously treated urothelial carcinoma of the urinary

S. Naz · Y. Wang · S. Chari · A. S. Thomas (✉)
Department of Gastroenterology, Hepatology & Nutrition, Division of Internal Medicine, The University of Texas MD Anderson Cancer Center, Houston, TX, USA
e-mail: SNaz@mdanderson.org; STChari@mdanderson.org; asthomas1@mdanderson.org

S. Yedururi
Department of Abdominal Imaging, The University of Texas MD Anderson Cancer Center, Houston, TX, USA
e-mail: SYedururi@mdanderson.org

Y. Wang
Department of Gastroenterology, Hepatology & Nutrition, The University of Texas MD Anderson Cancer Center, Houston, TX, USA
e-mail: YWang59@mdanderson.org

Y. Wang (ed.), *Challenging Cases in Immunotherapy Related Organ Toxicities*, https://doi.org/10.1007/978-3-031-83533-9_46

bladder on ICI therapy developed an asymptomatic elevation of lipase (1672 U/L) after 4 months of 2 cycles of combination immunotherapy i.e., nivolumab plus ipilimumab. Medical history was notable for childhood asthma, cataract and a pulmonary embolism.

Notably, there were no associated clinical symptoms of abdominal pain, nausea or emesis. Contrast enhanced computed tomography (CT) imaging of the abdomen did not demonstrate any evidence of peripancreatic edema or diffuse enlargement of the pancreas at the time of elevated serum lipase. However, at serial volumetry pancreatic volume has slightly increased (~19%) above pretreatment baseline at the time of pancreatic lipase elevation with subsequent decrease (~22%) below the pretreatment baseline at 2 year follow up study (Fig. 46.1). The elevated lipase levels continued to fluctuate over subsequent visits, but the patient remained asymptomatic. Given the asymptomatic nature of the lipase elevation and particularly the absence of clinical or imaging evidence of pancreatitis, ICI was continued.

Due to disease progression and eventual endocrinological irAE i.e., ICI related thyroiditis necessitating hormone replacement therapy, ICI was discontinued after 9 months of treatment, and the patient transitioned well to lxazomib with gemcitabine. Serial neck CT images in this patient before and immediately after stopping ICI treatment show diffuse thyroid atrophy.

At follow up, 2 years after exposure to ICI, the lipase levels were within normal limits. There was no clinical evidence of exocrine/ endocrine pancreatic insufficiency even though minimal pancreatic parenchymal volume loss was detected at serial pancreas volumetry. The patient passed away due to disease progression ~2 years of discontinuing treatment.

PATIENT 2: Asymptomatic lipase elevation with imaging evidence of pancreatitis.

A Caucasian male in 30 s with left upper back melanoma treated with wide local excision and sentinel lymph node biopsy followed by left axillary lymphadenectomy and adjuvant treatment completed 2 years back was recently diagnosed with peritoneal and retroperitoneal metastatic disease. Otherwise, medical history was notable for hypertension, asthma, and psoriasis. He was started on combination

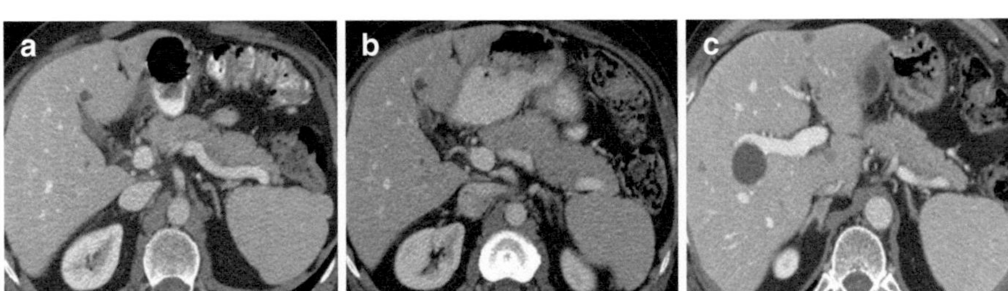

Fig. 46.1 Abdominal imaging of pancreas for patient 1. (**a**) at baseline before ICI initiation, (**b**) while receiving ICI treatment with lipase elevation and new mild enlargement of pancreas with mild peri-pancreatic edema, (**c**) 2 years post-peak lipase elevation shows diffuse pancreatic volume atrophy

immunotherapy treatment. A routine restaging contrast enhanced CT after 6 cycles of immunotherapy showed new mild peripancreatic fat stranding without peripancreatic fluid collections or necrosis concerning for acute interstitial pancreatitis (Fig. 46.2). Clinically, the patient was asymptomatic without reported abdominal pain, nausea, emesis or diarrhea. Routine labs showed an elevated lipase and amylase levels of 2098 U/L and 167 U/L respectively. Due to the asymptomatic nature of pancreatic enzyme elevation and imaging findings, immunotherapy was continued. A subsequent follow up CT after 2 years showed mild diffuse pancreatic volume loss on visual assessment. At serial pancreatic volumetry, the pancreatic volume has decreased slightly (~5%) from the pretreatment baseline at the time of elevated lipase and significantly more (~55%) at 2 year follow up.

At subsequent visits, lipase levels continued to fluctuate, and imaging changes resolved spontaneously. Cancer course was complicated by progression of disease with brain metastasis and leptomeningeal disease necessitating a brief course of targeted therapy with encorafenib and binimetinib with subsequent resumption of nivolumab monotherapy. Other immune related adverse events sustained included grade 1 hepatitis and colitis managed with steroids. At last visit, following 5 years

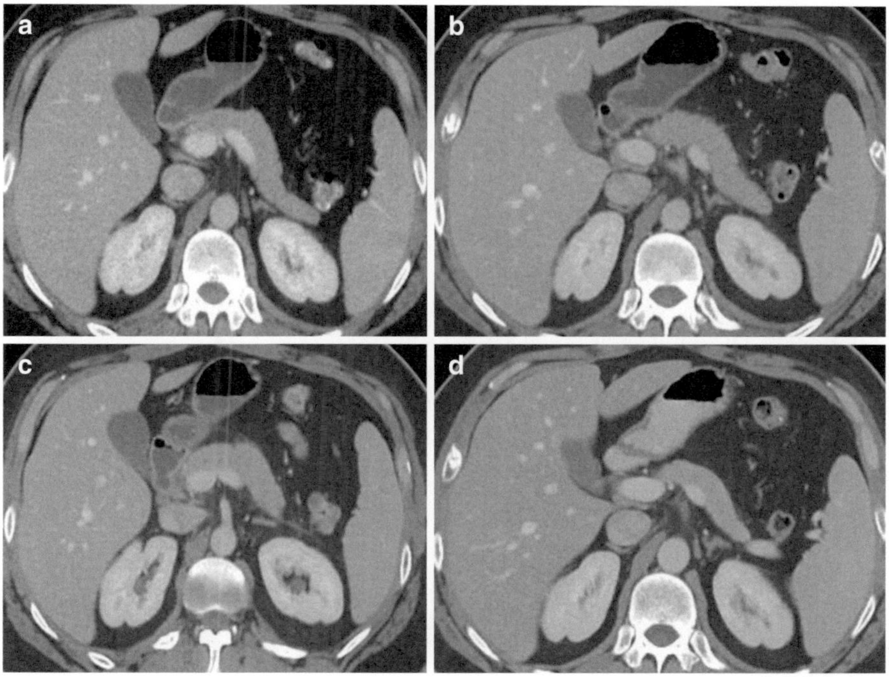

Fig. 46.2 Abdominal imaging of pancreas for patient 2. (**a**) at baseline before ICI initiation, (**b**) while receiving ICI treatment with elevation of lipase shows new mild peripancreatic fat stranding without peripancreatic fluid collections or necrosis, (**c**) On ICI treatment, at peak lipase elevation mild diffuse enlargement of pancreas with mild peripancreatic edema, (**d**) 2 years post-peak lipase elevation shows mild diffuse pancreatic volume loss

of immunotherapy, his cancer remains stable. His lipase levels have completely normalized; however, his pancreas shows persistent and grossly stable parenchymal atrophy.

PATIENT 3: Clinical pancreatitis with normal imaging.

A female in 50 s with melanoma of the right thigh previously treated with wide local excision presented with recurrence in the right inguinal lymph node and received combined immunotherapy with ipilimumab and nivolumab followed by surgical resection and nivolumab monotherapy maintenance.

Treatment course was complicated with grade 3 colitis requiring hospital admission after 17 cycles of immunotherapy necessitating initiation of systemic corticosteroids. Shortly thereafter, the patient was re-admitted with nausea, emesis and upper abdominal pain characteristic for pancreatitis. Both lipase and amylase levels were elevated at 2562 U/L and 134 U/L respectively. Contrast enhanced CT imaging performed 1 month later did not show any peripancreatic edema or pancreatic enlargement.

Immunotherapy was held and weight based steroid therapy was administered with consequential normalization of pancreatic enzymes. However, subsequent visits showed fluctuating lipase levels, without remarkable clinical symptoms.

Note was made of mild atrophy on follow up contrasted imaging of the abdomen about 2.5 years later (Fig. 46.3). Serial pancreatic volumetry from the studies acquired at ~4 months after starting immunotherapy, 1 month after detecting elevated serum lipase/amylase and 2.5 years later confirmed the findings at visual assessment with significant volume loss on the studies done 1 month (31%) and 2.5 years (45%) after the detection of elevated lipase/amylase.

Recurrence of malignant melanoma was managed with surgical intervention and adjuvant targeted therapy. While his disease course has been complicated with presumed drug induced elevated liver function tests (LFT), his cancer remains in remission. His lipase was normal at last follow up and he was noted to have persistent grossly stable pancreas volume loss on further follow up studies 5.5 years after initial lipase elevation upon visual assessment.

PATIENT 4: Clinical pancreatitis with imaging evidence of pancreatitis.

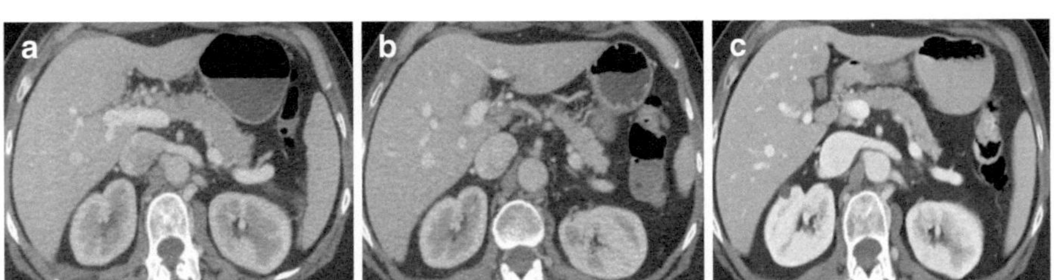

Fig. 46.3 Abdominal imaging of pancreas for patient 3. (**a**) 4 months after starting ICI, before serum lipase elevation shows mild diffuse enlargement of the pancreas with mild peripancreatic edema; (**b**) 16 months after starting ICI and 1 month after peak serum lipase elevation shows pancreatic volume loss; (**c**) 2.5 years post-peak lipase elevation shows diffuse pancreatic atrophy

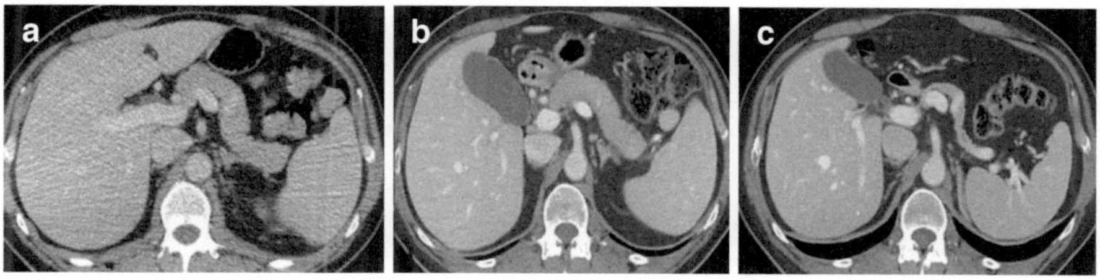

Fig. 46.4 Abdominal imaging of pancreas for patient 4. (**a**) at baseline before ICI initiation, (**b**) show diffuse enlargement of the pancreas at the time of elevated lipase with mild peripancreatic edema, (**c**) subsequent follow-up CT almost 2 years after peak lipase elevation shows diffuse pancreatic atrophy

A Caucasian female in 50 s with history of previously treated melanoma of the abdominal wall with wide local excision presented with breast metastasis and received combination immunotherapy with pembrolizumab and ipilimumab. Medical history was significant for hypothyroidism, anemia, and hypertension. Following the completion of 13 cycles of therapy, the patient developed type 3 autoimmune pancreatitis characterized by abdominal pain and nausea. Laboratory investigations revealed elevated lipase and amylase levels at 489 U/L and 226 U/L respectively. A non-contrast CT of the abdomen at the time of elevated pancreatic enzymes confirmed acute pancreatitis characterized by diffuse pancreatic enlargement and peripancreatic fat stranding (Fig. 46.4).

Weight based steroid treatment in conjunction with withholding ICI led to a clinical improvement. Serial CT imaging studies show diffuse enlargement of pancreas at the time of elevated lipase and follow up CT 2 years later showed no pancreatic atrophy on visual assessment. At serial pancreatic volumetry the pancreas volume increased to ~25% above pretreatment baseline on the CT at the time of elevated lipase and then decreased to 27% below the pretreatment baseline on the follow up CT acquired 2.3 years later. Biochemically, lipase levels remained elevated at 800 U/L in absence of clinical signs of pancreatitis. Cancer course was complicated by right lobular breast carcinoma status post surgery along with hormonal therapy and radiotherapy. At last follow up, her melanoma remains in remission, and the patient was under observation with no appreciable pancreas volume loss on imaging.

Discussion

Pancreatic injury has been reported as irAE related to ICI among cancer patients even severe necrotizing pancreatitis in rare cases (1–3). Our case series highlights varied clinical presentations of this irAE that can persist as mere biochemical abnormalities (Fig. 46.5) or show varying degree of anatomical changes suggestive of acute pancreatitis on CT exam at or around the time of elevated lipase levels. In addition, recently pancreatic volume loss has also been described as a long term

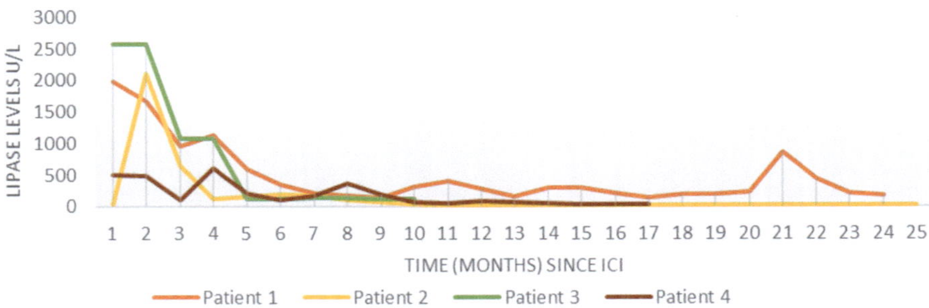

Fig. 46.5 Lipase levels (U/L) in our sample post ICI therapy

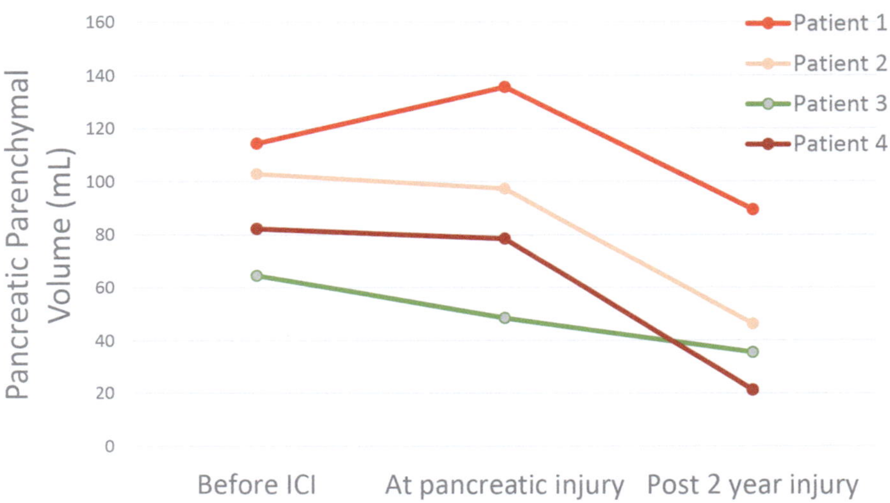

Fig. 46.6 Pancreatic volume in our sample with pancreatic irAEs

consequence (4) which is demonstrated among this cohort in Fig. 46.6. Due to the curvilinear orientation of pancreas closely aligned with the C-loop of duodenum, pancreatic volume loss is difficult to detect visually and necessitates detailed comparisons with pretreatment baseline studies. Owing to the limitations of visual assessment, serial volumetry can be used to establish pancreatic volume loss. A common pattern observed on serial imaging studies in patients on ICI therapy presenting with symptomatic or asymptomatic elevation of serum lipase is diffuse pancreatic enlargement on CTs around the time of peak lipase elevation followed by variable degree of pancreatic volume loss. Given the limited data in this field, further studies are needed to understand the risk of pancreatic insufficiency in these cases as well as appropriate ways to mitigate the long term sequelae [1–4].

References

1. Abu-Sbeih H, Tang T, Lu Y, Thirumurthi S, Altan M, Jazaeri AA, et al. Clinical characteristics and outcomes of immune checkpoint inhibitor-induced pancreatic injury. J Immunother Cancer. 2019;7:31.
2. Friedman CF, Clark V, Raikhel AV, Barz T, Shoushtari AN, Momtaz P, et al. Thinking critically about classifying adverse events: incidence of pancreatitis in patients treated with nivolumab + ipilimumab. J Natl Cancer Inst. 2017;109:djw260. Abu-Sbeih H, Tang T, Lu Y, et al. Clinical characteristics and outcomes of immune checkpoint inhibitor-induced pancreatic injury. J Immunother Cancer. 2019;7(1):31.
3. Khurana S, Chi Zhang H, Peng Y, Lu Y, Wang Y. Severe fistulizing pancreatitis in a patient with Merkel cell carcinoma treated with avelumab. Eur J Gastroenterol Hepatol. 2020;32(9):1266–7.
4. Thomas AS, Abreo M, Sayed SA, Yedururi YWS, Chari ST. Autoimmune pancreatitis secondary to immune checkpoint inhibitor therapy (type 3 AIP): insights into a new disease from serial pancreatic imaging. Gastroenterology. 2022;164(1):154–5.

Chapter 47
Necrotizing Pancreatitis Related to Immune Checkpoint Inhibitor Therapy

Sidra Naz, Sireesha Yedururi, Yinghong Wang, Suresh Chari, and Anusha S. Thomas

Abbreviations

CT	Computed tomography
ICI	Immune checkpoint inhibitor
irAEs	Immune related adverse events
TPN	Total Parenteral Nutrition

Case Presentation

A Caucasian male in 60 s with a history of stage 3 Merkel cell carcinoma of the right upper limb with wide local excision presented with right axillary lymph node metastases and received adjuvant immune checkpoint inhibitor (ICI) avelumab as treatment. Medical history was significant for hypertension, type 2 diabetes, and splenic vein thrombosis. Following the completion of 6 cycles of ICI, the patient developed necrotizing pancreatitis characterized by severe abdominal pain, nausea, vomiting,

S. Naz · Y. Wang · S. Chari · A. S. Thomas (✉)
Department of Gastroenterology, Hepatology & Nutrition, The University of Texas MD Anderson Cancer Center, Houston, TX, USA
e-mail: SNaz@mdanderson.org; YWang59@mdanderson.org; STChari@mdanderson.org; asthomas1@mdanderson.org

S. Yedururi
Department of Abdominal Imaging, The University of Texas MD Anderson Cancer Center, Houston, TX, USA
e-mail: SYedururi@mdanderson.org

Y. Wang (ed.), *Challenging Cases in Immunotherapy Related Organ Toxicities*,
https://doi.org/10.1007/978-3-031-83533-9_47

and constipation. Laboratory investigations revealed elevated amylase and lipase levels at 986 U/L and 600 U/L respectively (Table 47.1). A non-contrast CT scan of the abdomen at the time of elevated pancreatitis confirmed necrotizing pancreatitis characterized by peripancreatic fluid and fat stranding, and hypodense, liquified areas in the head, body, and tail of the pancreas (Fig. 47.1).

Table 47.1 Lab values

Test	Value at onset of GI symptoms	Value at resolution of GI symptoms
Amylase (30-110 U/L)	986 U/L	45 U/L
Lipase (5–60 IU/L)	>600 IU/L	11 IU/L
White blood count (4–11 K/uL)	16 K/uL	3.7 K/uL
Hgb (14–18 gm/dL)	15.3 gm/dL	10.5 gm/dL
Platelets (140–440 K/uL)	139 K/uL	163 K/uL
Albumin (3.4–5.4 g/dL)	2.9 g/dL	4.2 g/dL
Lactic acid (0.5–2.2 mmol/L)	2.7 mmol/L	0.9 mmol/L

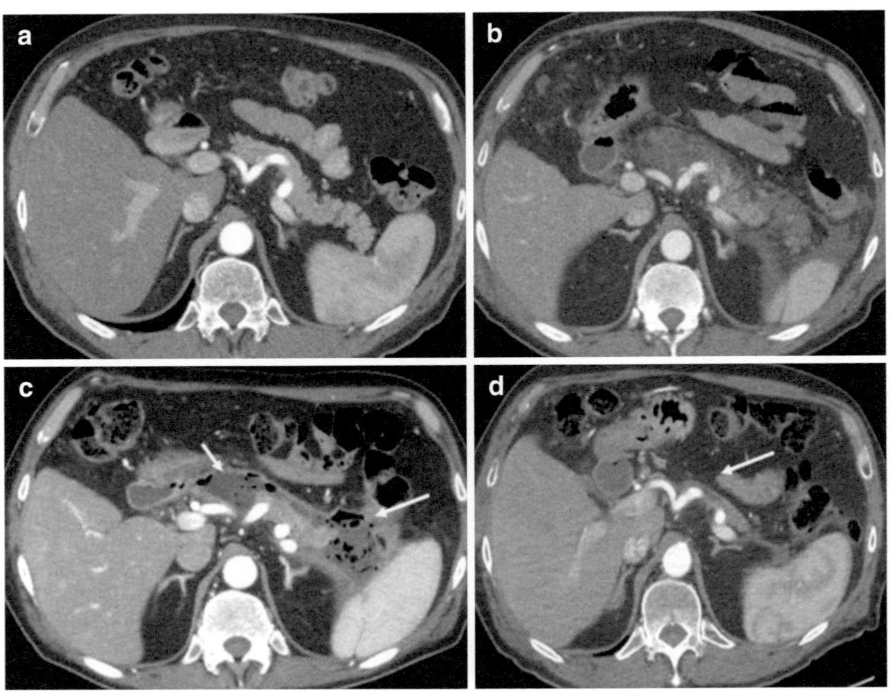

Fig. 47.1 (**a**) Abdominal imaging at baseline before ICI treatment, (**b**) CT imaging studies show diffuse enlargement of the pancreas associated with non-enhancing pancreatic parenchyma (arrow heads) at the time of elevated lipase consistent with necrotizing pancreatitis, (**c**) Follow-up CT 2 months later showed persistent pancreatic parenchymal necrosis, now showing multiple foci of air (arrows) consistent with abscess formation and this was drained. (**d**) Subsequent follow-up CT almost 1 year after peak lipase elevation shows diffuse pancreatic atrophy

Disease Course and Outcome

The patient was hospitalized and managed with weight-based steroids in conjunction with TPN and withholding ICI which led to the symptom improvement. The patient was advanced to low-fat diet and steroids on hospital discharge with eventual discontinuation of TPN. On intermittent hospital admissions due to sepsis related to necrotizing pancreatitis, serial CT scans with contrast showed increased peripancreatic fluid indicating pancreatic abscess and biochemically resolution of amylase and lipase elevation. The patient discharged on antibiotics and was continued on high dose steroids. Eight weeks follow-up imaging showed persistent pancreatic parenchymal necrosis and a fistulous communication between the pancreatic tail collection and the left colon. This required surgical intervention of pancreatic drain placement and restart on TPN for about 1 year. Notably, pancreatic enzyme levels remained within the normal range, and the patient did not report symptoms of steatorrhea. At 2-year follow-up, the CT scan findings were striking for marked pancreatic body/tail atrophy. His Merkel cell carcinoma remained in remission for 2 years of follow up despite off ICI since pancreatitis event.

Summary

This is a case with Merkel cell carcinoma, received 6 doses of avelumab with subsequent severe necrotizing pancreatitis. The disease course after steroid treatment was complicated with pancreatic abscess/fistula and sepsis requiring prolonged antibiotics, frequent drain placement and long term TPN. Patient ultimately recovered from the event after 1 year. Over the follow up of 2 years, patient developed asymptomatic pancreatic atrophy, with cancer in remission despite ICI termination. Summary of the events is depicted in Fig. 47.2.

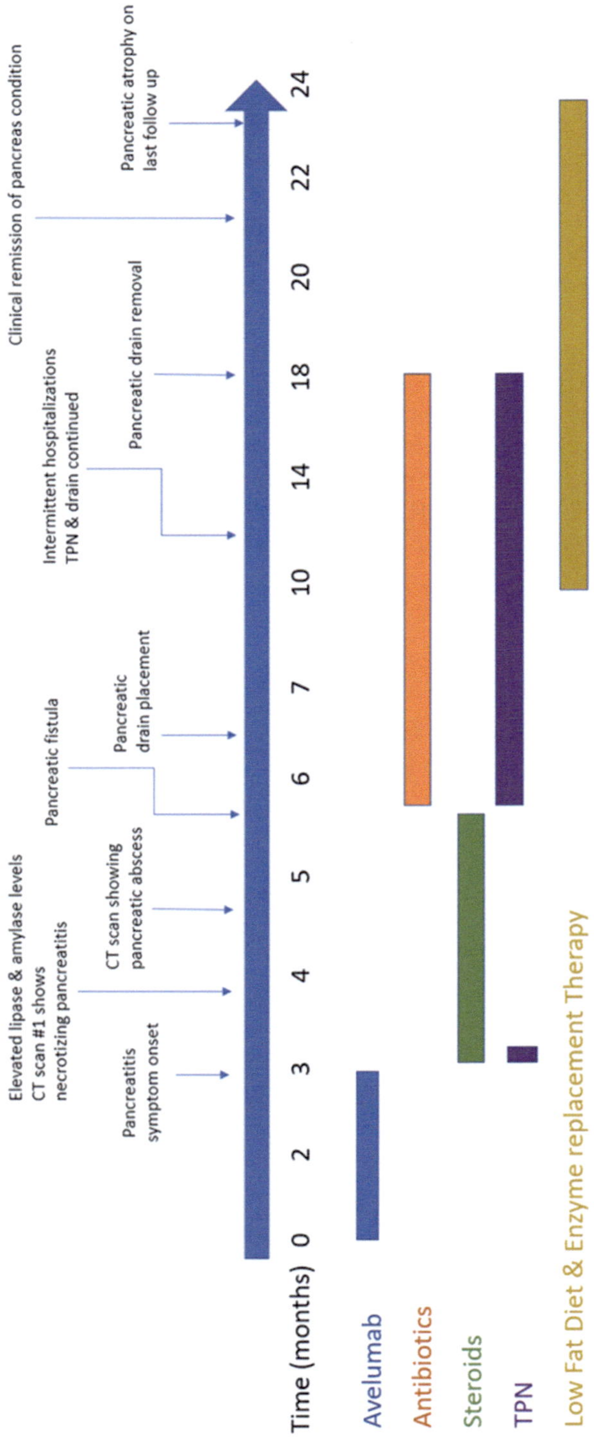

Fig. 47.2 Summary of timeline events (timepoint of 0 is the initiation of avelumab)

Discussion

Necrotizing pancreatitis, a severe form of pancreatitis characterized by tissue necrosis, is a rare but potentially life-threatening adverse event associated with ICI therapy [1]. ICI-induced pancreatic injury (ICIPI) has been previously reported with the incidence rate of 4–26.9% of ≥grade 3 elevation in amylase and lipase, respectively [2–4], however, only one-fifth of these patients (1.7% overall) developed symptomatic pancreatitis. Given the low incidence and variable onset of ICIPI, baseline testing with pancreatic enzyme levels during immunotherapy is not recommended [5]. The mechanism by which ICIs trigger necrotizing pancreatitis remains a subject of ongoing research. It is believed to be related to an immune-mediated inflammatory response against pancreatic tissue, resulting in tissue damage and necrosis. Understanding the underlying pathophysiology is essential for early recognition and management of this serious complication. This case emphasizes the significance of close monitoring and surveillance on clinical and biochemical labs of pancreas status during ICI therapy, early recognition of characteristic imaging findings, and prompt management. The decision to discontinue ICI therapy is often warranted in cases of necrotizing pancreatitis, as was done in this instance. However, it is essential to weigh the potential benefits and risks of discontinuation, considering the underlying malignancy's response to the treatment. Despite the rare incidence of necrotizing pancreatitis as irAE, this case underscores the high complexity of clinical management, the impact of cancer treatment interruption and quality of life, and significant morbidities associated with it.

Conclusion

Our case highlights the critical importance of recognizing ICI-induced necrotizing pancreatitis as a rare yet moderately severe adverse event. Early detection, and prompt management are crucial in mitigating the potential morbidity and mortality associated with this rare irAE [1]. As the use of ICIs continues to expand, clinicians must remain vigilant, and further research is needed to better understand the mechanisms and risk factors for such severe adverse events.

References

1. Khurana S, Chi Zhang H, Peng Y, Lu Y, Wang Y. Severe fistulizing pancreatitis in a patient with Merkel cell carcinoma treated with avelumab. Eur J Gastroenterol Hepatol. 2020;32(9):1266–7.
2. Motzer RJ, Penkov K, Haanen J, Rini B, Albiges L, Campbell MT, et al. Avelumab plus axitinib versus sunitinib for advanced renal-cell carcinoma. N Engl J Med. 2019;380:1103–15.
3. Friedman CF, Clark V, Raikhel AV, Barz T, Shoushtari AN, Momtaz P, et al. Thinking critically about classifying adverse events: incidence of pancreatitis in patients treated with nivolumab

+ ipilimumab. J Natl Cancer Inst. 2017;109:djw260. Abu-Sbeih H, Tang T, Lu Y, et al. Clinical characteristics and outcomes of immune checkpoint inhibitor-induced pancreatic injury. J Immunother Cancer. 2019;7(1):31.

4. Abu-Sbeih H, Tang T, Lu Y, Thirumurthi S, Altan M, Jazaeri AA, et al. Clinical characteristics and outcomes of immune checkpoint inhibitor-induced pancreatic injury. J Immunother Cancer. 2019;7:31.
5. Brahmer JR, Lacchetti C, Schneider BJ, Atkins MB, Brassil KJ, Caterino JM, et al. National Comprehensive Cancer Network. Management of immune-related adverse events in patients treated with immune checkpoint inhibitor therapy: American Society of Clinical Oncology clinical practice guideline. J Clin Oncol. 2018;36:1714–68.

Part XI
Pulmonology

Chapter 48
Immune Checkpoint Inhibitor Therapy Induced Relapsing Pneumonitis

Saad Farooq, Saadia A. Faiz, Vickie R. Shannon, and Ajay Sheshadri

Abbreviations

ALT	Alanine aminotransferase
ASCO	American Society of Clinical Oncology
AST	Aspartate aminotransferase
ATS	American Thoracic Society
BAL	Bronchoalveolar lavage
CT	Computed tomography
ESMO	European Society for Medical Oncology
ER	Estrogen receptor
HER 2	Human epidermal growth receptor 2
HIV	Human Immunodeficiency virus
ICI	Immune checkpoint inhibitors
PCR	Polymerase chain reaction
PFTS	Pulmonary function tests
PR	Progesterone receptor
RBC	Red cell count
WBC	White cell count

S. Farooq
Divisions of Critical Care, Pulmonary & Sleep Medicine, The University of Texas Houston, McGovern Medical School at UTHealth, Houston, TX, USA
e-mail: Saad.Farooq@uth.tmc.edu

S. A. Faiz · V. R. Shannon · A. Sheshadri (✉)
Department of Pulmonary Medicine, The University of Texas MD Anderson Cancer Center, Houston, TX, USA
e-mail: safaiz@mdanderson.org; vshannon@mdanderson.org; asheshadri@mdanderson.org

Y. Wang (ed.), *Challenging Cases in Immunotherapy Related Organ Toxicities*,
https://doi.org/10.1007/978-3-031-83533-9_48

Clinical Presentation

This is a Caucasian woman in her 60 s with a history of left, triple-negative (ER/PR-, HER2-), stage IIB breast cancer who presented to our hospital with dyspnea and cough. She completed curative intent neoadjuvant chemotherapy with four cycles of pembrolizumab, paclitaxel and carboplatin followed by additional cycles of pembrolizumab, doxorubicin and cyclophosphamide. Pembrolizumab was given for a total of twelve cycles but was held in between for 5 months while she was undergoing a left segmental mastectomy and subsequent radiation to the left breast. A sentinel lymph node biopsy showed pathological complete response.

Three months after her last radiation session and around the time of her tenth cycle of pembrolizumab, the patient developed progressive dyspnea and a dry cough. She also developed diarrhea around the same time, which resolved with the use of oral diphenoxylate/atropine pills. She received azithromycin and doxycycline and a 5-day course of prednisone at 40 mg/day as an outpatient, which initially ameliorated her dyspnea and cough, but her pulmonary symptoms recurred when she stopped the corticosteroids. Due to worsening of her cough and dyspnea, she was admitted to our hospital for further evaluation. Her last dose of pembrolizumab was less than a month prior to hospital admission, and further doses were held.

Upon evaluation by the pulmonary service, she was noted to have a dry cough and dyspnea that had been present for about a month, but she denied swelling in the legs, orthopnea, fevers, sore throat, skin rashes or abdominal pain. On exam, the patient was in no acute distress but required 2 liters of oxygen to maintain saturation above 90%; otherwise, vital signs were within normal limits. Breath sounds were equal and symmetric. There was no wheezing or use of accessory muscles, but rhonchi were present on the left lung base. The patient was alert and had a normal neurological exam. No jugular venous distention or peripheral edema were present. No skin rash was seen. Blood work was unremarkable and shown in Table 48.1.

A CT scan (Fig. 48.1a, b) of the chest was done and showed extensive, new consolidative opacities without cavitation affecting most of the left lung along with some new, irregular nodular opacities in the right upper and middle lobe as well. There was no mediastinal or hilar adenopathy. No evidence of metastatic disease was seen. Pulmonary function tests showed a symmetric reduction in FEV1 and FVC, moderate restriction with a total lung capacity of 61% of predicted, and a moderately reduced diffusing capacity of carbon monoxide at 52% of predicted (not corrected for hemoglobin) (Table 48.2). An echocardiogram showed normal left and right ventricular with no valvular abnormalities. There was no pericardial effusion and no evidence of diastolic dysfunction.

Table 48.1 Lab values

Variables	Value
WBC (4.1–10.5)	10.4 K/uL
Hgb (12.2–15.3)	**9.3 gm/dL (L)**
Hct (36.4–46.8)	**28.7% (L)**
Platelet count (160–397)	368 K/uL
Sodium (136–145)	140 mEq/L
Potassium (3.5–5.1)	4.5 mEq/L
Chloride (98–107)	105 mEq/L
CO2 (22–29)	27 mEq/L
BUN (6–23)	7 mg/dL
Creatinine (0.51–0.95)	**0.48 mg/dL (L)**
Glucose (70–99)	129 mg/dL
Calcium (8.4–10.2)	9.1 mg/dL
Magnesium (1.6–2.6)	2.1 mg/dL
Phosphorus (2.5–4.5)	3.8 mg/dL
Albumin (3.5–5.2)	2.4 gm/dL
ALT (≤33)	**46 U/L (H)**
AST (≤32)	17 U/L

Lab values in bold are abnormal. (H) = high, (L) = low

A bronchoscopy with BAL was performed in the right upper lobe posterior segment (B2). The returned lavage was cloudy with mucous plugs. The results are shown in Table 48.3. Infectious work-up including respiratory viral pane, COVID-19 PCR, sputum, BAL and blood cultures, fungitell, HIV, T-SPOT, urine pneumococcal and legionella antigens, were all negative.

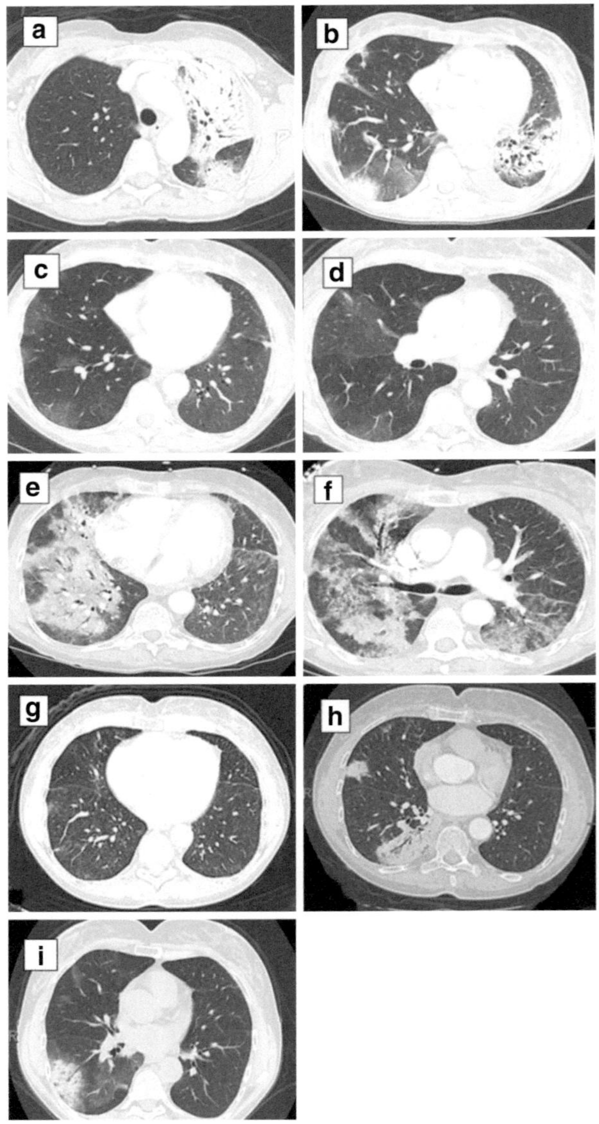

Fig. 48.1 Chest CT images. (**a**, **b**) Initial presentation showing extensive areas of consolidation especially in the left lung and some patchy, ground glass opacities in the right upper and middle lobes. (**c**, **d**): Repeat CT chest 2 months after her initial presentation to the hospital showing improvement in patchy ground glass and consolidative opacities. (**e**, **f**): Follow-up CT chest showing extensive mixed airspace and ground glass opacification throughout the right lung. Patchy ground glass opacification in the left lower lobe is also present. (**g**) CT scan done after starting corticosteroids back again 2 months after the above CT scan showing near complete resolution of extensive consolidative and ground glass opacities. (**h**) CT scan obtained at outside hospital showing right lower lobe consolidation with additional patchy consolidation in the right middle lobe. The left lung is clear. (**i**) Most recent CT scan showing new right lower lobe opacity

Table 48.2 Initial PFTS on presentation

FVC pre (2.2–3.4)	**1.25 L (L)**
FVC (% pred) pre	**44% (L)**
FEV1 pre (1.64–2.16)	**1.13 L (L)**
FEV1 (%pred) pre	**52% (L)**
FEV1/FVC pre (67.6-77.4)	90.1%
FEV1/FVC (% pred) pre	116%
TLC (3.39-5.36)	**2.68 L (L)**
TLC (% pred)	**61% (L)**
RV (1.22-2.37)	1.43 L
RV (% pred)	79%
RV/TLC (31-50)	**53% (H)**
RV/TLC (% pred)	132%
DLCO_SB (15.18)	**7.95 ml/(min*mmHg) (L)**

Lab values in bold are abnormal. (H)= high, (L)= low

Table 48.3 Bronchoscopy with BAL

Appearance	Bloody
Total cells	100
WBC	151/mcl
Lymphocytes	22%
Segmented neutrophils	41%
Eosinophils	12%
Histiocytes	22%
RBC	505
Other cells	3%

Differential Diagnosis and Treatment

Our patient had new opacities on CT chest with hypoxemia. Her CT pattern showed consolidation predominantly in the left lung, but some patchy ground glass opacities were also seen in the right lung. Organizing pneumonia and ground glass opacities are the most common patterns observed in ICI-pneumonitis but focal consolidations, nodules, septal thickening, or a combination of different patterns may be seen as well [1]. No single pattern is pathognomonic for pneumonitis, and therefore radiology alone is not sufficient to make a definitive diagnosis [2].

Our patient also had a history of radiation to the left breast which may cause pneumonitis and may present initially as ground glass opacities and later, as an organizing pneumonia pattern. Factors including the combination of chemotherapy and radiation, immunotherapy, tumor related factors such as volume of disease, and comorbid conditions such as smoking, may all increase the risk of developing radiation pneumonitis [3]. Lung involvement typically occurs in areas of irradiation, but our patient' infiltrates were not localized to the left chest only, and therefore our suspicion for radiation induced pneumonitis was low.

Table 48.4 Repeat PFTS

FVC pre (2.2–3.4)	2.48 L
FVC (% pred) pre	88%
FEV1 pre (1.64–2.16)	2.16 L
FEV1 (%pred) pre	100%
FEV1/FVC (%) pre (67.6–77.4)	87.2%
FEV1/FVC (% pred) pre	113%
TLC (3.39–5.36)	3.90 L
TLC (% pred)	89%
RV (1.22–2.37)	1.29 L
RV (% pred)	72%
RV/TLC (%) (31–50)	33%
RV/TLC (% pred)	82%
DLCO_SB (16.52)	15.14 ml/(min*mmHg)
DLCO_SB (% pred)	92

Given the lack of evidence for infection in our thorough workup, our leading diagnosis was ICI-related pneumonitis or radiation-induced pneumonitis. Patient was started on IV solumedrol 1 mg/kg/day. Her oxygen needs increased from 2 liters to 5 liters via nasal cannula, suggesting early failure of corticosteroid therapy, and therefore one dose of infliximab 5 mg/kg was also given with dramatic clinical improvement over a few days. She was discharged on a steroid taper over several weeks.

Two months later, our patient followed up in clinic and remained asymptomatic. She had recently stopped taking steroids after tapering over 6 weeks. A repeat CT chest (Fig. 48.1c, d) showed marked radiographic improvement. PFTS showed improvement as well (Table 48.4). Two weeks after stopping corticosteroids, the patient started developing tachypnea and noted a low oxygen saturation on her home pulse oximeter. She was admitted to an outside hospital and received IV antibiotics, several days of prednisone at dose of 60 mg/day and one dose of infliximab (5 mg/kg) with improvement in her symptoms. CT chest (Fig. 48.1e, f) showed new consolidative opacities predominantly affecting the right lung and ground glass opacities in the left lower lobe. The patient was discharged again on a prednisone taper over several weeks.

After this hospitalization, the patient followed up in our clinical where she remained asymptomatic on corticosteroid therapy at 10 mg/day. Repeat CT scan showed near complete resolution of extensive consolidative and ground glass opacities (Fig. 48.1g). Given the significant improvement in lung functional status, prednisone was tapered after careful assessment. However, 1 month after stopping corticosteroids for a second time, the patient had similar symptoms of cough and shortness of breath with low home pulse oximeter readings and was readmitted to an outside hospital. CT chest showed showing right lower lobe consolidation with additional patchy consolidation in the right middle lone (Fig. 48.1h). She was restarted on prednisone which improved her symptoms. She followed up in clinic 2 months after this hospitalization and was taking 5 mg prednisone per day. She was clinically doing better but her CT showed a new right lower lobe opacity, therefore her prednisone was increased to 10 mg/day again (Fig. 48.1i). She was tapered off the prednisone very slowly over the next few months (taper by 5 mg every 4 to 8 weeks, then half the dose for another 4 weeks, then stopped) to prevent further relapse. She had both radiographic and clinical improvement. Her steroids were discontinued, and she did not have any subsequent relapse.

Case Summary

We present a patient with breast cancer who received neoadjuvant chemotherapy and radiation along with pembrolizumab which led to ICI related pneumonitis. Despite the favorable response of clinical symptoms and radiological evidence from treatment of prednisone and infliximab, she had multiple subsequent pneumonitis recurrence when steroid was tapered off that led to several hospital admissions and multiple courses of steroid treatment and additional doses of infliximab. The novelty of this case is the use of infliximab early during severe pneumonitis, as well as the requirement for infliximab when pneumonitis recurred.

Discussion

ICI-pneumonitis can develop in 10–19% of patients in a real world setting [1]. ICI-pneumonitis often presents with non-specific symptoms such as cough, dyspnea, fevers, chest pain, fatigue, many of which mimic underlying cancers. The timing of ICI-pneumonitis is highly variable and can occur after the first dose or even a few months after treatment. Most commonly, cases occur within the first 2 months of treatment [2–4]. The probability of developing pneumonitis depends on several factors such as the type of cancer (which may in part be a reflection of the exposures that lead to a given cancer (such as smoking tobacco products), type of immunotherapy, the presence of preexisting lung disease, the timing and dose of thoracic radiation, concurrent chemotherapy and perhaps other comorbidities [2]. There are no diagnostic tests to confirm ICI-pneumonitis. Bronchoscopy with BAL is recommended by several professional societies but the diagnostic yield is variable, ranging from 22 to 61% [5–7]. BAL lymphocytosis may be associated with interstitial lung diseases, but the utility has not been evaluated specifically ICI pneumonitis [8]. Per American Thoracic Society (ATS) guidelines, BAL lymphocyte threshold of 20, 30 and 40% has sensitivities of 95%, 88% and 76% and specificity of 26%, 43%, 61% respectively for hypersensitivity pneumonitis [9]. The potential benefit of bronchoscopy to evaluate for infection is highest when done as early as possible [10]. Transbronchial biopsies are generally not required when the clinical picture is consistent with pneumonitis [11].Currently the management of ICI-pneumonitis is driven by expert guidelines [11, 12]· with few randomized controlled trials

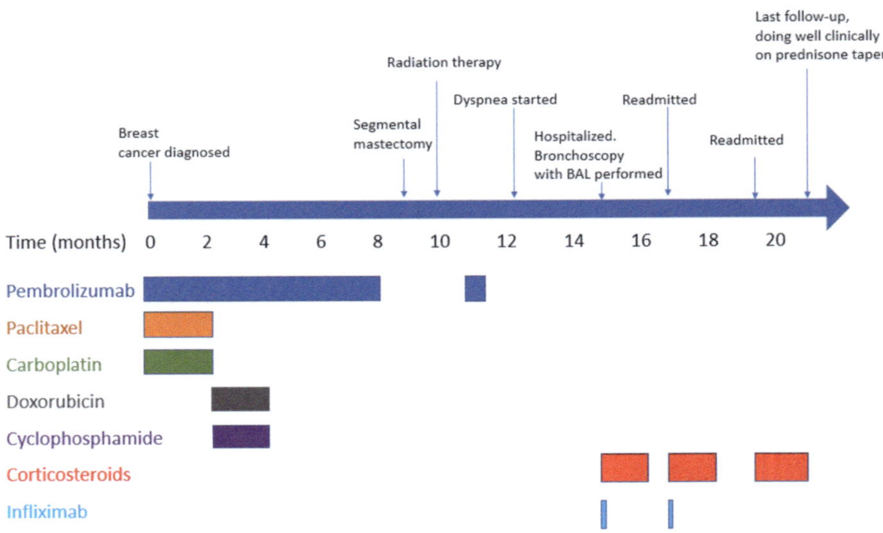

Fig. 48.2 Summary of pneumonitis disease course with timeline (timepoint of 0 is the breast diagnosis)

comparing therapeutic approaches. The mainstay of therapy for ICI-pneumonitis is systemic corticosteroids. Patients with grade 3 or higher pneumonitis should permanently discontinue ICI [13]. When there is not a sufficient response to corticosteroids, infliximab, cyclophosphamide, or mycophenolate can be considered as well. What constitutes an insufficient response is not well defined, and therefore when and in whom these therapies should be instituted is not optimally clear. Furthermore, in those who have recurrent pneumonitis, the duration of systemic immunosuppression and the utility of non-steroidal treatments (e.g., infliximab) is not clear. Infliximab was given in this setting due to clinical deterioration on corticosteroids. Another important consideration is therapeutic ICI re-challenge in patients with symptomatic pneumonitis since the rate of pneumonitis is higher than in a *de novo* setting [14]. In general, re-challenge is not attempted in patients with grade 3 or 4 pneumonitis, as per most guidelines [11, 12].

Our institutional practice is to use corticosteroids as first line and add on infliximab if there is lack of improvement on corticosteroids alone within 24 to 72 h. In a retrospective study from our institute, 94 patients were admitted for grade 3 or higher pneumonia and 11% required infliximab in addition to corticosteroids and antibitics [15]. Of the nine patients included in the study, 4 had sustained clinical improvements whereas 5 patients died [15]. Further data is still needed to optimize the use of infliximab and other second-line therapies in atypical ICI-pneumonitis cases (Fig. 48.2). In our case, her pneumonitis relapsed and required another round of corticosteroids and infliximab. Eventually a very slow and deliberate taper helped to prevent further relapse. In other cases, additional agents may be used, but this is an arena in need of further study and more evidence-based data.

References

1. Bade BC, Possick JD. Pulmonary complications of immunotherapy. Clin Chest Med. 2020;41(2):295–305. https://doi.org/10.1016/j.ccm.2020.02.012.
2. Palma DA, Senan S, Haasbeek CJA, Verbakel WFAR, Vincent A, Lagerwaard F. Radiological and clinical pneumonitis after stereotactic lung radiotherapy: a matched analysis of three-dimensional conformal and volumetric-modulated arc therapy techniques. Int J Radiat Oncol Biol Phys. 2011;80(2):506–13. https://doi.org/10.1016/j.ijrobp.2010.02.032.
3. Delaunay M, Prévot G, Collot S, Guilleminault L, Didier A, Mazières J. Management of pulmonary toxicity associated with immune checkpoint inhibitors. Eur Respir Rev. 2019;28(154):190012. https://doi.org/10.1183/16000617.0012-2019.
4. Altan M, Soto F, Zhong LL, et al. Incidence and risk factors for pneumonitis associated with checkpoint inhibitors in advanced non-small cell lung cancer: a single center experience. Oncologist. 2023;28:oyad118. https://doi.org/10.1093/oncolo/oyad118.
5. Joos L, Chhajed PN, Wallner J, et al. Pulmonary infections diagnosed by BAL: a 12-year experience in 1066 immunocompromised patients. Respir Med. 2007;101(1):93–7. https://doi.org/10.1016/j.rmed.2006.04.006.
6. Choo R, Naser NSH, Nadkarni NV, Anantham D. Utility of bronchoalveolar lavage in the management of immunocompromised patients presenting with lung infiltrates. BMC Pulm Med. 2019;19(1):51. https://doi.org/10.1186/s12890-019-0801-2.
7. Affolter K, Schumann DM, Tamm M, et al. Multiplex PCR on the Bronchoalveolar lavage fluid of Immunocompromised patients. Chest. 2018;154(3):722–5. https://doi.org/10.1016/j.chest.2018.06.018.
8. Meyer KC, Raghu G, Baughman RP, et al. An official American Thoracic Society clinical practice guideline: the clinical utility of Bronchoalveolar lavage cell analysis in interstitial lung disease. Am J Respir Crit Care Med. 2012;185(9):1004–14. https://doi.org/10.1164/rccm.201202-0320ST.
9. Raghu G, Remy-Jardin M, Ryerson CJ, et al. Diagnosis of hypersensitivity pneumonitis in adults: an official ATS/JRS/ALAT clinical practice guideline. Am J Respir Crit Care Med. 2020;202(3):e36–69. https://doi.org/10.1164/rccm.202005-2032ST.
10. Ramirez JA, Musher DM, Evans SE, et al. Treatment of community-acquired pneumonia in Immunocompromised adults. Chest. 2020;158(5):1896–911. https://doi.org/10.1016/j.chest.2020.05.598.
11. Schneider BJ, Naidoo J, Santomasso BD, et al. Management of Immune-Related Adverse Events in patients treated with immune checkpoint inhibitor therapy: ASCO guideline update. J Clin Oncol. 2021;39(36):4073–126. https://doi.org/10.1200/JCO.21.01440.
12. Haanen J, Obeid M, Spain L, et al. Management of toxicities from immunotherapy: ESMO clinical practice guideline for diagnosis, treatment and follow-up. Ann Oncol Off J Eur Soc Med Oncol. 2022;33(12):1217–38. https://doi.org/10.1016/j.annonc.2022.10.001.
13. Brahmer JR, Lacchetti C, Schneider BJ, et al. Management of Immune-Related Adverse Events in patients treated with immune checkpoint inhibitor therapy: American Society of Clinical Oncology clinical practice guideline. J Clin Oncol. 2018;36(17):1714–68. https://doi.org/10.1200/JCO.2017.77.6385.
14. Zhong L, Altan M, Shannon VR, Sheshadri A. Immune-related adverse events: pneumonitis. Immunotherapy. 2020;1244:255–69. https://doi.org/10.1007/978-3-030-41008-7_13.
15. Lai KA, Sheshadri A, Adrianza AM, et al. Role of infliximab in immune checkpoint inhibitor-induced pneumonitis. J Immunother Precis Oncol. 2020;3(4):172–4. https://doi.org/10.36401/JIPO-20-22.

Chapter 49
Pneumonitis and COVID-19 Pneumonia Post Immune Checkpoint Inhibitor Therapy

Saad Farooq, Saadia A. Faiz, Vickie R. Shannon, and Ajay Sheshadri

Abbreviations

ALT	Alanine aminotransferase
AST	Aspartate aminotransferase
BAL	Bronchoalveolar lavage
COPD	Chronic obstructive pulmonary disease
CT	Computed tomography
ICI	Immune checkpoint inhibitor
NAAT	Nucleic acid amplification test
PCR	Polymerase chain reaction
PFT	Pulmonary Function Tests
RP-1	Vusolimogene oderparepvec
RV	Residual volume
SCC	Squamous cell carcinoma
TLC	Total lung capacity

Clinical Presentation

This is a Caucasian man in his 60s with a history of metastatic squamous cell carcinoma of the scalp came in to be evaluated for shortness of breath. He was a former smoker (25 pack-years) but with no prior history of chronic obstructive pulmonary

S. Farooq
Divisions of Critical Care, Pulmonary & Sleep Medicine, The University of Texas Houston, McGovern Medical School at UTHealth, Houston, TX, USA
e-mail: Saad.Farooq@uth.tmc.edu

S. A. Faiz · V. R. Shannon · A. Sheshadri (✉)
Department of Pulmonary Medicine, The University of Texas MD Anderson Cancer Center, Houston, TX, USA
e-mail: safaiz@mdanderson.org; vshannon@mdanderson.org; asheshadri@mdanderson.org

Y. Wang (ed.), *Challenging Cases in Immunotherapy Related Organ Toxicities*,
https://doi.org/10.1007/978-3-031-83533-9_49

disease (COPD). Other medical history was significant for hypertension and hyperlipidemia. Squamous cell carcinoma (SCC) of the scalp was initially treated with Mohs resection followed by right-sided modified radical neck dissection and carboplatin-based chemoradiation 2 years later for biopsy-proven disease recurrence. Approximately 5 months later, the patient was enrolled in a randomized controlled clinical trial of cemiplimab with or without RP-1 (Vusolimogene oderparepvec) (CERPASS trial) for disease progression and unresectable SCC.

Rash following the first cycle of therapy resolved with simple skin moisturization. Following the third cycle of therapy, the patient noted progressive paroxysmal nocturnal dyspnea, dry cough, and dyspnea, prompting hospitalization.

At presentation, the patient reported dyspnea at rest and required 3–4 L of supplemental oxygen to maintain oxygen saturations above 90%. The patient denied cough, fevers, chills, sore throat, rash, leg swelling or abdominal pain.

On physical examination, the patient was in no acute respiratory distress. He was afebrile. Other vital signs were within normal limits. Chest examination was remarkable for equal and symmetric breath sounds with bibasilar rales. No wheezes were noted. Other components of the examination including cardiac, neurologic, abdominal, and dermatologic assessments were within normal limits. No jugular venous distention or peripheral edema were present. Laboratory values showed mild anemia, no leukocytosis, and normal electrolytes (Table 49.1). A baseline echocardiogram performed 3 months prior was within normal limits (Fig. 49.1).

Table 49.1 Lab values

Variables	Value
WBC (4.1–10.5)	6.4 K/μL
Hgb (12.2–15.3)	**10.3 gm/dL (L)**
Hct (36.4–46.8)	**31.7% (L)**
Platelet count (160–397)	232 K/μL
Sodium Lvl (136–145)	136 mEq/L
Potassium Lvl (3.5–5.1)	4.4 mEq/L
Chloride (98–107)	99 mEq/L
CO_2 (22–29)	25 mEq/L
BUN (6–23)	11 mg/dL
Creatinine (0.51–0.95)	0.77 mg/dL
Glucose level (70–99)	112 mg/dL
Calcium Lvl (8.4–10.2)	9.2 mg/dL
Magnesium (1.6–2.6)	2.0 mg/dL
Phosphorus (2.5–4.5)	3.3 mg/dL
Albumin (3.5–5.2)	3.9 gm/dL
ALT (<=33)	19 U/L
AST (<=32)	15 U/L
NT-ProBNP (<125)	106 Pg/mL

Lab values in bold are abnormal. (H): High, (L): Low

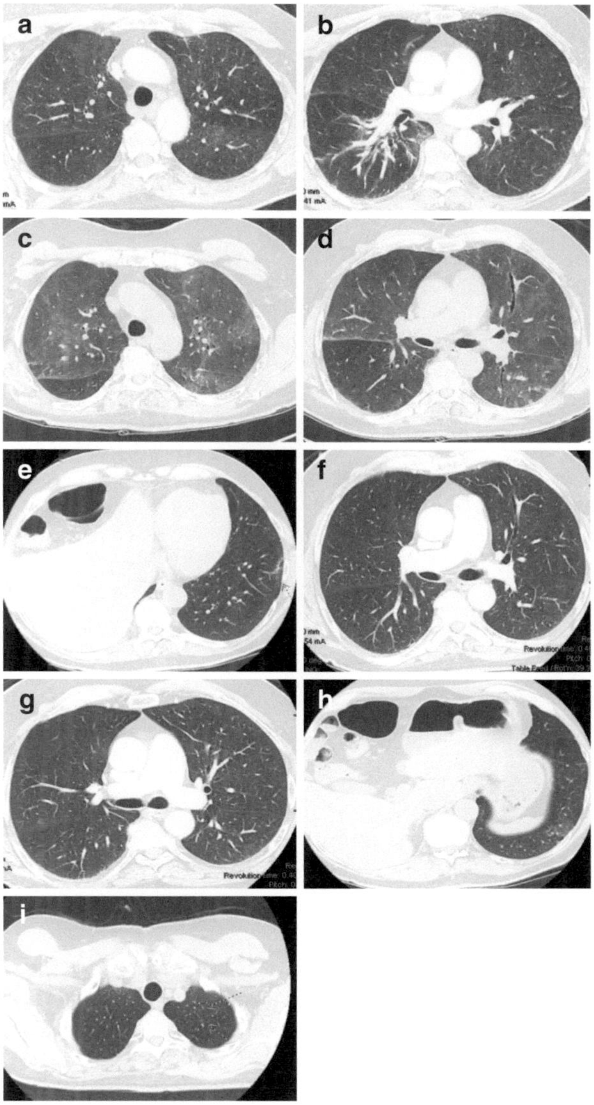

Fig. 49.1 Bronchoscopy images showing thin, frothy secretions in the main and secondary carina

An admitting chest CT showed diffuse ground glass opacities (Fig. 49.2a, b). No hilar or mediastinal lymphadenopathy was seen. Supraclavicular lymphadenopathy appeared stable when compared to prior studies, however, slightly increased axillary lymph nodes were noted. The presenting history and workup suggested Cemiplimab-related pneumonitis and the drug was placed on hold. Pulmonary consultation was ordered. The patient underwent bronchoscopic examination with bronchoalveolar lavage (BAL) in the left upper lobe for evaluation of the infiltrates. Copious amounts of thin, frothy clear secretions were noted in the distal airways bilaterally (Fig. 49.1). BAL fluid analysis revealed a lymphocyte-predominant

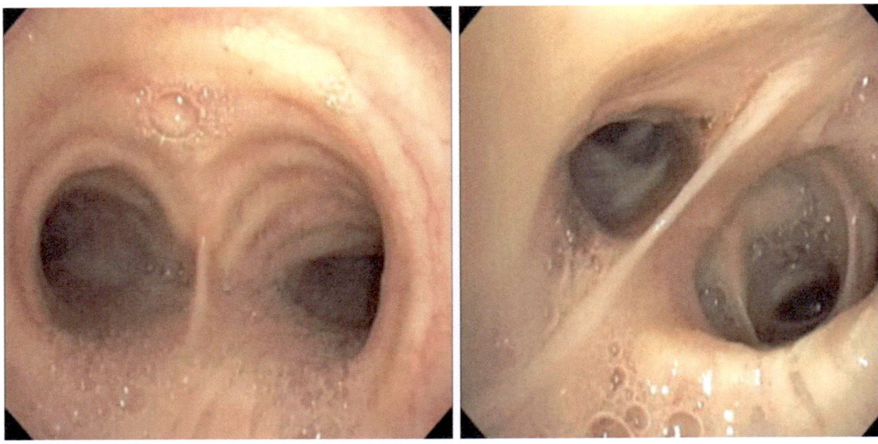

Fig. 49.2 CT chest images during the disease course. (**a**, **b**) Initial CT scan showing diffuse ground glass opacities in both lungs. (**c**, **d**) CT scan on second hospital admission showing worsened diffuse bilateral ground glass opacities off steroids. (**e**, **f**) Repeat CT scan done shortly after starting corticosteroids again on the second hospital admission. (**g**, **h**, **i**) Most recent CT Chest showing resolution of prior ground glass opacities but new peripheral ground glass/consolidative opacities in the left lower lobe and lingula were seen along with new scattered ground glass opacities in the left upper lobe

Table 49.2 Bronchoscopy with BAL

Appearance	Hazy
Total cells	100
WBC	309/mcl
Lymphocytes	53%
Segmented neutrophils	6%
Eosinophils	24%
Histiocytes	10%
RBC	33%
Other cells	7%

alveolitis with increased eosinophils (Table 49.2). No malignant cells were identified. Cultures of BAL fluid were negative. Iron stains and GMS stains for fungi, pneumocystis, and CMV were also negative. The NAAT for COVID-19 was positive therefore he was treated with remdesivir. He was also started on prednisone 80 mg daily with taper down by 10 mg every 3 days and eventually discharged with 3 L of oxygen at home.

In the following month, two weeks after the prednisone taper off, he presented to the emergency room with dyspnea again. He reported fatigue but had no other symptoms like cough, fever, wheezing or chills etc. His oxygen saturations were measured at 88% despite supplemental oxygen, and he was now requiring 5 L/min

Table 49.3 Pulmonary function testing (PFTS) 1 month apart

FVC (3.39–4.29 L) pre	**2.467 (L)**	**2.435(L)**
FVC (% pred) pre	58	57
FEV1 (2.42–3.18 L) pre	**1.659 (L)**	**1.589 (L)**
FEV1 (%pred) pre	52	50
FEV1/FVC (%) pre (64.5–74.2)	67.26	65.23
FEV1/FVC (% pred) pre	91	88
TLC (5.67–7.97 L)	5.674	6.019
TLC (% pred)	83	88
RV (1.85–3.20 L)	3.044	**3.509 (H)**
RV (% pred)	121	139
RV/TLC (%)	**53.648 (L)**	**58.299 (L)**
RV/TLC (31–49) (% pred)	**134 (H)**	**145 (H)**
DLCO_SB ml/(min*mmHg)	**10.391(L)**	**10.401 (L)**
Lab values in bold are abnormal. (H): High, (L): Low		

to maintain saturations above 90%. In the emergency room his vital signs were stable apart from the low oxygen saturations. A repeat CT chest (Fig. 49.3) showed diffuse ground glass opacities, similar in appearance but increased from prior. Due to these findings, there was concern for relapse of pneumonitis off steroids along with concern for possible bacterial pneumonia. He was started on vancomycin, cefepime and 1 mg/kg/day of oral prednisone along with sulfamethoxazole and trimethoprim.

Pulmonary function testing done 2 weeks after admission showed no evidence of obstruction. Increased RV/TLC ratio was noted suggesting possible air trapping. There was moderately reduced diffusion capacity (Table 49.3).

Differential Diagnosis

Our patient received cemiplimab, a PD-1/PD-L1 antibody that causes pneumonitis in 2.6% of patients who were enrolled in clinical trials of the agent [1]. He also tested positive for COVID-19. Although PCR testing of respiratory samples can help ascertain the diagnosis of prior COVID-19 lower respiratory infection, it cannot exclude concomitant immune-related pneumonitis. It can also not determine whether such an infection is active or simply reflects viral shedding [2]. Despite careful examination of timing and the natural history of the lung disease, it is not often possible to determine whether a new respiratory impairment is due to SARS-CoV-2 pneumonia in patients receiving ICIs, ICI pneumonitis in patients exposed to SARS-CoV-2 in the past, or concurrent SARS-CoV-2 pneumonia with ICI pneumonitis. Especially since NAAT testing cannot determine acute infection and no biomarker for ICI pneumonitis exists. Furthermore, radiologic findings cannot distinguish between these two entities [1]. SARS-CoV-2 pneumonia typically presents with peripheral ground-glass opacities, which can mimic the organizing pneumonia, and organizing pneumonia is the most common radiographic pattern seen in ICI-pneumonitis [3]. Acute COVID-19 improves with anti-inflammatory therapies such as corticosteroids, and SARS-CoV-2 can also trigger organizing pneumonia after acute infection [4, 5]. Given that our patient deteriorated while weaning corticosteroids and had CT findings supporting pneumonitis, we suspected that the patient had an overlap of both ICI pneumonitis and post-COVID-19 organizing pneumonia.

Management Options

During the initial hospitalization, our patient was treated for both acute SARS-CoV-2 pneumonia and ICI pneumonitis. He was on remdesivir and started on a prednisone taper. However, symptoms recurred while tapering off corticosteroids, we restarted prednisone and noted improvement. Cemiplimab was held for a total of 3 months during the time our patient was hospitalized and while he was on corticosteroids.

Follow-Up and Outcome

Cemiplimab was ultimately resumed under close monitoring once our patient was off corticosteroids and dyspnea had improved. During the most recent pulmonary clinic follow-up, almost a year after resumption of cemiplimab therapy, the patient remained symptom free. A neck CT showed a slight decrease in the size of rim-enhancing right neck lesion and biopsy of that lesion showed focal squamous cell cancer with necrosis. His follow up CT chest showed improvement, though with residual ground-glass opacities and consolidation in the left lower lobe (Fig. 49.2c, d). A 6-min walk examination showed the ability to walk an acceptable distance (497 m), but he desaturated from 94% to 87% at peak exercise, necessitating supplemental oxygen with exercise. PFTs showed improvement (Table 49.4). He continues to receive cemiplimab at the last follow up 1 month ago with stable cancer condition.

Table 49.4 PFTS almost a year after hospitalization and on cemiplimab therapy

FVC (3.25–4.12 L) pre	**2.71 (L)**
FVC (% pred) pre	66
FEV1 (2.31–3.04 L) pre	**1.77 (L)**
FEV1 (%pred) pre	58
FEV1/FVC (64.3–74.0%) pre	65.42
FEV1/FVC (% pred) pre	74
TLC (5.51–7.81 L)	6.56
TLC (% pred)	98
RV (1.84–3.19 L)	**3.78 (H)**
RV (31–49) % pred	**150 (H)**
RV/TLC (%)	58
RV/TLC (% pred)	**142 (H)**
DLCO_SB ml/(min*mmHg)	**13.63 (L)**
DLCO_SB (% pred)	**60 (L)**

Lab values in bold are abnormal. (H): High, (L): Low

Summary Paragraph

This is a case of ICI-induced pneumonitis and concurrent COVID-19 infection. The unique feature of this case is to illustrate the difficulty of distinguishing between ICI pneumonitis and SARS-CoV-2 pneumonia, as well as post-COVID-19 organizing pneumonia, since imaging and clinical findings are often similar. Most importantly, after adequate treatment, he was successfully re-challenged with cemiplimab, and he did not develop recurrent pneumonitis or respiratory symptoms again.

Discussion

Patients with cancer are not only at a higher risk for developing COVID-19 but also develop more severe illness, possibly due to immunosuppression and anticancer treatments [6, 7]. In a retrospective study of 121 patients with solid malignancies and COVID-19 infection, unvaccinated patients were 10 times more likely to be admitted to an intensive care unit when compared to vaccinated patients. Interestingly, patients who were being treated with ICIs had increased mortality compared to the same type of patients treated with chemotherapy alone [3]. The CDC recommends COVID-19 vaccination including 1 or 2 doses of the updated vaccine to everyone aged 6 months and older who is moderately or severely immunocompromised such as patients with cancer [8]. Another study evaluating 3920 patients from the COVID-19 and Cancer Consortium (CCC-19) registry showed that 30-day mortality is 18% in patients who underwent immunotherapy within

1–3 months prior to COVID-19 but this was not adjusted for cancer stage or type [9]. Though causality is not clear in these studies, they indicate that patients being treated with ICI therapies are at high risk for adverse outcomes after SARS-CoV-2 infection.

Usually, a bronchoscopy is advised for patients suspected to have ICI pneumonitis. However, in patients with COVID-19, there is an increased risk of transmission to staff through aerosolization. Disposable bronchoscopes, proper personal protective equipment, negative pressure rooms and other precautions should be used to minimize transmission risk [10].

For treatment, an attractive option for both COVID-19 pneumonia and ICI pneumonitis is anti-IL-6 therapy such as tocilizumab. IL-6 is often implicated in acute lung injury [11]. In patients with COVID-19 pneumonia who are not on mechanical ventilation, IL-6 inhibition with tocilizumab reduced likelihood of progression to the composite outcome of mechanical ventilation or death [12]. In ICI pneumonitis, the use of IL-6 inhibitors is guided primarily by anecdotal case reports [13]. Additional prospective studies are warranted to further evaluate the efficacy of anti-IL-6 therapy in the treatment of ICI pneumonitis with and without concurrent lung COVID infection. Because our patient had grade 3 pneumonitis and improved after corticosteroid therapy, additional immunosuppression was not warranted.

It remains to be an important decision when and if cemiplimab could be safely restarted after SARS-CoV-2 infection. Some experts recommend two negative COVID-19 tests and clinical stability before considering resumption of therapy [14]. However, these patients often have prolonged shedding of the virus therefore may not achieve a negative PCR [2]. Cycle threshold values are sometimes used to guide decision making, but it is not currently advised to do so[11]. Overall, there is not sufficient data to guide the optimal time window for resumption of ICI therapy after SARS-CoV-2 pneumonia. In terms of recurrence risk, in clinical trials involving cemiplimab, 40% of patients with pneumonitis had recurrence after restarting cemiplimab, and guidelines recommend the permanently discontinuation of therapy in patients who develop grade 3 or 4 pneumonitis [15, 16]. Professional societies recommend that therapeutic rechallenge may be attempted in select patients with grade 3 pneumonitis in whom benefits outweigh the risk [16, 17]. This remains an area of ongoing research and currently therapeutic rechallenge may be attempted on a case-by-case basis with the appropriate precautions [13]. It is not as critical or feasible to determine if the cause of pneumonitis was organizing pneumonia after SARS-CoV-2 infection or due to ICI, since in theory both are treated similarly, and in theory both could flare with ICI resumption.

Timeline of Events

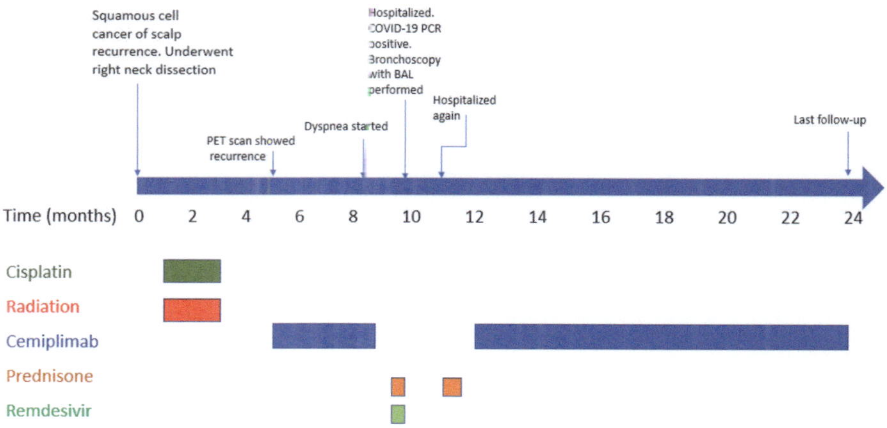

Fig. 49.3 Summary of pneumonitis disease course with timeline (timepoint of 0 is the point when squamous cell cancer recurred)

References

1. LIBTAYO® (cemiplimab-rwlc). LIBTAYO HCP. https://www.libtayohcp.com/. Accessed 12 Aug 2023.
2. Aydillo T, Gonzalez-Reiche AS, Aslam S, et al. Shedding of viable SARS-CoV-2 after immunosuppressive therapy for cancer. N Engl J Med. 2020;383(26):2586–8. https://doi.org/10.1056/NEJMc2031670.
3. Hatic H, Hearld KR, Das D, Deshane J. Clinical outcomes in COVID-19 patients treated with immunotherapy. Cancers. 2022;14(23):5954. https://doi.org/10.3390/cancers14235954.
4. Bazdyrev E, Panova M, Zherebtsova V, et al. The hidden pandemic of COVID-19-induced organizing pneumonia. Pharmaceuticals. 2022;15(12):1574. https://doi.org/10.3390/ph15121574.
5. Anon. Dexamethasone in hospitalized patients with Covid-19. N Engl J Med. 2021;384(8):693–704. https://doi.org/10.1056/NEJMoa2021436.
6. Bertini CD, Khawaja F, Sheshadri A. Coronavirus Disease-2019 in the Immunocompromised host. Clin Chest Med. 2023;44(2):395–406. https://doi.org/10.1016/j.ccm.2022.11.012.
7. Dumoulin DW, Gietema HA, Paats MS, Hendriks LEL, Cornelissen R. Differentiation of COVID-19 pneumonitis and ICI induced pneumonitis. Front Oncologia. 2020;10:577696. Accessed 12 Aug 2023. https://doi.org/10.3389/fonc.2020.577696.
8. CDC. COVID-19 Vaccination. Centers for Disease Control and Prevention. Published February 11, 2020. https://www.cdc.gov/coronavirus/2019-ncov/vaccines/recommendations/immuno.html. Accessed 14 Oct 2023.
9. Wise-Draper TM, Desai A, Elkrief A, et al. LBA71 systemic cancer treatment-related outcomes in patients with SARS-CoV-2 infection: a CCC19 registry analysis. Ann Oncol. 2020;31:S1201–2. https://doi.org/10.1016/j.annonc.2020.08.2312.
10. Alhazzani W, Møller MH, Arabi YM, et al. Surviving sepsis campaign: guidelines on the management of critically Ill adults with coronavirus disease 2019 (COVID-19). Crit Care Med. 2020;46:854. https://doi.org/10.1097/CCM.0000000000004363.
11. Rosas IO, Bräu N, Waters M, et al. Tocilizumab in hospitalized patients with severe Covid-19 pneumonia. N Engl J Med. 2021;384(16):1503–16. https://doi.org/10.1056/NEJMoa2028700.

12. Salama C, Han J, Yau L, et al. Tocilizumab in patients hospitalized with Covid-19 pneumonia. N Engl J Med. 2021;384(1):20–30. https://doi.org/10.1056/NEJMoa2030340.
13. Zhong L, Altan M, Shannon VR, Sheshadri A. Immune-related adverse events: pneumonitis. Immunotherapy. 2020;1244:255–69. https://doi.org/10.1007/978-3-030-41008-7_13.
14. Sullivan RJ, Johnson DB, Rini BI, et al. COVID-19 and immune checkpoint inhibitors: initial considerations. J Immunother Cancer. 2020;8(1):e000933. https://doi.org/10.1136/jitc-2020-000933.
15. Brahmer JR, Abu-Sbeih H, Ascierto PA, et al. Society for Immunotherapy of cancer (SITC) clinical practice guideline on immune checkpoint inhibitor-related adverse events. J Immunother Cancer. 2021;9(6):e002435. https://doi.org/10.1136/jitc-2021-002435.
16. Thompson JA, Schneider BJ, Brahmer J, et al. NCCN guidelines insights: Management of Immunotherapy-Related Toxicities, version 1.2022, NCCN clinical practice guidelines in oncology. J Natl Compr Cancer Netw. 2022 Apr;20(4):387–405.
17. Haanen J, Ernstoff M, Wang Y, et al. Rechallenge patients with immune checkpoint inhibitors following severe immune-related adverse events: review of the literature and suggested prophylactic strategy. J Immunother Cancer. 2020;8(1):e000604. https://doi.org/10.1136/jitc-2020-000604.

Chapter 50
Immune Checkpoint Inhibitor Associated Pneumonitis in a Patient with Interstitial Lung Abnormalities

Saad Farooq, Saadia A. Faiz, Vickie R. Shannon, and Ajay Sheshadri

Abbreviations

ALT	Alanine aminotransferase
AST	Aspartate aminotransferase
BAL	Bronchoalveolar lavage
CT	Computed tomography
ICI	Immune checkpoint inhibitors
ILA	Interstitial lung abnormalities
ILD	Interstitial lung disease
IPF	Idiopathic pulmonary fibrosis
NSCLC	Non-small cell lung cancer
PCR	Polymerase chain reaction
PFTS	Pulmonary function tests
RBC	Red cell count
WBC	White cell count

S. Farooq
Divisions of Critical Care, Pulmonary & Sleep Medicine, The University of Texas Houston, McGovern Medical School at UTHealth, Houston, TX, USA
e-mail: Saad.Farooq@uth.tmc.edu

S. A. Faiz · V. R. Shannon · A. Sheshadri (✉)
Department of Pulmonary Medicine, The University of Texas MD Anderson Cancer Center, Houston, TX, USA
e-mail: safaiz@mdanderson.org; vshannon@mdanderson.org; asheshadri@mdanderson.org

Y. Wang (ed.), *Challenging Cases in Immunotherapy Related Organ Toxicities*,
https://doi.org/10.1007/978-3-031-83533-9_50

Clinical Presentation

This is a man in his 60s who was diagnosed with stage 3 esophageal adenocarcinoma and subsequently received proton radiation (5040 RBEcGy) in 28 fractions to the esophagus for 1 month (Fig. 50.1) followed by pembrolizumab, oxaliplatin and 5 fluorouracil, followed by docetaxel and 5 fluorouracil alone. His other medical history was significant for gastroesophageal reflux disease. He was a non-smoker and had no prior known lung disease. Three weeks after his last treatment, he presented to the emergency department for shortness of breath progressing over 1–2 weeks. At presentation, the patient reported dyspnea at rest and required 4 L/min of supplemental oxygen to maintain oxygen saturations above 90%. He also complained of a dry cough, fatigue, and difficulty swallowing. He denied fevers, chills, sore throat, rash, leg swelling or abdominal pain.

On physical examination, the patient was not in acute respiratory distress and did not require use of accessory muscles to breathe. He was afebrile. Other vital signs were within normal limits. Chest auscultation was remarkable for equal and symmetric breath sounds with end-expiratory rhonchi. Cardiac, neurologic, abdominal, and dermatologic assessments revealed no abnormalities. No jugular venous distention or peripheral edema were present. Laboratory values were unremarkable apart from a slightly decreased albumin (Table 50.1).

Our patient had a baseline CT scan done at an outside hospital a few months before he was started on any treatment which showed diffuse subpleural ground glass opacities along with some scattered small pulmonary nodules (Fig. 50.2a, b). These were not worked up before, and he had no clinical diagnosis of interstitial lung disease. A chest CT for this hospital admission showed development of extensive, bilateral, heterogenous opacities predominantly in the left upper lobes and both lower lobes (Fig. 50.2c, d). In addition, he was noted to have prominent bilateral hilar lymphadenopathy.

The presenting history and workup suggested pneumonitis, but it was not clear whether it was induced by radiation, aspiration, or immune checkpoint inhibitor therapy. The patient was started on empiric antibiotics and solumedrol 60 mg every 12 h for 24 h and was eventually decreased to 50 mg daily. Bronchoscopy with bronchoalveolar lavage was not done as his initial oxygen requirements were too

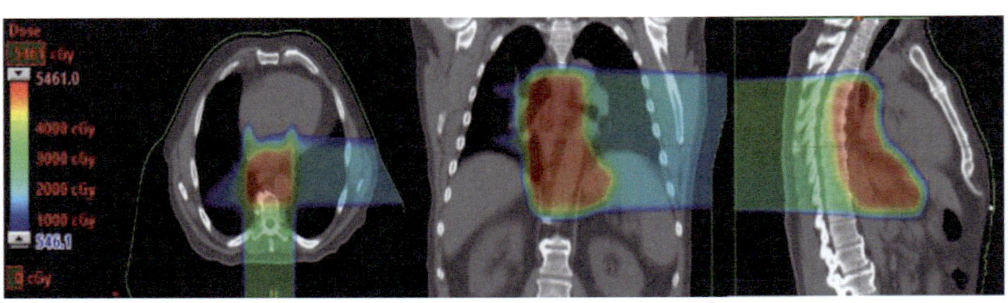

Fig. 50.1 Proton radiation field showing the areas targeted by radiation

Table 50.1 Lab values at the time of event

Variables	Value
WBC (4.1–10.5)	10.4 K/uL
Hgb (12.2–15.3)	14.7 gm/dL
Hct (36.4–46.8)	42.3%
Platelet count (160–397)	237 K/uL
Sodium Lvl (136–145)	**134 mEq/L (L)**
Potassium Lvl (3.5–5.1)	4.3 mEq/L
Chloride (98–107)	98 mEq/L
CO2 (22–29)	24 mEq/L
BUN (6–23)	21 mg/dL
Creatinine (0.51–0.95)	0.93 mg/dL
Glucose level (70–99)	99 mg/dL
Calcium Lvl (8.4–10.2)	8.7 mg/dL
Magnesium (1.6–2.6)	2.4 mg/dL
Phosphorus (2.5–4.5)	3.3 mg/dL
Albumin (3.5–5.2)	**2.9 gm/dL (L)**
ALT (≤33)	**49 U/L (H)**
AST (≤32)	39 U/L

Lab values in bold are abnormal. (H) = high, (L) = low

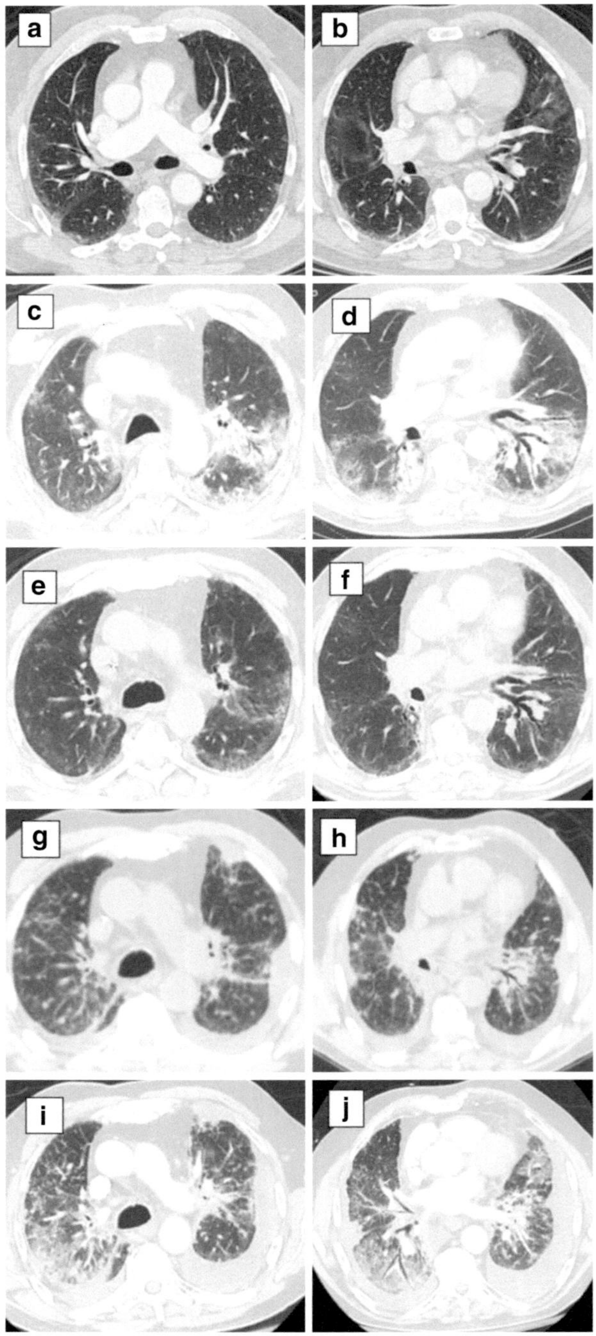

Fig. 50.2 CT scan of the chest at different timepoints. (**a**, **b**) Baseline CT scan before any treatments for esophageal adenocarcinoma showing diffuse subpleural ground glass opacities. (**c**, **d**) CT scan on initial admission to the hospital showing extensive, bilateral heterogeneous lung opacities, predominantly in the left upper lobe and both lower lobes. (**e**, **f**) Repeat CT scan 6 months after hospitalization showing residual peripheral pulmonary opacities. (**g**, **h**) CT scan more than a year after hospitalization showing nodular thickening of the interlobular septa and peribronchovascular soft tissue in both lungs suspicious for lymphangitic neoplastic disease and hematogenous metastases. In addition, there are scattered consolidative and ground glass opacities in the lungs predominantly in the lower lobes. (**i**, **j**) CT scan on the last hospital admission showing worsening multifocal bilateral ground glass and consolidative opacities, thickening of the interlobular septa and peribronchial soft tissue thickening, suspicious for metastatic disease with lymphangitic spread of tumor along with worsening of moderate left pleural effusion and small right pleural effusion

Table 50.2 Pulmonary function test

	At baseline before hospitalization	9 months later
FVC pre (3.61–4.52)	3.19 L	**1.79 (L)**
FVC (% pred) pre	70%	**40% (L)**
FEV1 pre (2.61–3.38)	2.66 L	**1.59 (L)**
FEV1 (%pred) pre	79%	**48% (L)**
FEV1/FVC pre (65.2–74.8)	83.6	74.6
FEV1/FVC (% pred) pre	112%	119%
TLC (5.83–8.13)	**4.50 L (L)**	**3.38 L (L)**
TLC (% pred)	**64% (L)**	**48% (L)**
RV (1.81–3.16)	1.31 L	1.53 L
RV (% pred)	53%	61%
RV/TLC (30–48)	**29 (L)**	45
RV/TLC (% pred)	75%	115%
DLCO_SB (23.1)	22.1 mL/(min*mmHg)	**11.1 mL/(min*mmHg) (L)**
DLCO_SB (% pred)	96%	**52% (L)**
Lab values in bold are abnormal. (H) = high, (L) = low		

high, and he improved rapidly with steroids. He was eventually discharged with a prednisone taper over 5 weeks and on supplemental oxygen at 3 L/min along with trimethoprim/sulfamethoxazole for pneumocystis carinii pneumonia prophylaxis.

At follow-up, he had been off of corticosteroids for 2 weeks and had self-titrated himself off of supplemental oxygen. He felt markedly better and denied shortness of breath, cough, or wheezing. Repeat imaging showed residual reticular opacities bilaterally with a predominance in the left lung base which were improved from the acute episode of pneumonitis (Fig. 50.2e, f). His repeat pulmonary function test (PFT) showed severe restriction along with reduction in diffusion capacity (Table 50.2), but he did not desaturate on exertion during a 6-min walk test, indicating the lack of need for supplemental oxygen therapy.

Differential Diagnosis

Our patient developed pneumonitis due to either immune checkpoint inhibitor therapy, radiation, or a combination of both. Since he had active esophageal cancer, there was concern for aspiration pneumonitis as well. In addition, he received oxaliplatin, which has been associated rarely with pneumonitis based on limited case studies [1]. The opacities were most dense in the radiation field, but because these opacities were present on the contralateral side, we believed there was some contribution from pembrolizumab therapy. However, radiation pneumonitis is occasionally associated with opacities contralateral to the site of treatment, and therefore the location of opacities relative to the location of radiation therapy is only suggestive of the etiology of pneumonitis but not confirmatory [2, 3].

Management Options

Our patient was treated with corticosteroids and improved significantly after starting therapy. While he received antibiotics initially, microbiological studies did not reveal infection. Notably, he did not undergo bronchoalveolar lavage for a definitive assessment of infectious pneumonia; although that could be considered if his initial oxygen requirements were lower or he did not show improvement on corticosteroids. He did not require any secondary immunosuppressive agents such as infliximab since he had early improvement with corticosteroids alone. He made a full recovery from this episode of pneumonitis and was back to his pre-treatment baseline at his follow up examination.

Follow-Up and Outcome

Sixteen months after the initial episode of pneumonitis, our patient reported a worsening cough and dyspnea for a few weeks without any fever or chills. In this interval, he had worsening metastatic disease and had received palliative radiotherapy to his cervical spine. We repeated a CT scan (Fig. 50.2g, h) which showed increased thickening of interlobular septa and more reticular opacities noted in the left lung mid-field, most suggestive of lymphangitic neoplastic disease. In addition, he had ground glass and consolidative opacities in both lungs, predominantly in the lower lobes, concerning for superimposed aspiration pneumonia. He was given antibiotics as an outpatient and restarted on prednisone 40 mg with some improvement in symptoms, but again required admission to the emergency room due to worsening dyspnea. He denied any fevers or chills, but required high flow oxygen to maintain oxygen saturations. He received IV methylprednisolone and scheduled nebulized therapies, with partial improvement. Repeat imaging (Fig. 50.2i, j) showed worsening multifocal bilateral ground glass and consolidative opacities, more pronounced in the right lower lobe, along with worsening of bilateral numerous bilateral lung nodules, thickening of the interlobular septa and peribronchial soft tissue thickening, suspicious for metastatic disease with lymphangitic spread of tumor. The left pleural effusion was also worse from prior. An infectious workup, including respiratory viral panel, serum fungitell, and blood cultures, were negative. The patient was started on intravenous antibiotics (cefepime, vancomycin, treatment dose trimethoprim/sulfamethoxazole) as well as steroids on admission. Unfortunately, these interventions did not improve the patient's respiratory status, and he expired during the same admission.

Summary Paragraph

We present a case with pneumonitis most likely due to combined immune checkpoint inhibitor and radiation therapy, with potential additional injury from oxaliplatin. Unfortunately, despite recovering from index pneumonitis, he eventually developed progressive lymphangitic spread of cancer with worsening hypoxemic respiratory failure and died due to his cancer. Summary of the timeline event is shown in Fig. 50.3.

Discussion

There are several factors that may increase the risk of ICI pneumonitis. Our patient had received thoracic radiation for esophageal adenocarcinoma, which, when given together with ICI therapies, can increase the risk for pneumonitis [4]. Administering ICI with concurrent chemoradiation (CRT) may induce higher pulmonary toxicity than monotherapy with ICI or chemoradiation alone [4]. In the KEYNOTE 590 trial evaluating pembrolizumab and chemotherapy vs chemotherapy alone in locally advanced esophageal cancer, pneumonitis occurred in 5% of the patients in ICI given with chemotherapy, whereas none of the patients in the chemotherapy alone group had pneumonitis [5].

Our patient also had areas of peripheral ground glass opacities on his initial CT scan before any treatment for his cancer had begun. Interstitial lung abnormalities (ILAs) are areas of increased density seen on CT chest in patients with no known ILD and may be present in 7–10% of elderly population [6]. These ILAs are more

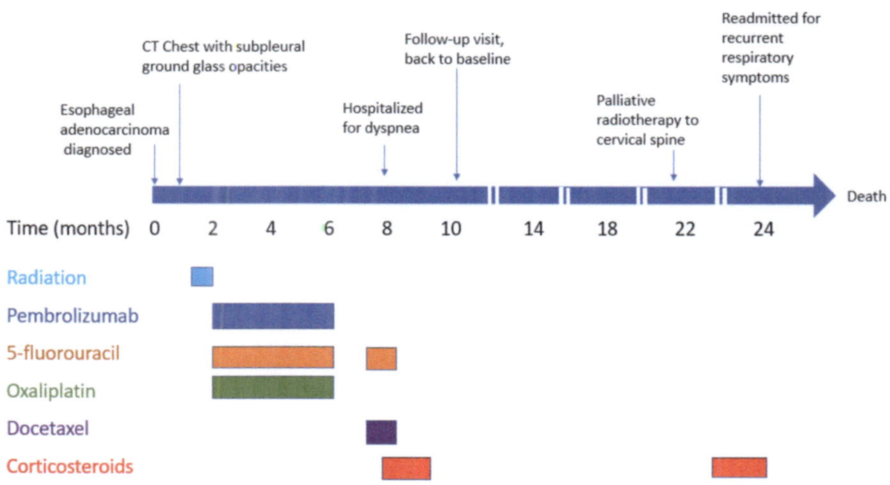

Fig. 50.3 Summary of pneumonitis disease course with timeline (timepoint of 0 is the point when esophageal adenocarcinoma was diagnosed)

commonly seen in smoking populations and may herald the development of ILD in some patients, though many never develop lung disease [6–8]. Patents with ILA and ILD may have increased risk of pneumonitis from ICI therapy. In two studies from our institution, we found that ILD increased the risk for pneumonitis in patients treated with ICI alone or in the setting of concurrent chemoradiotherapy [9, 10]. In a retrospective study from Japan, among 83 patients with non-small cell lung cancer, ICI-related pneumonitis was significantly higher in patients with ILAs, and ground glass opacities particularly increased the risk for ICI pneumonitis [11]. This association has also been reported in non-lung cancers [12]. In a retrospective study of 199 patients with non-lung cancers, the authors found that ground glass opacities and reticulation, but not honeycombing or traction bronchiectasis, were risk factors for ICI-related ILD. The authors postulated that this represented active inflammation in areas of reticulation and ground-glass opacities, whereas honeycombing or traction bronchiectasis reflect destruction of lung tissue and fibrosis [12]. This is also consistent with the notion that idiopathic pulmonary fibrosis may be associated with less lung inflammation than other ILDs [13]. However, another study of 209 patients with solid tumors found no association between preexisting ILAs and ICI-induced pneumonitis, though smoking was found to be risk factor for ICI pneumonitis [14]. Because smoking is associated with a risk for ILAs, the modeling of pneumonitis risk should carefully consider causal inference pathways in order to minimize the introduction of bias. Further studies are urgently needed to evaluate the best strategies to mitigate the risk for developing therapy induced pneumonitis. Importantly, preexisting ILD or ILA should not exclude these patients from ICI therapy, but risk and benefit discussions with patients are paramount before therapy is begun.

References

1. Moskovitz M, Wollner M, Haim N. Oxaliplatin-induced pulmonary toxicity in gastrointestinal malignancies: two case reports and review of the literature. Case Rep Oncol Med. 2015;2015:341064. https://doi.org/10.1155/2015/341064.
2. Hassaballa HA, Cohen ES, Khan AJ, Ali A, Bonomi P, Rubin DB. Positron emission tomography demonstrates radiation-induced changes to nonirradiated lungs in lung cancer patients treated with radiation and chemotherapy. Chest. 2005;128(3):1448–52. https://doi.org/10.1378/chest.128.3.1448.
3. Makimoto T, Tsuchiya S, Hayakawa K, Saitoh R, Mori M. Risk factors for severe radiation pneumonitis in lung cancer. Jpn J Clin Oncol. 1999;29(4):192–7. https://doi.org/10.1093/jjco/29.4.192.
4. Azhar M, Abrencillo R, Gandhi S, Altan M, Sheshadri A. Immunotherapy-related pneumonitis and the synergic impact of thoracic radiation and preexisting interstitial lung disease. Curr Opin Pulm Med. 2023;29(4):248–55. https://doi.org/10.1097/MCP.0000000000000975.
5. Sun JM, Shen L, Shah MA, et al. Pembrolizumab plus chemotherapy versus chemotherapy alone for first-line treatment of advanced oesophageal cancer (KEYNOTE-590): a randomised, placebo-controlled, phase 3 study. Lancet. 2021;398(10302):759–71. https://doi.org/10.1016/S0140-6736(21)01234-4.

6. Axelsson GT, Gudmundsson G. Interstitial lung abnormalities—current knowledge and future directions. Eur Clin Respir J. 2021;8(1):1994178. https://doi.org/10.1080/20018525.2021.1994178.
7. King TE. Smoking and subclinical interstitial lung disease. N Engl J Med. 2011;364(10):968–70. https://doi.org/10.1056/NEJMe1013966.
8. Washko GR, Hunninghake GM, Fernandez IE, et al. Lung volumes and emphysema in smokers with interstitial lung abnormalities. N Engl J Med. 2011;364(10):897–906. https://doi.org/10.1056/NEJMoa1007285.
9. Altan M, Soto F, Zhong LL, et al. Incidence and risk factors for pneumonitis associated with checkpoint inhibitors in advanced non-small cell lung cancer: a single center experience. Oncologist. 2023;28:oyad118. https://doi.org/10.1093/oncolo/oyad118.
10. Altan M, Soto F, Xu T, et al. Pneumonitis after concurrent Chemoradiation and immune checkpoint inhibition in patients with locally advanced non-small cell lung cancer. Clin Oncol R Coll Radiol G B. 2023;35(10):630–9. https://doi.org/10.1016/j.clon.2023.07.003.
11. Nakanishi Y, Masuda T, Yamaguchi K, et al. Pre-existing interstitial lung abnormalities are risk factors for immune checkpoint inhibitor-induced interstitial lung disease in non-small cell lung cancer. Respir Investig. 2019;57(5):451–9. https://doi.org/10.1016/j.resinv.2019.05.002.
12. Shimoji K, Masuda T, Yamaguchi K, et al. Association of preexisting interstitial lung abnormalities with immune checkpoint inhibitor–induced interstitial lung disease among patients with nonlung cancers. JAMA Netw Open. 2020;3(11):e2022906. https://doi.org/10.1001/jamanetworkopen.2020.22906.
13. Schafer MJ, White TA, Iijima K, et al. Cellular senescence mediates fibrotic pulmonary disease. Nat Commun. 2017;8(1):14532. https://doi.org/10.1038/ncomms14532.
14. Horiuchi K, Ikemura S, Sato T, et al. Pre-existing interstitial lung abnormalities and immune checkpoint inhibitor-related pneumonitis in solid tumors: a retrospective analysis. Oncologist. 2023;29:oyad187. https://doi.org/10.1093/oncolo/oyad187.

Chapter 51
Tracheobronchitis Related to Pembrolizumab Therapy

Shaun Pienkos, Gerald Berry, Kaissa de Boer, and Nathaniel Myall

Abbreviations

CT	Computed tomography
FEV1	Forced expiratory volume in the first second
FVC	Forced vital capacity
ICI	Immune checkpoint inhibitor
NSCLC	Non-small cell lung cancer
PCR	Polymerase chain reaction

Clinical Presentation

This is a female in her 60s with a history of thyroid cancer treated with radiation therapy 16 years ago, stage I non-small cell lung cancer (NSCLC) surgically resected 32 years ago, and recently diagnosed pT3N0 lung adenocarcinoma who underwent left-sided lobectomy and segmentectomy with mediastinal lymph node dissection approximately 1 year prior to presentation. She underwent four cycles of

S. Pienkos (✉) · K. de Boer
Department of Medicine, Division of Pulmonary and Critical Care Medicine, Stanford University, Stanford, CA, USA
e-mail: spienkos@stanford.edu; kdeboer@stanford.edu

G. Berry
Department of Pathology, Stanford University, Stanford, CA, USA
e-mail: gerald.berry@stanford.edu

N. Myall
Department of Medicine, Division of Oncology, Stanford University, Stanford, CA, USA
e-mail: nmyall@stanford.edu

Y. Wang (ed.), *Challenging Cases in Immunotherapy Related Organ Toxicities*,
https://doi.org/10.1007/978-3-031-83533-9_51

adjuvant carboplatin, pemetrexed, and pembrolizumab, followed by consolidative therapy with pembrolizumab alone. On the day of cycle 13 of pembrolizumab, the patient reported mild intermittent cough and throat irritation which was thought to be due to environmental allergies. Approximately 1 month later, her cough began to worsen, and by 2 months after the first report of cough, she had begun producing green sputum. Notably, there was no leukocytosis or dyspnea, however new exertional hypoxemia was observed at an outpatient oncology visit, so she was admitted to the hospital for diagnostic evaluation.

Upon hospitalization, a computed tomography (CT) with pulmonary angiography was performed, which showed new mild soft tissue thickening of the trachea and central bronchi. There was no pulmonary embolism, no new opacities in the lung parenchyma, and several stable sub-centimeter pulmonary nodules were seen. Reverse transcriptase PCR was performed on a nasopharyngeal swab specimen which was negative for influenza A/B, respiratory syncytial virus, and SARS-CoV-2. The following day, her oxygen saturation by pulse oximetry was 99% without supplemental oxygen, suggesting the hypoxemia noted at her outpatient visit may have been spurious. She was discharged home with a five-day course of antibiotics for possible bacterial bronchitis, inhaled albuterol, and oral benzonatate.

At outpatient follow up 1 week later, her cough was minimally improved, and still productive of green sputum. Four weeks after her hospitalization, she continued to experience productive cough, and had developed intermittent trace hemoptysis, so a repeat CT scan was performed. This showed similar circumferential thickening of the trachea and central bronchi, with soft tissue stranding adjacent to these large airways, but no other new findings (Fig. 51.1). She underwent further evaluation with bronchoscopy, revealing diffuse erythema of the tracheal and mainstem bronchial mucosa, and mild edema of the left and right lobar bronchi. Cell count and differential analysis of a bronchoalveolar lavage from the right upper lobe revealed elevations in neutrophil and lymphocyte proportions (Table 51.1). Cultures from this lavage were negative for bacterial, mycobacterial, and fungal pathogens, and cytology showed no malignant cells. Histopathology from a tracheal biopsy specimen demonstrated infiltrating lymphocytes, plasma cells, occasional eosinophils and mast cells, and no malignant cells (Fig. 51.2). Due to her negative studies for pulmonary infection, biopsy findings, and imaging correlates of large airway inflammation, the patient was diagnosed with pembrolizumab-induced tracheobronchitis.

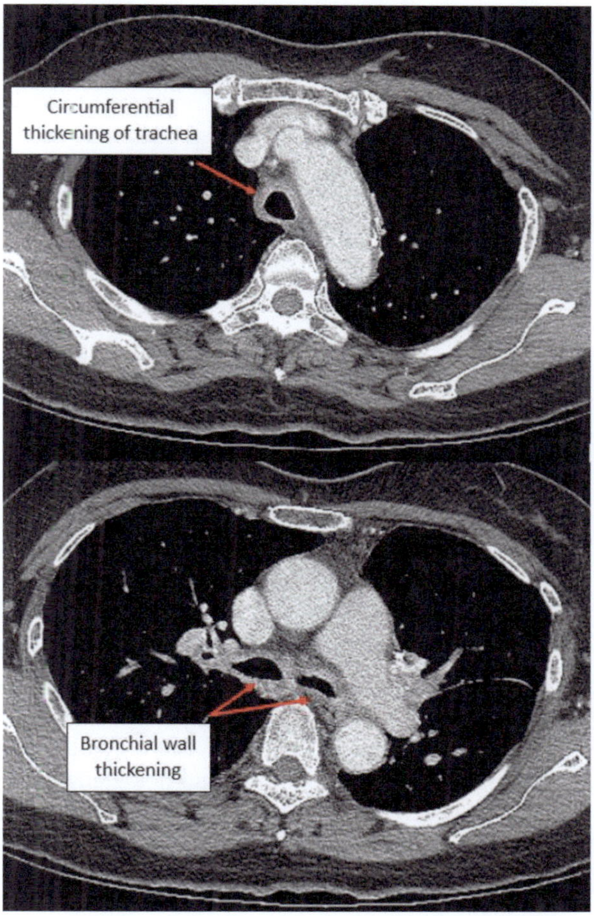

Fig. 51.1 Circumferential thickening and soft-tissue stranding adjacent to (**a**) trachea and (**b**) bilateral mainstem bronchi

Table 51.1 Bronchoalveolar Lavage Cell Count/Differential

Parameters (reference range)	
Nucleated cell count	28 cells/uL
Monocytes/macrophages (**>85%**)	35%
Neutrophils (**≤3%**)	44%
Lymphocytes (**10–15%**)	20%
Eosinophils (**≤1%**)	1%
Red blood cells	19,625 cells/uL

Differential Diagnosis

The differential diagnosis for this case is largely categorized by infectious and non-infectious inflammatory conditions and guided by the anatomical structures noted to be abnormal on cross-sectional imaging. Radiologic signs of inflammation surrounding the large airways points toward a tracheobronchitis as the etiology of this

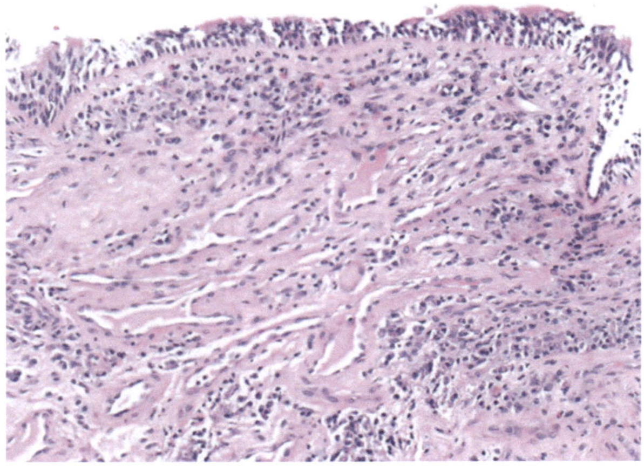

Fig. 51.2 High power magnification showing tracheal biopsy with chronic inflammation composed of lymphocytes, plasma cells and rare eosinophils and mast cells. The lymphocytes are dispersed in the mucosal and submucosal layers

patient's symptoms. Due to the absence of significant abnormalities in the lung parenchyma, pneumonia can be eliminated from consideration.

The most common causes of acute bronchitis in adults are respiratory viruses such as the influenza viruses, rhinovirus, and parainfluenza viruses [1]. Since the year 2020, SARS-CoV-2 has risen to prominence as one of the most common causes of bronchitis [2]. Despite the frequent use of antibacterial agents for bronchitis, bacteria are an infrequent finding on sputum isolates of patients hospitalized with acute respiratory illness, especially in those without a clinical diagnosis of pneumonia or underlying lung disease [3]. When bacteria are identified, atypical organisms such as mycoplasma pneumoniae and bordetella pertussis may be responsible. In regions where tuberculosis is endemic, endobronchial tuberculosis should be considered [4], and immunocompromised host status should raise concern for opportunistic infections such as aspergillosis and herpes viruses.

Common etiologies of large airway inflammation which may not have a clear microbiologic cause include asthma, chronic obstructive pulmonary disease, chronic bronchitis, and bronchiectasis. Less common causes of tracheal and/or bronchial inflammation include autoimmune disease such as inflammatory bowel disease [5], relapsing polychondritis, granulomatosis with polyangiitis, and sarcoidosis. Medication-induced tracheobronchitis appears to be rare given a paucity of published cases.

Treatment, Follow Up and Outcome

The patient was started on prednisone 20 mg daily for ICI-induced tracheobronchitis. One week later, her cough was greatly improved. Pulmonary function tests were performed shortly after prednisone initiation, showing new mild airflow obstruction but preserved diffusion capacity of carbon monoxide (Table 51.2).

Table 51.2 Initial Pulmonary Function Test

Parameters (reference range)	
Forced expiratory volume in 1 s (FEV1) (1.49–2.49 L)	1.50 L (74% predicted)
Forced vital capacity (FVC) (1.90–3.12 L)	2.25 L (90% predicted)
FEV1/FVC (≥69%)	67%
Diffusion capacity of carbon monoxide (13.24–23.93 mL/min/mmHg)	18.00 mL/min/mmHg (102% predicted)

Table 51.3 Repeat Pulmonary Function Test After Treatment

Parameters (reference range)	
Forced expiratory volume in 1 s (FEV1) (1.49–2.49 L)	1.53 L (76% predicted)
Forced vital capacity (FVC) (1.90–3.12 L)	2.22 L (88% predicted)
FEV1/FVC (≥69%)	69%
Diffusion capacity of carbon monoxide (13.22–23.95 mL/min/mmHg)	17.89 mL/min/mmHg (101% predicted)

Approximately 3 weeks after initiation of prednisone, another CT scan showed reduced circumferential thickening of the large airways and her respiratory symptoms continued to improve. The prednisone taper was completed in 5 weeks. Repeat pulmonary function testing after her corticosteroid course was relatively stable, but technically showed resolution of the previously observed airflow obstruction due to an increase in FEV1/FVC ratio (Table 51.3).

Summary

This is a case with lung adenocarcinoma who received approximately 8 months of pembrolizumab therapy and developed tracheobronchitis as a rare adverse event. Her diagnosis was established with pulmonary function tests, cross-sectional imaging, bronchoscopic visualization and tracheal biopsy, all of which assisted in excluding alternative etiologies. Her respiratory symptoms greatly improved with cessation of pembrolizumab and initiation of systemic corticosteroid therapy. Summary of the timeline events is shown in Fig. 51.3.

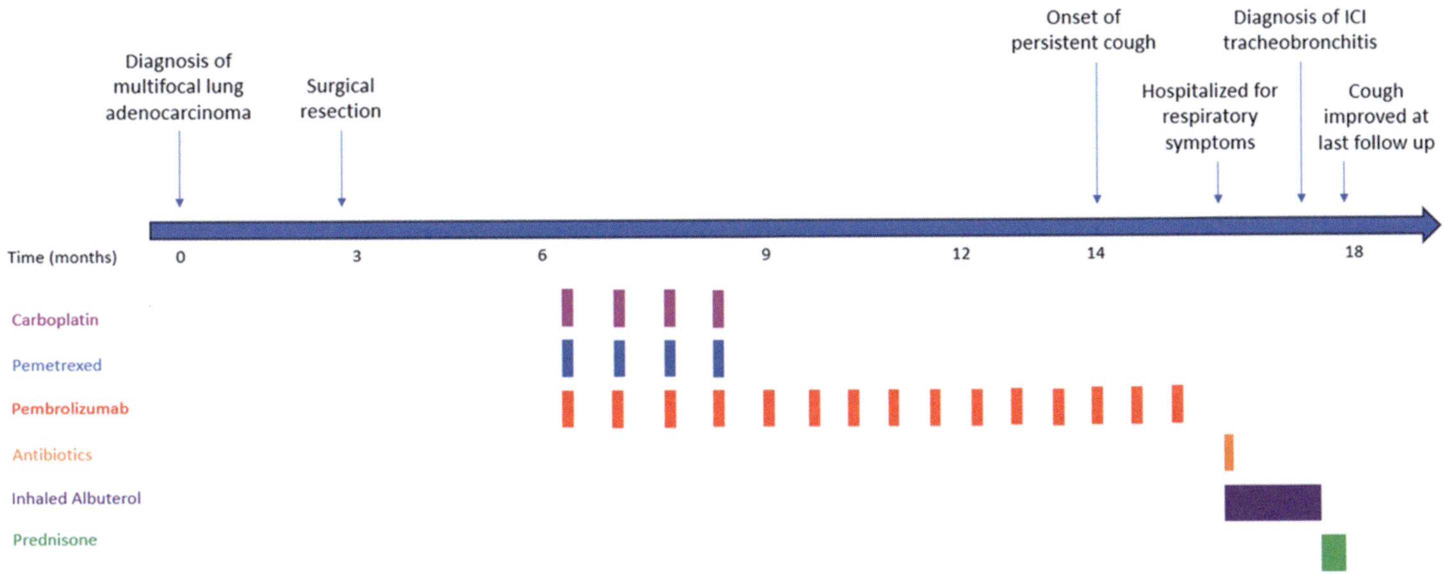

Fig. 51.3 Summary of timeline events (timepoint of 0 is the diagnosis of lung cancer)

Discussion

Immune checkpoint inhibitors have been known to carry risk of pulmonary toxicity since early clinical trials of these agents in renal cell carcinoma, melanoma, NSCLC, and others [6]. Pneumonitis, characterized by dyspnea, cough, parenchymal lung opacities, and impaired oxygen exchange, is the most common manifestation, occurring in approximately 5% of patients who receive these therapies [7]. Airways disease is an uncommon manifestation of ICI toxicity, however, only previously described in case reports which have noted a variety of disease subtypes. For example, eosinophilic tracheitis has also been described in the setting of nivolumab therapy with similar presentation to the case we presented here [8]. Two additional cases which primarily affected the large bronchi were characterized by an obstructive pattern on pulmonary function tests, elevated lymphocyte and eosinophil cell differential on bronchoalveolar lavage, as well as lymphocyte and eosinophil infiltration on endobronchial biopsy specimens [9]. Maeno et al. describe a case of reversible airflow obstruction, high fraction of exhaled nitric oxide (a marker of eosinophilic airway inflammation), and elevated serum immunoglobin E, all supportive of a new diagnosis of eosinophilic asthma while on nivolumab [10]. Small airways disease has been associated with ICI therapy as well, as a patient with an obstructive pulmonary function test pattern, diffuse micronodules of the lung on CT, and lymphocytic infiltration of the bronchioles found on transbronchial biopsy received a diagnosis of ICI-associated bronchiolitis [11].

There are no society or consensus guidelines for management of ICI-induced airways disease. Cessation of the offending agent and consideration of immunosuppression are the primary strategies utilized for other ICI toxicities. For those who suffer ICI pneumonitis of grade II or higher (toxicity causing pulmonary symptoms and involving >25% of the lung parenchyma), oral or intravenous corticosteroid therapy can lead to clinical and radiographic improvement [12]. There is likely some shared pathology between airway and parenchymal lung toxicity, and we posit that corticosteroids should also be utilized for airway disease. Inhaled corticosteroids may be useful as systemic corticosteroid doses are tapered, and clinicians may consider serial spirometry to evaluate treatment response and timing of immunosuppression taper/discontinuation. In prior cases of ICI airway disease, systemic glucocorticoid doses of up to prednisone 2 mg/kg daily, and fluticasone propionate 500 μg daily have been reported [8, 10].

Given the efficacy and increasing use of ICI for numerous malignancies, it is probable that new manifestations of pulmonary toxicity will continue to emerge. Though airway inflammation induced by these agents appears to be rare, it may be underdiagnosed, and clinicians should consider this diagnosis when faced with patients whose pulmonary symptoms are not explained by more common etiologies. While experience with ICI-induced tracheobronchitis is lacking, rechallenge with the offending agent may be reasonable in the absence of life-threatening hemoptysis or other severe airway complications.

References

1. Wenzel RP, Fowler AA. Clinical practice. Acute bronchitis N Engl J Med. 2006;355(20):2125–30. http://www.ncbi.nlm.nih.gov/pubmed/17108344.
2. Diseases. NC for I and R. Respiratory Disease Season Outlook—Summary. [Internet]. [cited 2023 Sep 25]. https://www.cdc.gov/respiratory-viruses/whats-new/2023-2024-season-outlook.html#print.
3. Clark TW, Medina M, Batham S, Curran MD, Parmar S, Nicholson KG. Adults hospitalised with acute respiratory illness rarely have detectable bacteria in the absence of COPD or pneumonia; viral infection predominates in a large prospective UK sample. J Infect. 2014;69(5):507–15. http://www.ncbi.nlm.nih.gov/pubmed/25108123
4. Jung S-S, Park H-S, Kim J-O, Kim S-Y. Incidence and clinical predictors of endobronchial tuberculosis in patients with pulmonary tuberculosis. Theatr Res Int. 2015;20(3):488–95. http://www.ncbi.nlm.nih.gov/pubmed/25620110.
5. Camus P, Piard F, Ashcroft T, Gal AA, Colby TV. The lung in inflammatory bowel disease. Medicine (Baltimore). 1993;72(3):151–83. http://www.ncbi.nlm.nih.gov/pubmed/8502168.
6. Nishino M, Giobbie-Hurder A, Hatabu H, Ramaiya NH, Hodi FS. Incidence of programmed cell death 1 inhibitor-related pneumonitis in patients with advanced cancer: a systematic review and meta-analysis. JAMA Oncol. 2016;2(12):1607–16. http://www.ncbi.nlm.nih.gov/pubmed/27540850.
7. Naidoo J, Wang X, Woo KM, Iyriboz T, Halpenny D, Cunningham J, et al. Pneumonitis in patients treated with anti-programmed Death-1/programmed death ligand 1 therapy. J Clin Oncol. 2017;35(7):709–17. http://www.ncbi.nlm.nih.gov/pubmed/27646942.
8. Tellez-Garcia E, Valdivia Padilla A, Grosu H. Immunotherapy-induced eosinophilic tracheitis. Cureus. 2022;14(4):e24130. http://www.ncbi.nlm.nih.gov/pubmed/35573537.
9. Mitropoulou G, Daccord C, Sauty A, Pasche A, Egger B, Aedo Lopez V, et al. Immunotherapy-induced airway disease: a new pattern of lung toxicity of immune checkpoint inhibitors. Theatr Res Int. 2020;99(2):181–6. http://www.ncbi.nlm.nih.gov/pubmed/31914436.
10. Maeno K, Fukuda S, Oguri T, Niimi A. Nivolumab-induced asthma in a patient with non-small-cell lung cancer. Ann Oncol. 2017;28(11):2891. http://www.ncbi.nlm.nih.gov/pubmed/28945837.
11. Yamaya T, Hee HM, Aoyagi T, Ogimoto T, Yamada N, Ishikawa R, et al. Pembrolizumab-associated bronchiolitis in an elderly lung cancer patient required the treatment with an inhaled corticosteroid, erythromycin and bronchodilators. Respir Med Case Rep. 2019;28:100866. http://www.ncbi.nlm.nih.gov/pubmed/31198678.
12. Schneider BJ, Naidoo J, Santomasso BD, Lacchetti C, Adkins S, Anadkat M, et al. Management of Immune-Related Adverse Events in patients treated with immune checkpoint inhibitor therapy: ASCO guideline update. J Clin Oncol. 2021;39(36):4073–126. http://www.ncbi.nlm.nih.gov/pubmed/34724392.

Part XII
Rheumatology

Chapter 52
Inflammatory Arthritis Post Immune Checkpoint Inhibitor Therapy

Savannah Bowman, Rodabe N. Amaria, and Huifang Lu

Abbreviations

CCP	Cyclic cirtrullinated peptide
CRP	C-reactive protein
ICI	immune checkpoint inhibitor
irAE	Immune related adverse event
SSZ	Sulfasalazine

Case Presentation

The patient is a Caucasian female in her 60 s diagnosed with T4N0 left sinonasal malignant melanoma who was initially treated with neoadjuvant immune checkpoint inhibitors (ICI) nivolumab and ipilimumab with subsequent endoscopic resection of the tumor. After two cycles of ICI, she developed colitis and was treated with oral prednisone at 1 mg/kg twice daily with taper and infliximab once at 5 mg/kg. She presented to the hospital 3 days after the first infliximab infusion, with bilateral knee joint pain and swelling. Her only other past medical history is allergic rhinitis

S. Bowman
Department of Allergy, Immunology & Rheumatology, Department of Internal Medicine, Baylor College of Medicine, Houston, TX, USA
e-mail: savannah.bowman@bcm.edu

R. N. Amaria
Department of Melanoma Medical Oncology, Division of Cancer Medicine, The University of Texas MD Anderson Cancer Center, Houston, TX, USA

H. Lu (✉)
Department of Rheumatology and Immunology, Division of Internal Medicine, The University of Texas MD Anderson Cancer Center, Houston, TX, USA
e-mail: hlu@mdanderson.edu

Y. Wang (ed.), *Challenging Cases in Immunotherapy Related Organ Toxicities*,
https://doi.org/10.1007/978-3-031-83533-9_52

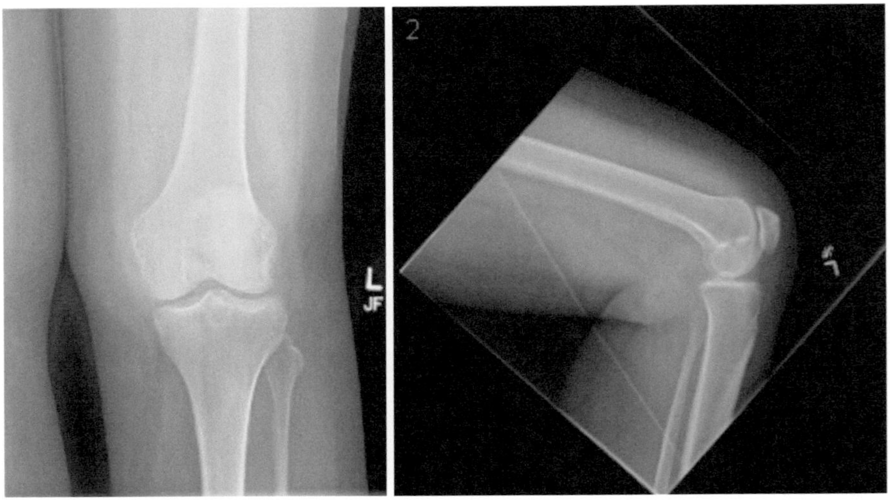

Fig. 52.1 Left knee X-ray with no acute fractures, dislocations, or joint abnormality. There is soft tissue swelling about the knee with a suprapatellar space concerning for joint effusion

for which she takes cetirizine. She also takes vitamin B6 and vitamin C supplements. Physical exam showed tenderness, warmth, and large effusion of bilateral knees. Knee X-rays showed bilateral joint effusions (Fig. 52.1). The patient denied prior join pain or swelling. Her inflammatory c-reactive protein (CRP) was elevated at 79.37 mg/L (Table 52.1). Rheumatoid factor and anti-CCP antibodies were negative. Infectious work up was unrevealing. She declined arthrocentesis of her knee.

Differential Diagnosis

Given her new onset bilateral knee joint pain and swelling, several differential diagnoses were considered. These include septic arthritis, crystal arthritis, or ICI induced inflammatory oligoarthritis. The patient declined arthrocentesis. X-ray of her knees showed no sign of CPPD or osteoarthritis, but joint fluid effusion. Because of her uncontrolled diarrhea, she received the second dose of infliximab infusion and solumedrol 1 mg/kg twice daily intravenously, her knee pain and swelling rapidly improved. The symmetry and rapid improvement with steroid and infliximab, making a septic arthritis diagnosis unlikely. Considering the onset of her knee joint swelling after her ICI therapy, she was given the diagnosis of ICI-induced inflammatory arthritis.

Table 52.1 Laboratory findings

Laboratory test	Value
White blood count	$8.1 \times 10^3/\mu L$
Hemoglobin	12.7 g/dL
Platelet count Sodium Potassium Chloride Carbon dioxide Blood urea nitrogen Creatinine	$256 \times 10^3/\mu L$ **132 mEq/L** **3.2 mEq/L** **94 mEq/L** 24 mEq/L 13 mg/dL 0.67 mg/dL
Glucose Calcium ALT AST Alkaline phosphatase Total bilirubin Total protein Albumin International normalization ratio	93 mg/dL 8.8 mg/dL 11 U/L 17 U/L 70 U/L 0.2 mg/dL **6.3 g/dL** **3.4 g/dL** 1.09
Blood culture (2 sets)	Negative
Urine culture	Negative
CRP	**79.37 mg/L**
Rheumatoid factor	12 IU/mL
CCP antibody	<15. 6 units

Abbreviations: *AST* aspartate aminotransferase, *ALT* alanine transaminase, *CRP* C reactive peptide, *CCP* cyclic citrullinated peptide

Laboratory reference values: sodium 136–145 mEq/L, potassium 3.5–5.1 mEq/L, chloride 98–107 mEq/L, total protein 6.4–8.3 g/dL, albumin 3.5–5.2 g/dL, CRP Less than or equal to 10.00 mg/L

Abnormal lab values are in bold

Hospital Course and Management

The knee arthritis improved with adding intravenous methylprednisolone 1 mg/kg two times a day for 3 days, which was given for her uncontrolled diarrhea symptom and then she was transitioned to oral prednisone 60 mg twice a day. Her diarrhea resolved within a week of this regimen. Her bilateral knee synovitis also improved with this regimen within a week and she was discharged home.

Case Outcome

She followed up with rheumatology outpatient and the prednisone was slowly tapered and was ultimately able to be stopped over 4 months. Her arthritis was in remission for 5 weeks while off prednisone. She then developed bilateral synovitis

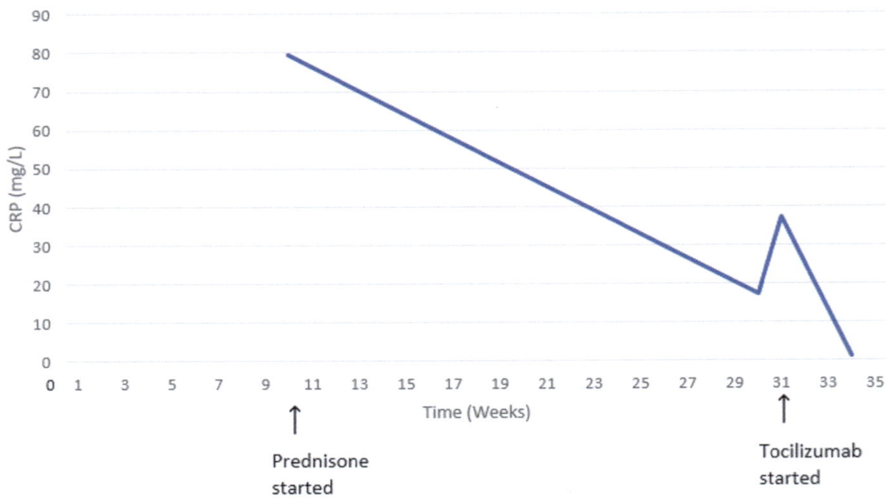

Fig. 52.2 Trend of C reactive protein (CRP) before and after treatment with tocilizumab. CRP normalized after initiation of tocilizumab

in knees, ankles, and left wrist. Prednisone was re-started, and she was also started on sulfasalazine as a steroid sparing agent. She remained without diarrhea, however continued to have frequent relapses of the arthritis requiring escalating doses of prednisone. She was then started on tocilizumab subcutaneous injections every other week. Her CRP normalized after initiation of tocilizumab (Fig. 52.2). After 3 doses of tocilizumab, the arthritis achieved remission. Given the cancer recurrence, she received talimogene laherparepvec intralesional treatment for 6 months, and resumed nivolumab monotherapy treatment for over 2 more years for a total of 70 infusions without flaring of her arthritis, while on bi-weekly tocilizumab concurrent treatment. About 6 months after she was off nivolumab, she was tapered off tocilizumab successfully. She remained cancer free and without flares of her arthritis at her last follow up 6 months after she was off tocilizumab.

Summary

This is a case of a patients with T4N0 sinonasal malignant melanoma who had received two cycles of ipilimumab and nivolumab who subsequently developed inflammatory arthritis of bilateral knees related to ICI treatment. This patient received corticosteroids and sulfasalazine with no response, but achieved complete remission on tocilizumab. This therapeutic effect sustained over 2 years despite patient resumed nivolumab monotherapy for cancer recurrence while receiving tocilizumab as concurrent treatment. The summary of the disease course is depicted in Fig. 52.3.

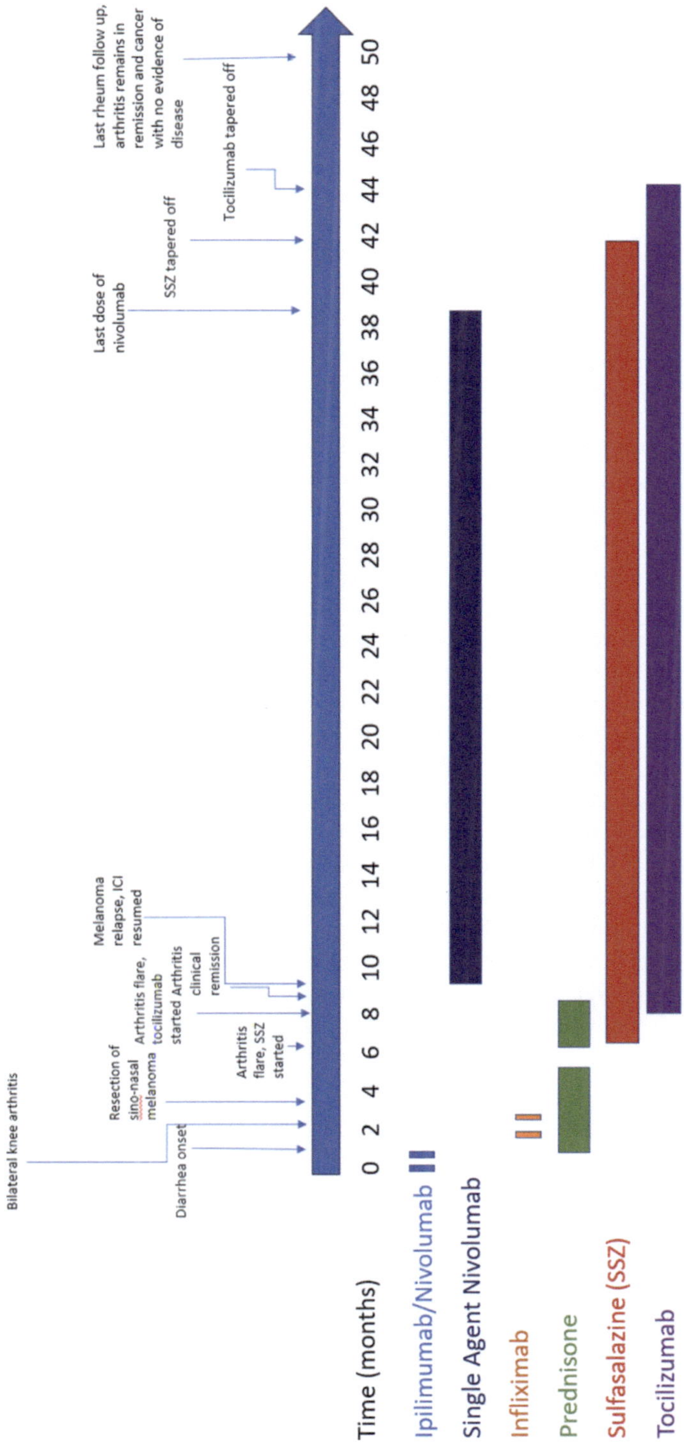

Fig. 52.3 Timeline representation of events and medications used in the case. (Time point of 0 is initiation if ICI)

Discussion

This case illustrates a typical case of ICI-induced inflammatory arthritis. Arthralgia and arthritis represent the most frequent rheumatic immune-related adverse events (irAEs) following treatment with immune checkpoint inhibitors [1, 2]. Clinical studies have indicated that approximately 10.0–13.3% of patients develop inflammatory arthralgia, while 1.8–10.0% experience arthritis after receiving programmed cell death 1 (PD-1) inhibitors, either alone or in combination with cytotoxic T-lymphocyte-associated antigen 4 (CTLA-4) inhibitors [3–5].

ICI-induced arthritis patterns include monoarthritis, reactive arthritis-like oligoarthritis, rheumatoid arthritis (RA)-like polyarthritis, remitting seronegative symmetrical synovitis with pitting edema (RS3PE), and undifferentiated arthritis, with the knee being the most frequently impacted joint, followed by small joints [6, 7]. While the majority of irAEs manifest within the first 12 weeks following initial ICI therapy [8], arthritis-irAE tends to occur later. Monoarthritis typically arises around a median of 9 months after the first infusion, while oligoarthritis and polyarthritis tend to develop around a median of 3 months of initial ICI therapy [6]. Specific markers, as anti-CCP antibodies, rheumatoid factor, and ANA are often negative [9].

Importantly, patients treated with combination ICI who develop arthritis irAE are often more resistant to steroids than patients treated with anti-PD-1 monotherapy [7]. Given these cases are often steroid refractory and arthritis-irAE can significantly impact the quality of life, these patients should be treated early on and often require disease modifying anti-rheumatic drugs or biologics. Options include sulfasalazine, methotrexate, anti-IL6 receptor blockers (tocilizumab), and TNF-α inhibitors (infliximab). Recent studies have shown that combined blockade of either IL-6 or TNF and PD-1 elicits synergistic anti-tumor responses [10, 11]. As demonstrated in our case, biologics can control the arthritis effectively and it is safe for patients to continue the ICI despite developing arthritis-irAE. However, a subsequent retrospective multicenter observational study found that while time to arthritis control was significantly faster for TNF inhibitors compared to methotrexate, time to cancer progression was significantly shorter. Neither outcome was statistically significant when comparing methotrexate to IL-6 receptor blockers [12]. Further studies are still warranted in this field.

References

1. Ramos-Casals M, Lambotte O, Kostine M, Calabrese L, Suarez-Almazor M, Bingham C, Radstake TR, Baldini C, Schaeverbeke T, Gottenberg J-E. THU0649 phenotypic clusters of rheumatic/systemic immune-related adverse events induced by cancer immunotherapies (Immunocancer international registry). Noida: BMJ Publishing Group Ltd; 2019.
2. Calabrese LH, Calabrese C, Cappelli LC. Rheumatic immune-related adverse events from cancer immunotherapy. Nat Rev Rheumatol. 2018;14(10):569–79.

3. Robert C, Schachter J, Long GV, Arance A, Grob JJ, Mortier L, Daud A, Carlino MS, McNeil C, Lotem M. Pembrolizumab versus ipilimumab in advanced melanoma. N Engl J Med. 2015;372(26):2521–32.
4. Postow MA, Chesney J, Pavlick AC, Robert C, Grossmann K, McDermott D, Linette GP, Meyer N, Giguere JK, Agarwala SS. Nivolumab and ipilimumab versus ipilimumab in untreated melanoma. N Engl J Med. 2015;372(21):2006–17.
5. Buder-Bakhaya K, Benesova K, Schulz C, Anwar H, Dimitrakopoulou-Strauss A, Weber TF, Enk A, Lorenz H-M, Hassel JC. Characterization of arthralgia induced by PD-1 antibody treatment in patients with metastasized cutaneous malignancies. Cancer Immunol Immunother. 2018;67(2):175–82.
6. Pundole X, Abdel-Wahab N, Suarez-Almazor ME. Arthritis risk with immune checkpoint inhibitor therapy for cancer. Curr Opin Rheumatol. 2019;31(3):293–9.
7. Cappelli LC, Brahmer JR, Forde PM, Le DT, Lipson EJ, Naidoo J, Zheng L, Bingham CO III, Shah AA. Clinical presentation of immune checkpoint inhibitor-induced inflammatory arthritis differs by immunotherapy regimen. In: Semin Arthritis Rheum, vol. 48; 2018. p. 553–7.
8. Boutros C, Tarhini A, Routier E, Lambotte O, Ladurie FL, Carbonnel F, Izzeddine H, Marabelle A, Champiat S, Berdelou A. Safety profiles of anti-CTLA-4 and anti-PD-1 antibodies alone and in combination. Nat Rev Clin Oncol. 2016;13(8):473–86.
9. Cappelli LC, Gutierrez AK, Baer AN, Albayda J, Manno RL, Haque U, Lipson EJ, Bleich KB, Shah AA, Naidoo J. Inflammatory arthritis and sicca syndrome induced by nivolumab and ipilimumab. Ann Rheum Dis. 2017;76(1):43–50.
10. Tsukamoto H, Fujieda K, Miyashita A, Fukushima S, Ikeda T, Kubo Y, Senju S, Ihn H, Nishimura Y, Oshiumi H. Combined blockade of IL6 and PD-1/PD-L1 signaling abrogates mutual regulation of their immunosuppressive effects in the tumor microenvironment. Cancer Res. 2018;78(17):5011–22.
11. Bertrand F, Montfort A, Marcheteau E, Imbert C, Gilhodes J, Filleron T, Rochaix P, Andrieu-Abadie N, Levade T, Meyer N. TNFα blockade overcomes resistance to anti-PD-1 in experimental melanoma. Nat Commun. 2017;8(1):2256.
12. Bass AR, Abdel-Wahab N, Reid PD, Sparks JA, Calabrese C, Jannat-Khah DP, Ghosh N, Rajesh D, Aude CA, Gedmintas L. Comparative safety and effectiveness of TNF inhibitors, IL6 inhibitors and methotrexate for the treatment of immune checkpoint inhibitor-associated arthritis. Ann Rheum Dis. 2023;82(7):920–6.

Chapter 53
Sicca Syndrome Induced by Immune Checkpoint Inhibitor Therapy

Yuanteng Jeff Li, Sang T. Kim, Nizar M. Tannir, and Huifang Lu

Abbreviations

ANA	Antinuclear Antibody
Anti-CCP	Anti cyclic citrullinated peptide antibody
Anti-MPO	Anti-myeloperoxidase antibody
Anti- PR3	Anti-proteinase-3 antibody
C3 and C4	Complement 3 and Complement 4
CBC	Complete blood count
CMP	Comprehensive metabolic profile
CRP	C-reactive protein
CT	Computed tomography
ESR	Erythrocyte sedimentation rate
HIV	Human immunodeficiency virus
ICI	Immune checkpoint inhibitor
RF	Rheumatoid Factor

Y. J. Li · H. Lu (✉)
Department of Rheumatology and Immunology, Division of Internal Medicine, The University of Texas MD Anderson Cancer Center, Houston, TX, USA
e-mail: yli61@mdanderson.org; hlu@mdanderson.org

S. T. Kim
Department of Rheumatology, Allergy & Immunology, Yale University, New Haven, CT, USA
e-mail: sangtaek.kim@yale.edu

N. M. Tannir
Department of Genitourinary Medical Oncology, Division of Cancer Medicine, UT MD Anderson Cancer Center, Houston, TX, USA
e-mail: Ntannir@mdanderson.org

Y. Wang (ed.), *Challenging Cases in Immunotherapy Related Organ Toxicities*,
https://doi.org/10.1007/978-3-031-83533-9_53

Clinical Presentation

This is a female in 60 s with a history of stage 4 clear cell kidney carcinoma presenting to rheumatology clinic for evaluation of dry eyes and dry mouth that developed after initiating nivolumab. Ten months prior to the initial rheumatology evaluation, patient was started on nivolumab as her cancer had progressed despite being on everolimus and pazopanib. At the time of the evaluation, she had already developed hypothyroidism and pneumonitis related to nivolumab, which required 6 weeks of prednisone treatment and nivolumab stoppage. A few days after patient finished prednisone for her pneumonitis, she developed dry eyes, dry mouth, and bilateral parotid gland enlargement, suggesting sicca syndrome. Her past medical history included hypertension, asthma, sinusitis, and hyperlipidemia. Her past surgical history included cholecystectomy, left radical nephrectomy, L5–S1 laminectomy, tonsillectomy, mammoplasty, and cesarean section. Her outpatient medications included albuterol inhaler 180 μg every 6 h as needed, amlodipine 5 mg daily, atenolol 25 mg nightly, and levothyroxine 112 μg daily. Patient was not taking any antihistamine related medications on a routine basis.

Evaluations

Her CMP and CBC were unremarkable and stable (Table 53.1). Her infectious disease and autoimmune work up revealed a negative HIV, ANA, anti-SSA, anti-SSB, anti-MPO, anti-PR3, anti-CCP autoantibodies, and cryoglobulin. Her C3 and C4 were normal. Interestingly, her rheumatoid factor was moderately elevated (Table 53.2). CT soft tissue neck revealed non-specific, mild prominence and heterogeneity of the bilateral parotid glands (Fig. 53.1).

Treatment

Patient was started on prednisone 20 mg daily and pilocarpine 5 mg three times a day. She tapered off prednisone over a period of 7 weeks with gradual improvement in her dry eyes and dry mouth. Her symptoms remained stable until 3 weeks after she stopped her prednisone when she developed a flare of sicca syndrome and new inflammatory joint pain in her shoulders. Prednisone was restarted, and hydroxychloroquine 200 mg twice daily was added as a steroid sparing agent. It is important to note that patient did not feel improvement in her sicca syndrome until 1 week into her treatment.

Table 53.1 Laboratory findings at SICCA symptom onset

Laboratory test	Value
White blood count	$8.7 \times 10^3/\mu L$
Hemoglobin	12.4 g/dL
Platelet count	$287 \times 10^3/\mu L$
Sodium	137 mmol/L
Potassium	4.6 mmol/L
Chloride	98 mmol/L
Carbon dioxide	29 mmol/L
Blood urea nitrogen	13 mg/dL
Creatinine	0.64 mg/dL
Glucose	93 mg/dL
Calcium	9.8 mg/dL
ALT	40 U/L
AST	36 U/L
Alkaline phosphatase	101 U/L

Laboratory reference values: White blood count 6.0–11.0 × 10³/uL hemoglobin 12.0–16.0gm/dL, platelet count 140–440 K/uL, sodium 136–145 mEq/L, potassium 3.5–5.0 mEq/L, chloride 98–107 mEq/L, carbon dioxide 23–30 mEq/L, blood urea nitrogen 8 = 20 mg/dL, creatinine 0.60–1.00 mg/dL, ALT 7–56 U/L, AST 15–46 U/L, alkaline phosphatase 38–126 U/L
Abnormal lab values are in bold

Table 53.2 Autoimmune and infectious disease laboratory findings

Laboratory test	Value
ANA titer	< 1:40
Anti-SSA	< 0.2 unit
Anti-SSB	< 0.2 unit
RF	**50.8 IU/mL**
Anti-CCP ab	< 15.6 units
Anti-MPO ab	< 0.2 units
Anti- PR3 ab	< 0.2 units
C3	135 mg/dL
C4	21 mg/dL
Cryoglobulin	Negative
ESR	15 mm/hour
CRP	**5.03 mg/L**
HIV	Non-reactive

Laboratory reference values: ANA titer <1:40, anti-SSA < 1 unit, anti-SSB < 1 unit, RF 0.0–15.9 IU/mL, anti-CCP ab <20 units, anti-MPO ab <0.4 units, anti-PR3 ab <0.4 units, C3 75–175 mg/dL, C4 14–40 mg/dL, cryoglobulin negative, ESR 0–20 mm/h, CRP > 3.0 mg/L, HIV non-reactive
Abnormal lab values are in bold

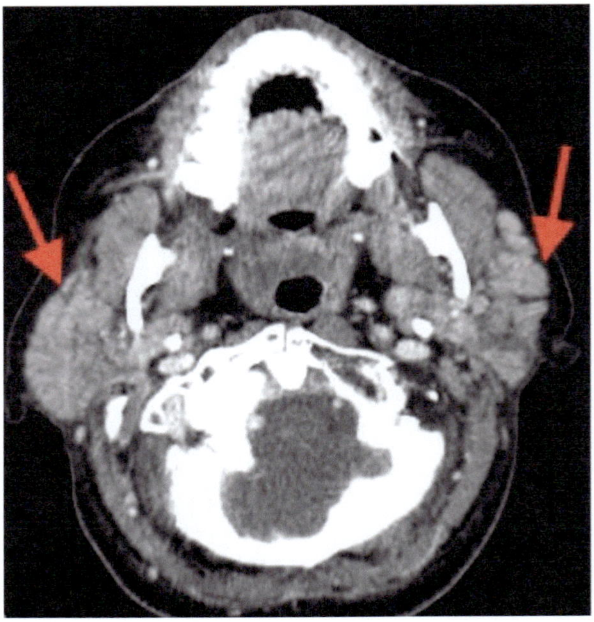

Fig. 53.1 CT axial soft tissue neck. Mild prominence of the bilateral parotid glands, more conspicuous on the right than left. No cystic changes or calcifications are identified. No focal parotid mass lesions

Case Outcome

In total, patient required 26 weeks of prednisone treatment before her sicca syndrome went quiescent. She remained on hydroxychloroquine monotherapy for an additional 12 weeks, and her sicca syndrome stayed in remission (Fig. 53.2). Throughout the course, her inflammatory markers were not significantly elevated. Finally, her cancer remained stable with no progression even though nivolumab was never restarted.

Summary

This is a case with a clear cell kidney carcinoma patient on nivolumab treatment who developed ICI related sicca syndrome. Her sicca syndrome was successfully treated with a combination of prednisone and hydroxychloroquine, which were eventually tapered off. Her cancer remained in remission while on an immunosuppressant for 26 weeks for sicca syndrome and other immune related adverse events.

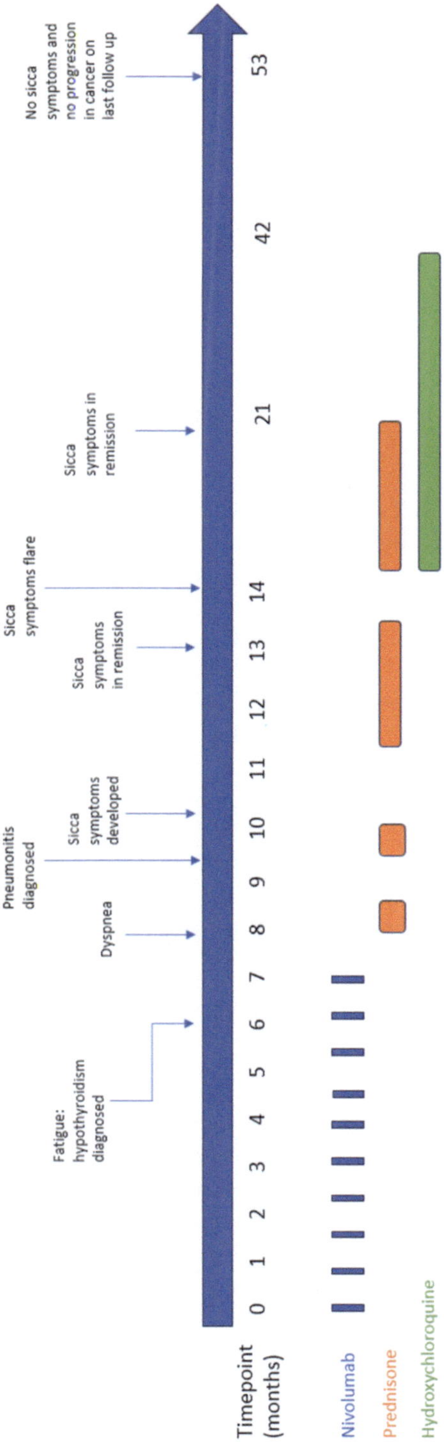

Fig. 53.2 Timeline of SICCA symptom onset after treatment of nivolumab and response to prednisone and hydroxychloroquine

Discussion

Primary Sjogren's disease and ICI-induced sicca syndrome appear to be two different diseases despite having similar clinical presentations. For instance, although anti-SSA and anti-SSB autoantibodies play an important role in diagnosing primary Sjogren's syndrome, most patients with ICI-induced sicca syndrome test negative for anti-SSA and anti-SSB autoantibodies [1–4]. Moreover, other autoantibodies such as ANA and rheumatoid factor are negative in most ICI-induced sicca syndrome patients [1–4]. The histopathology behind the two diseases is also vastly different. In primary Sjogren's disease, the affected exocrine glands are characterized by periductal mononuclear infiltration mainly and $CD20^+$ B cells [4–6]. In contrast, ICI-induced sicca syndrome has histology characteristically showing only a few $CD20^+$ B cells and mostly T cells with more $CD4^+$ T cells than $CD8^+$ T cells [1, 7].

The use of immunosuppressants to treat primary Sjogren's dry eyes and dry mouth symptoms is generally not recommended [8]. However, as Sjogren's and ICI-induced sicca syndrome may be different based on histopathology, it is not entirely clear if immunosuppressant such as prednisone would be beneficial for ICI-induced sicca syndrome. One study reported that in 12 out of the 20 ICI-induced sicca syndrome patients whose ICI were stopped and/or corticosteroids were used, 10 patients reported moderate or significant improvement, but not completely abated [1]. Furthermore, in those patients who had subjectively responded to steroids, objective measures only showed mild benefit [1]. Other case reports and case series have also shown mixed results with the use of prednisone for the treatment of this indication [9–11]. Furthermore, when compared to holding ICI, prednisone appeared to have a lesser effect on controlling ICI-induced sicca syndrome [2]. In our case, a combination of prednisone and hydroxychloroquine appears to be effective. Perhaps this is due to the early introduction of prednisone in the disease course which may suggest that prednisone's utility may be dictated by its early use.

Conclusion

Current management of ICI-induced sicca syndrome is mostly symptom based. Glucocorticoids may be considered early on and in severe cases though its role in eradicating symptoms is dubious with mixed results. Further research is still needed to expand the knowledge in managing ICI induced sicca syndrome.

References

1. Warner BM, Baer AN, Lipson EJ, et al. Sicca syndrome associated with immune checkpoint inhibitor therapy. Oncologist. 2019;24(9):1259–69.
2. Ortiz Brugues A, Sibaud V, Herbault-Barres B, et al. Sicca syndrome induced by immune checkpoint inhibitor therapy: optimal management still pending. Oncologist. 2020;25(2):e391–e5.
3. Ramos-Casals M, Maria A, Suarez-Almazor ME, et al. Sicca/Sjogren's syndrome triggered by PD-1/PD-L1 checkpoint inhibitors. Data from the international ImmunoCancer registry (ICIR). Clin Exp Rheumatol. 2019;37 Suppl 118(3):114–22.
4. Burbelo PD, Ferre EMN, Chaturvedi A, et al. Profiling autoantibodies against salivary proteins in Sicca conditions. J Dent Res. 2019;98(7):772–8.
5. Costa S, Schutz S, Cornec D, et al. B-cell and T-cell quantification in minor salivary glands in primary Sjogren's syndrome: development and validation of a pixel-based digital procedure. Arthritis Res Ther. 2016;18:21.
6. Alessandri C, Ciccia F, Priori R, et al. CD4 T lymphocyte autophagy is upregulated in the salivary glands of primary Sjogren's syndrome patients and correlates with focus score and disease activity. Arthritis Res Ther. 2017;19(1):178.
7. Higashi T, Miyamoto H, Yoshida R, et al. Sjogren's syndrome as an immune-related adverse event of Nivolumab treatment for gastric cancer. Intern Med. 2020;59(20):2499–504.
8. Harris JA, Huang K, Miloslavsky E, Hanna GJ. Sicca syndrome associated with immune checkpoint inhibitor therapy. Oral Dis. 2022;28(8):2083–92.
9. Cappelli LC, Gutierrez AK, Baer AN, et al. Inflammatory arthritis and sicca syndrome induced by nivolumab and ipilimumab. Ann Rheum Dis. 2017;76(1):43–50.
10. Richter MD, Pinkston O, Kottschade LA, et al. Brief report: cancer immunotherapy in patients with preexisting rheumatic disease: the Mayo Clinic experience. Arthritis Rheumatol. 2018;70(3):356–60.
11. Narvaez J, Juarez-Lopez P, LLuch J, et al. Rheumatic immune-related adverse events in patients on anti-PD-1 inhibitors: fasciitis with myositis syndrome as a new complication of immunotherapy. Autoimmun Rev. 2018;17(10):1040–5.

Chapter 54
Polymyalgia Rheumatica-Like Syndrome Post Immune Checkpoint Inhibitor Therapy

Huifang Lu, Savannah Bowman, N. P. Linda Bobby, Sang T. Kim, Pavlos Msaouel, and Jean Tayar

Abbreviations

CCP	Cyclic citrullinated peptide
CRP	C-reactive protein
ESR	Erythrocyte sedimentation rate
ICI	Immune checkpoint inhibitor
IL-6	Interleukin-6
PD-1	Programmed cell death protein-1
PMR	Polymyalgia rheumatica

H. Lu (✉) · N. P. Linda Bobby · J. Tayar
Department of Rheumatology and Immunology, Division of Internal Medicine,
The University of Texas MD Anderson Cancer Center, Houston, TX, USA
e-mail: hlu@mdanderson.edu; jhtayar@mdanderson.org

S. Bowman
Department of Allergy, Immunology & Rheumatology, Department of Internal Medicine,
Baylor College of Medicine, Houston, TX, USA
e-mail: savannah.bowman@bcm.edu

S. T. Kim
Department of Rheumatology, Allergy & Immunology, Yale University,
New Haven, CT, USA
e-mail: sangtaek.kim@yale.edu

P. Msaouel
Department of Genitourinary Medical Oncology, Division of Cancer Medicine,
The University of Texas MD Anderson Cancer Center, Houston, TX, USA
e-mail: pmsaouel@mdanderson.org

Y. Wang (ed.), *Challenging Cases in Immunotherapy Related Organ Toxicities*,
https://doi.org/10.1007/978-3-031-83533-9_54

Case Presentation

This is a Caucasian male in 70 s diagnosed with clear cell metastatic renal cell carcinoma, status post treatment with surgery, radiation, and first-line combination immune checkpoint inhibitor (ICI) therapy with ipilimumab plus nivolumab. After the third cycle of combination therapy, the patient developed pain and stiffness of his neck and proximal muscle groups in bilateral shoulders and hips. He had morning stiffness for 2 h every day. His other past medical history included obstructive sleep apnea, hypertension, hyperlipidemia, and chronic kidney disease stage 2 (baseline creatinine 1.3 mg/dL). His medications included ezetimibe and lisinopril.

Evaluations

Physical examination showed impaired range of motion of his shoulders with abduction and flexion are limited to 75 degrees. His elbows also had impaired range of motion with extension to only 80 degrees with no joint effusion. Flexion and extension were also limited in his knees to approximately 75 degrees each with no joint effusion. His shoulder and hip muscles were sore but there was no tenderness on exam, and the joints had no effusion. He did not have headache, blurry vision, vision loss, or jaw claudication. Laboratory work up showed negative rheumatoid factor and anti-cyclic citrullinated peptide (CCP) antibodies. Infectious work up was unrevealing. Inflammatory markers were mildly elevated with sedimentation rate of 30 mm/h. (normal range 0–9 mm/h) and c-reactive protein of 10.93 (normal range < 10.00 mg/L) (Table 54.1).

Diagnosis

This presentation of the neck, and bilateral shoulder and hip girdle pain, along with normal muscle enzymes levels and lack of joint tenderness or swelling on exam he was diagnosed with polymyalgia rheumatica (PMR)-like syndrome.

Treatment

He was empirically started on prednisone 20 mg for (PMR)-like syndrome with resolution of symptoms within 3 days. After prednisone 20 mg daily for 2 weeks, he was then tapered by 5 mg every 2 weeks. When he got below prednisone 10 mg daily, his proximal muscle and joint pain and stiffness flared. He was the started on Sarilumab, an interleukin-6 receptor antagonist, 200 mg subcutaneous injections

Table 54.1 Laboratory findings

Laboratory test	Value
White blood count	6.6 × 10^3/μL
Hemoglobin	**11.5 g/dL**
Platelet count	291 × 10^3/μL
Sodium	141 mEq/L
Potassium	4.5 mEq/L
Chloride	101 mEq/L
Carbon dioxide	26 mEq/L
Blood urea nitrogen	**21 mg/dL**
Creatinine	**1.34 mg/dL**
Glucose	93 mg/dL
Calcium	9.1 mg/dL
ALT	9 U/L
AST	14 U/L
Alkaline phosphatase	75 U/L
Total bilirubin	0.1 mg/dL
Total protein	7.9 g/dL
Albumin	4.4 g/dL
International normalization ratio	0.93
ESR	**30 mm/h**
CRP	**10.93 mg/L**
Rheumatoid factor	<10 IU/mL
CCP antibody	<15. 6 units

Abbreviations: *AST* aspartate aminotransferase, *ALT* alanine transaminase, *ESR* erythrocyte sedimentation rate, *CRP* C reactive peptide, *CCP* cyclic citrullinated peptide
Laboratory reference values: Hemoglobin 14.0–18.0 g/dL, blood urea nitrogen 6–23 mg/dL, creatinine 0.67–1.17 mg/dL, ESR 0–9 mm/h, CRP less than or equal to 10.00 mg/L
Abnormal lab values are in bold

every 2 weeks as a steroid sparing agent with good control of his symptoms allowing further slow tapering of his prednisone.

Case Outcome

The combination ICI was resumed, and he was able to complete the intended treatment course of 4 cycles of combination therapy and 2 more cycles of maintenance nivolumab monotherapy. Since then, his cancer has been in remission without recurrence for over 4 years. His prednisone was tapered off slowly over the next 5 months after starting sarilumab. Two weeks after stopping prednisone, while still on sarilumab bi-weekly injection, he began experiencing knee and shoulder pain again with morning stiffness lasting 1–2 h. His symptoms quickly resolved by adding 10 mg of prednisone daily. Over the next 13 weeks his prednisone was again tapered off this time without symptoms flaring. Unfortunately, over the next 6 months he had a consistent down trending of his absolute neutrophil count and his sarilumab was held. He was restarted on 20 mg prednisone daily. His neutrophil count normalized after being off sarilumab for 7 months, at that time sarilumab was restarted and prednisone was tapered down to 7.5 mg daily to maintain good control of his symptoms.

Case Summary

This is a case with metastatic clear cell renal cell carcinoma, who developed PMR-like syndrome after 3 cycles of combination ICI therapy of ipilimumab and nivolumab. Clinically, he had the classic presentation of neck and proximal muscle pain and stiffness, although his inflammation markers were only mildly elevated. He responded well to 20 mg of prednisone, however he failed several attempts at tapering prednisone off despite adding sarilumab, but finally able to achieve clinical remission with combination of sarilumab and low dose maintenance prednisone at 7.5 mg daily. Summary of timeline events is shown in Fig. 54.1.

Discussion

This case illustrates a typical case of ICI-induced PMR-like syndrome in a patient who experienced profound antitumor efficacy to ICI with his metastatic cancer remaining in remission for over 4 years now. It is unclear if ICI induced PMR-like syndrome is its own clinical entity or the same disease as traditional PMR [1]. The prevalence of ICI induced PMR-like syndrome is reported as 0.2–2.1% [2]. Our patient fits the classic age for developing PMR, which is similar between traditional and ICI induced condition in the seventh decade of life [3, 4]. Like the symptoms reported in this case, hip girdle and shoulder girdle stiffness and pain without

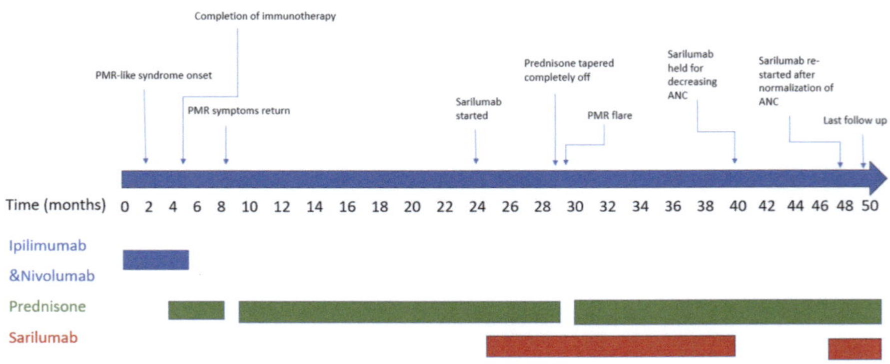

Fig. 54.1 Timeline representation of events and medications used in the case. Time point of 0 is initiation if ICI

objective tenderness or weakness are the classic symptoms in both traditional PMR and ICI induced PMR-like syndrome. However, ICI included PMR-like syndromes may include several disease entities that differ from traditional PMR. In a study of 20 patients on ICI therapy with PMR-like syndrome, several had more severe symptoms or atypical features including concurrent arthritis in knees or hands, sicca symptoms, and lack of ESR and CRP elevation [5]. This is similar to our case who had only mildly elevated ESR and CRP, rather than the significant elevations that are typically seen in classic PMR. Although not performed in our case, cases like this without classic presentation including elevated inflammatory markers can benefit from addtional imaging modalities including ultrasound or MRI of affected areas to evaluate for bursitis and tendinosis [6].

ICI related PMR-like syndrome typically arises around a median of 3.3 months after the first infusion of immunotherapy [4]. It is often more difficult to treat than traditional PMR, and many patients require higher dose glucocorticoids (>20 mg) than are traditionally used in PMR [5]. As in this case, many patients will require a steroid sparing agent to achieve remission of disease. Recent studies have shown that combined blockade of IL-6 and PD-1 elicits synergistic anti-tumor responses [7]. Sarilumab, an IL-6 receptor blocker, was approved by the FDA to treat steroid resistant PMR [8], thus has been used as steroid sparing agent for ICI induced PMR-like syndromes. As demonstrated in our case, biologics such as IL-6 blocker can control the PMR-like syndrome effectively while preserving long-term antitumor efficacy despite ICI discontinuation.

References

1. Manzo C, Isetta M, Natale M, Castagna A. Identification and classification of polymyalgia rheumatica (PMR) and PMR-like syndromes following immune checkpoint inhibitors (ICIs) therapy: discussion points and grey areas emerging from a systematic review of published literature. Medicines. 2020;7(11):68.
2. Le Burel S, Champiat S, Mateus C, Marabelle A, Michot J-M, Robert C, Belkhir R, Soria J-C, Laghouati S, Voisin A-L. Prevalence of immune-related systemic adverse events in patients treated with anti-programmed cell death 1/anti-programmed cell death-ligand 1 agents: a single-Centre pharmacovigilance database analysis. Eur J Cancer. 2017;82:34–44.
3. Raheel S, Shbeeb I, Crowson CS, Matteson EL. Epidemiology of polymyalgia rheumatica 2000–2014 and examination of incidence and survival trends over 45 years: a population-based study. Arthritis Care Res. 2017;69(8):1282–5.
4. Abdel-Wahab N, Suarez-Almazor ME. Frequency and distribution of various rheumatic disorders associated with checkpoint inhibitor therapy. Rheumatology. 2019;58(Supplement_7): vii40–8.
5. Calabrese C, Cappelli LC, Kostine M, Kirchner E, Braaten T, Calabrese L. Polymyalgia rheumatica-like syndrome from checkpoint inhibitor therapy: case series and systematic review of the literature. RMD Open. 2019;5(1):e000906.
6. Calabrese C, Kirchner E, Kontzias A, Velcheti V, Calabrese L. Rheumatic immune-related adverse events of checkpoint therapy for cancer: case series of a new nosological entity. RMD Open. 2017;3(1):e000412.

7. Tsukamoto H, Fujieda K, Miyashita A, Fukushima S, Ikeda T, Kubo Y, Senju S, Ihn H, Nishimura Y, Oshiumi H. Combined blockade of IL6 and PD-1/PD-L1 signaling abrogates mutual regulation of their immunosuppressive effects in the tumor microenvironment. Cancer Res. 2018;78(17):5011–22.
8. Spiera RF, Unizony S, Warrington KJ, Sloane J, Giannelou A, Nivens MC, Akinlade B, Wong W, Bhore R, Lin Y. Sarilumab for relapse of polymyalgia rheumatica during glucocorticoid taper. N Engl J Med. 2023;389(14):1263–72.

Chapter 55
Large Vessel Vasculitis Occurring After Exposure to Immune Checkpoint Inhibitor Therapy

Joshua O. Hendin, P. Scott Pollock, Pratyusha D. Banik, Scott C. DeRoo, Patricia J. Papadopoulos, Kelly D. Smith, Maria T. Nelson, and Namrata Singh

Abbreviations

FDG	Fluorodeoxyglucose
G-CSF	Granulocyte-colony stimulating factor
ICI	Immune checkpoint inhibitor
LVV	large vessel vasculitis
PET	Positron emission tomography
TNF	Tumor necrosis factor-alpha

J. O. Hendin · P. S. Pollock · P. D. Banik · N. Singh (✉)
Division of Rheumatology, Department of Medicine, University of Washington, Seattle, WA, USA
e-mail: joshua.hendin@mercy.net; pspolloc@uw.edu; pbanik24@uw.edu; nasingh@uw.edu

S. C. DeRoo
Division of Cardiac Surgery, University of Washington, Seattle, WA, USA
e-mail: sderoo@uw.edu

P. J. Papadopoulos
MultiCare Rheumatology Specialists, Tacoma, WA, USA
e-mail: trish.papadopoulos@multicare.org

K. D. Smith · M. T. Nelson
Department of Pathology, University of Washington, Seattle, WA, USA
e-mail: kelsmith@uw.edu; mnelson8@uw.edu

Y. Wang (ed.), *Challenging Cases in Immunotherapy Related Organ Toxicities*,
https://doi.org/10.1007/978-3-031-83533-9_55

Clinical Presentation

A Hispanic female in her 40 s had a diagnosis of BRCA2 positive bilateral breast cancer (invasive ductal carcinoma, triple negative on the right; invasive ductal carcinoma, ER+, PR+, HER2+ on the left). She was started on a regimen of neoadjuvant chemotherapy with pembrolizumab (200 mg every 3 weeks), paclitaxel, and carboplatin. Granulocyte-colony stimulating factor (G-CSF) was also administered for neutropenia related to chemotherapy. 5 months later, she presented to the emergency room (index presentation) with left-sided pleuritic chest pain, shortness of breath, and a productive cough. In the emergency room, a CT scan of the chest with contrast was notable for new onset of marked wall thickening and inflammatory changes surrounding the thoracic aorta from the mid-ascending aorta through the mid-descending aorta. Blood work showed an erythrocyte sedimentation rate of 130 mm/h. (upper limit of normal 20 mm/h) and a C-reactive protein level of 23.2 mg/dL (ULN 1.0 mg/dL).

She was diagnosed with large vessel vasculitis (LVV). Due to suspicion for an immune mediated adverse event related to immune checkpoint inhibitor (ICI) therapy, pembrolizumab was stopped after the patient had received 4 doses. Further testing for other autoimmune and infectious causes of LVV was unrevealing, including anti-nuclear antibody, anti-neutrophil cytoplasmic antibody, IgG4, rheumatoid factor, as well as screening tests for syphilis and tuberculosis. She was treated with 500 mg of intravenous methylprednisolone for 3 days followed by prednisone 80 mg daily with a plan for a slow taper over 6–12 months guided by serial evaluations. Her chest pain resolved over the next few days. 1 week later, a repeat CT scan of the chest, abdomen, and pelvis with contrast showed an interval decrease in wall thickening and surrounding inflammatory changes. The dose of prednisone was slowly tapered. 2 weeks later she underwent bilateral mastectomy with sentinel lymph node biopsies.

10 weeks after her diagnosis of vasculitis she was started on a chemotherapy regimen of cyclophosphamide, methotrexate, and 5-fluorouracil (CMF), which achieved cancer remission and resolution of vasculitis on repeat PET-FDG 6 months later.

However, 2 months after that, she developed recurrent chest pain. A CT scan of the chest with contrast showed new moderate to severe narrowing of the proximal left subclavian artery prior and proximal left vertebral artery (Fig. 55.1). The prednisone dose was increased from 20 mg daily to 40 mg daily. She completed the planned course of CMF 2 weeks later. 2 months later intravenous tocilizumab 8 mg/kg every 4 weeks was started for the persistent vasculitis despite prednisone. While on tocilizumab, she reported no new symptoms, and the dose of prednisone was weaned to 10 mg daily.

About 18 months after her diagnosis of index vasculitis, a CT scan of the chest, abdomen, and pelvis with contrast, ordered for monitoring of vasculitis, showed a proximal ascending aortic aneurysm 50 mm in diameter, new compared to imaging 6 months prior (Fig. 55.1). Prednisone was increased to 30 mg daily and she was

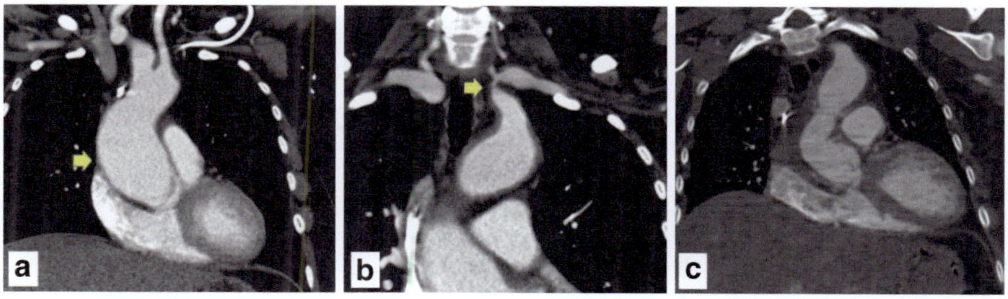

Fig. 55.1 Representative contrast enhanced CT images showing proximal aortic aneurysm (**a**) and left subclavian artery stenosis (**b**). Representative image of aorta after surgical repair (**c**)

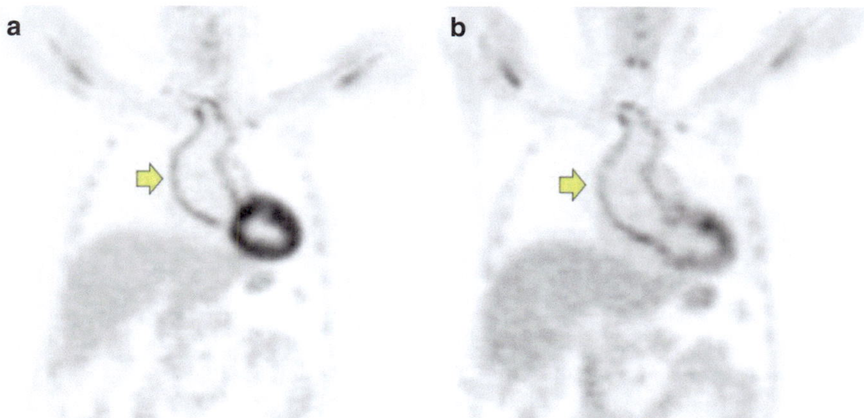

Fig. 55.2 Representative PET-FDG scan images showing ascending aortic aneurysm with associated FDG uptake before (**a**) and after (**b**) treatment with cyclophosphamide for 6 doses (EURO-LUPUS protocol). There is physiologic FDG uptake in the left ventricular myocardium

referred to a cardiothoracic surgeon. Further evaluation with a PET-FDG scan showed intense FDG uptake associated with the ascending aortic aneurysm (Fig. 55.2). FDG uptake was also seen involving the aortic arch and great vessel origins.

Tocilizumab was deemed a treatment failure and was stopped. Given CMF had previously led to resolution of aortic inflammation, 20 months after her diagnosis of vasculitis she was started on cyclophosphamide 500 mg IV every 2 weeks for a total of 6 doses (EURO-LUPUS protocol). Prednisone was weaned to 15 mg daily. At the conclusion of 3 months of therapy, a repeat PET-FDG scan showed decreased but persistent FDG uptake in a similar distribution when compared to the prior PET-FDG scan (Fig. 55.2). The proximal ascending aortic aneurysm had continued to grow to 56 mm in diameter.

Due to the persistently enlarging aortic aneurysm, 24 months after her initial diagnosis of vasculitis, the patient underwent ascending aorta hemiarch replacement. Under direct visualization in the operating room, the aorta was noted to be

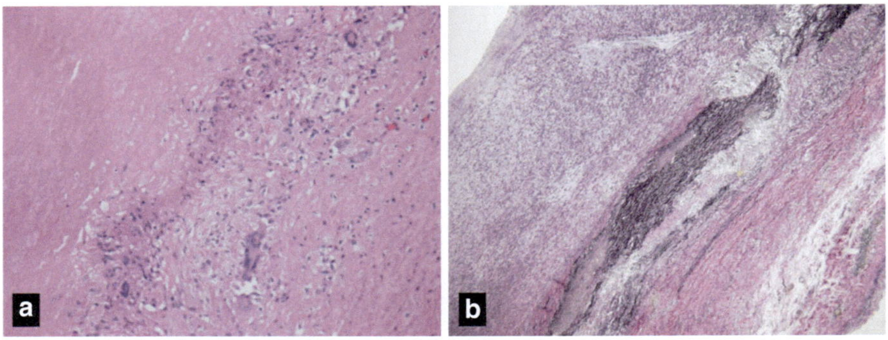

Fig. 55.3 Biopsy specimen of the aorta. On hematoxylin and eosin staining at 20x magnification, (**a**) there are multinucleated giant cells with surrounding histiocyte rich inflammation. On Verhoeff stain at 4× magnification (**b**), which stains elastic fibers black, there is disruption and destruction of the elastic media

thickened with areas of nodularity, with adhesions to peri-aortic tissues. Furthermore, there was profound atherosclerotic disease on the inner surface of the aorta, with near circumferential plaque and ulceration. All of this was felt to be consistent with a severe inflammatory state associated with the aorta. Her postoperative course was noted for hypoxemic respiratory failure and elevated liver enzymes, both of which had resolved at the time of her discharge home after 8 days in the hospital.

Pathology review of aortic tissue showed marked medial granulomatous inflammation with extensive destruction of the elastic media, necrosis and surrounding histiocyte rich inflammation with multinucleated giant cells (Fig. 55.3). Based on this, her rheumatology team planned to treat the patient with intravenous infliximab although at the time of writing, this had not yet been started.

Summary of the Case

This is a case with bilateral breast cancer who underwent treatment with pembrolizumab and subsequently developed LVV. She underwent several lines of treatments including tocilizumab and 2 courses of cyclophosphamide. In addition, she required continuous steroids and was unable to wean below 10 mg of prednisone daily. Despite this, she had ongoing aortitis and enlarging proximal aortic aneurysm that ultimately underwent surgical repair. Histologic examination of aortic tissue demonstrating marked granulomatous inflammation. Treatment with infliximab was planned post surgery however had not been started at the time of writing. Timeline events are summarized in Fig. 55.4.

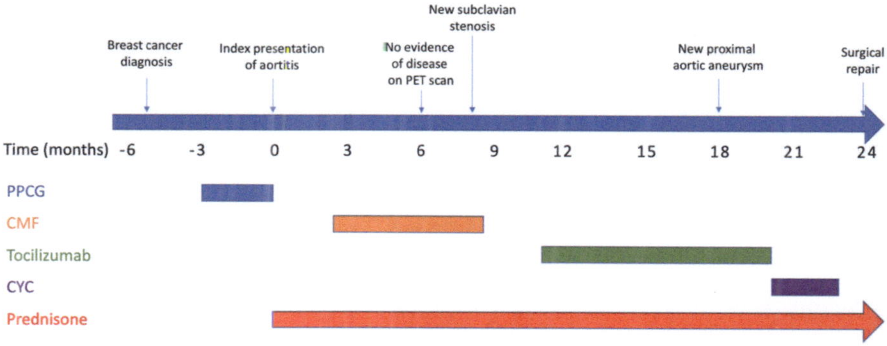

Fig. 55.4 Clinical course and timeline of events. Timepoint 0 is the index presentation for vasculitis. PPCG: Pembrolizumab 200 mg every 3 weeks, paclitaxel 80 mg/m^2 of body surface area weekly, carboplatin dosing by Calvert method every 3 weeks, and G-CSF 5 mg/kg of body weight daily as needed. CMF: cyclophosphamide 100 mg PO daily, methotrexate 40 mg/m^2 of body surface area every 7 days, 5-fluorouracil 600 mg/m^2 of body surface area every 7 days. Tocilizumab given 8 mg/kg IV every 4 weeks. CYC: cyclophosphamide 500 mg IV every 2 weeks for 6 doses

Discussion

There is a growing body of literature describing vasculitis as a complication of immune checkpoint inhibitor (ICI) exposure. Among cases of ICI associated vasculitis, the most common phenotype is giant cell arteritis [1]. Medium vessel and ANCA associated vasculitis have also been reported [2–4]. Treatment strategies for various types of vasculitis have involved courses of steroids with good response and low rates of relapse [5–7]. The exception to this is ICI associated ANCA vasculitis, where reported treatments have included rituximab and/or cyclophosphamide, similar to typical treatment of non-ICI associated ANCA vasculitis [2, 4]. The few case reports of aortitis associated with ICI exposure have responded well to steroids without recurrence [5]. G-CSF has also been reported as a cause of aortitis, however this type of LVV typically goes into remission within 14 days and has not been reported to persist longer than 3 months [8]. This contrasts with the case presented here, which more closely resembles Takayasu arteritis (TA) or giant cell arteritis (GCA), which have high rates of relapse [9–12]. Furthermore, disease monitoring proved challenging in this patient. Treatment with tocilizumab makes inflammatory markers unreliable [13]. PET-CT has been proposed as a useful tool for monitoring of LVV activity, although the optimal use of this technology is still unknown [14–17]. Despite the absence of ongoing clinical symptoms of LVV, our patient developed a rapidly enlarging aortic aneurysm requiring surgical repair. Thoracic aneurysms related to ICI have been rarely reported [18]. They are also an uncommon but well described complication of TA and GCA [10, 19]. The pathology from the aortic specimen showed marked granulomatous inflammation. Tumor necrosis factor-alpha (TNF) plays a central role in granuloma formation and maintenance [20], and treatment with TNF inhibitors are effective for several inflammatory diseases with prominent granulomatous inflammation, including Takayasu arteritis [21–23]. On this basis, treatment with a tumor necrosis factor inhibitor was planned, however the outcome of this treatment strategy for our patient is unknown at this time.

Conclusion

In summary, here we present a case of LVV that was temporally associated with ICI exposure and was complicated by a rapidly expanding proximal aortic aneurysm requiring surgical repair. LVV is an uncommon complication of ICI exposure, and typically responds well to steroids without recurrence. The optimal management for relapsed ICI associated LVV is unknown at this time, as is the optimal monitoring strategy for relapse of LVV.

References

1. Boland P, Heath J, Sandigursky S. Immune checkpoint inhibitors and vasculitis. Curr Opin Rheumatol. 2020;32(1):53–6. https://doi.org/10.1097/BOR.0000000000000672.
2. Aqeel F, Monroy-Trujillo J, Geetha D. Immune checkpoint inhibitors as potential triggers for ANCA vasculitis. RMD Open. 2022;8(2):e002500. https://doi.org/10.1136/rmdopen-2022-002500.
3. Oishi H, Morimoto R, Shimoyama Y, Kuroda K, Urata T, Kondo T, Okumura T, Bando YK, Akiyama M, Murohara T. Myocardial Vasculitis associated with the immune checkpoint inhibitor Pembrolizumab. JACC Case Rep. 2020;2(12):1937–41. https://doi.org/10.1016/j.jaccas.2020.07.028.
4. Qureshi S, Arani N, Parvathareddy V, Tchakarov A, Abdelrahim M, Suarez-Almazor M, Zhang J, Gibbons DL, Heymach J, Altan M, Abudayyeh A. Case report: immune checkpoint inhibitor-induced multiorgan vasculitis successfully treated with rituximab. Front Nephrol. 2023;3:1168614. https://doi.org/10.3389/fneph.2023.1168614.
5. Daxini A, Cronin K, Sreih AG. Vasculitis associated with immune checkpoint inhibitors—a systematic review. Clin Rheumatol. 2018;37:2579–84. https://doi.org/10.1007/s10067-018-4177-0.
6. Henderson D, Eslamian G, Poon D, Crabb S, Jones R, Sankey P, Kularatne B, Linch M, Josephs D. Republished: immune checkpoint inhibitor induced large vessel vasculitis. Drug Ther Bull. 2021;59(2):29–31. https://doi.org/10.1136/dtb.2020.233496rep.
7. Tominaga K, Takeuchi K, Takakuma S, et al. Immune checkpoint inhibitors associated granulomatous small vessel vasculitis accompanied with tubulointerstitial nephritis: a case report. BMC Nephrol. 2023;24:48. https://doi.org/10.1186/s12882-023-03091-8.
8. Hoshina H, Takei H. Granulocyte-colony stimulating factor-associated aortitis in cancer: a systematic literature review. Cancer Treat Res Commun. 2021;29:100454. https://doi.org/10.1016/j.ctarc.2021.100454. Epub 2021 Sep 12.
9. Comarmond C, Biard L, Lambert M, Mekinian A, Ferfar Y, Kahn JE, Benhamou Y, Chiche L, Koskas F, Cluzel P, Hachulla E, Messas E, Resche-Rigon M, Cacoub P, Mirault T, Saadoun D, French Takayasu Network. Long-term outcomes and prognostic factors of complications in Takayasu arteritis: a multicenter study of 318 patients. Circulation. 2017;136(12):1114–22. https://doi.org/10.1161/CIRCULATIONAHA.116.027094.

10. Schmidt J, Kermani TA, Bacani AK Crowson CS, Cooper LT, Matteson EL, Warrington KJ. Diagnostic features, treatment, and outcomes of Takayasu arteritis in a US cohort of 126 patients. Mayo Clin Proc. 2013;88(8):822–30. https://doi.org/10.1016/j.mayocp.2013.04.025.
11. Kermani TA, Warrington KJ, Cuthbertson D, Carette S, Hoffman GS, Khalidi NA, Koening CL, Langford CA, Maksimowicz-McKinnon K, McAlear CA, Monach PA, Seo P, Merkel PA, Ytterberg SR. Vasculitis clinical research consortium. Disease relapses among patients with Giant cell arteritis: a prospective, longitudinal cohort study. J Rheumatol. 2015;42(7):1213–7. https://doi.org/10.3899/jrheum.141347.
12. Labarca C, Koster MJ, Crowson CS, Makol A, Ytterberg SR, Matteson EL, Warrington KJ. Predictors of relapse and treatment outcomes in biopsy-proven giant cell arteritis: a retrospective cohort study. Rheumatology (Oxford). 2016;55(2):347–56. https://doi.org/10.1093/rheumatology/kev348.
13. Nishimoto N, Takagi N. Assessment of the validity of the 28-joint disease activity score using erythrocyte sedimentation rate (DAS28-ESR) as a disease activity index of rheumatoid arthritis in the efficacy evaluation of 24-week treatment with tocilizumab: subanalysis of the SATORI study. Mod Rheumatol. 2010;20(6):539–47. https://doi.org/10.1007/s10165-010-0328-0.
14. Galli E, Muratore F, Mancuso P, Boiardi L, Marvisi C, Besutti G, Spaggiari L, Casali M, Versari A, Giorgi Rossi P, Salvarani C. The role of PET/CT in disease activity assessment in patients with large vessel vasculitis. Rheumatology (Oxford). 2022;61(12):4809–16. https://doi.org/10.1093/rheumatology/keac125.
15. Grayson PC, Alehashemi S, Bagheri AA, Civelek AC, Cupps TR, Kaplan MJ, Malayeri AA, Merkel PA, Novakovich E, Bluemke DA, Ahlman MA. [18] F-Fluorodeoxyglucose-positron emission tomography as an imaging biomarker in a prospective, longitudinal cohort of patients with large vessel vasculitis. Arthritis Rheumatol. 2018;70(3):439–49. https://doi.org/10.1002/art.40379.
16. Slart RHJA, Nienhuis PH, Glaudemans AWJM, Brouwer E, Gheysens O, van der Geest KSM. Role of ^{18}F-FDG PET/CT in large vessel Vasculitis and polymyalgia Rheumatica. J Nucl Med. 2023;64(4):515–21. https://doi.org/10.2967/jnumed.122.265016.
17. van der Geest KSM, Treglia G, Glaudemans AWJM, Brouwer E, Sandovici M, Jamar F, Gheysens O, Slart RHJA. Diagnostic value of [18F]FDG-PET/CT for treatment monitoring in large vessel vasculitis: a systematic review and meta-analysis. Eur J Nucl Med Mol Imaging. 2021;48(12):3886–902. https://doi.org/10.1007/s00259-021-05362-8.
18. Ninomiya R, Kinehara Y, Tobita S, Konaka H, Jokoji R, Shintani T, Tachibana I. Inflammatory thoracic aortic aneurysm in a patient with advanced lung adenocarcinoma treated with Pembrolizumab. Intern Med. 2022;61(15):2339–41. https://doi.org/10.2169/internalmedicine.8688-21.
19. Evans JM, O'Fallon WM, Hunder GG. Increased incidence of aortic aneurysm and dissection in giant cell (temporal) arteritis. A population-based study. Ann Intern Med. 1995;122(7):502–7. https://doi.org/10.7326/0003-4819-122-7-199504010-00004.
20. Ehlers S. Role of tumour necrosis factor (TNF) in host defence against tuberculosis: implications for immunotherapies targeting TNF. Ann Rheum Dis. 2003;62(Suppl 2(Suppl 2)):ii37–42. https://doi.org/10.1136/ard.62.suppl_2.ii37.
21. Baughman RP, Drent M, Kavuru M, Judson MA, Costabel U, du Bois R, Albera C, Brutsche M, Davis G, Donohue JF, Müller-Quernheim J, Schlenker-Herceg R, Flavin S, Lo KH, Oemar B, Barnathan ES, Sarcoidosis Investigators. Infliximab therapy in patients with chronic sarcoidosis and pulmonary involvement. Am J Respir Crit Care Med. 2006;174(7):795–802. https://doi.org/10.1164/rccm.200603-402OC.
22. Colombel JF, Sandborn WJ, Reinisch W, Mantzaris GJ, Kornbluth A, Rachmilewitz D, Lichtiger S, D'Haens G, Diamond RH, Broussard DL, Tang KL, van der Woude CJ, Rutgeerts P, SONIC Study Group. Infliximab, azathioprine, or combination therapy for Crohn's disease. N Engl J Med. 2010;362(15):1383–95. https://doi.org/10.1056/NEJMoa0904492.
23. Hoffman GS, Merkel PA, Brasington RD, Lenschow DJ, Liang P. Anti-tumor necrosis factor therapy in patients with difficult to treat Takayasu arteritis. Arthritis Rheum. 2004;50(7):2296–304. https://doi.org/10.1002/art.20300.

Part XIII
Multi-organ Toxicity

Chapter 56
A Case of Persistent, Delayed Multisystem Toxicities After Anti-PD-1 Therapy

Rachel S. Goodman, Hannah Burnette, and Douglas B. Johnson

Abbreviations

BSA	Body surface area
ICI	Immune checkpoint inhibitor
IrAE	Immune related adverse event
PD-1	Programmed cell death protein −1

Case Presentation and Disease Course

This is a male in 70 s with no history of autoimmune disease or skin disorders presented with a localized melanoma (Breslow depth 1.1 mm, +ulceration) on the lower extremity and received wide local excision and sentinel lymph node biopsy. Five months later, he developed recurrent localized in-transit disease. The patient began (neo)adjuvant therapy with nivolumab (480 mg q4weeks). After surgical resection of the in-transit lesion, and 2 months after starting nivolumab, he developed oral ulcers treated with dexamethasone mouth rinse. He then developed hypothyroidism and levothyroxine was initiated. CT imaging throughout his course revealed no evidence of cancer. He continued to experience oral ulcerations largely controlled with topical corticosteroids.

Eleven months into his treatment course, he developed erythematous papules on his arms, controlled with triamcinolone cream. Six weeks later (2 weeks after

R. S. Goodman
Vanderbilt University School of Medicine, Nashville, TN, USA
e-mail: rachel.s.goodman@vanderbilt.edu

H. Burnette · D. B. Johnson (✉)
Department of Hematology/Oncology, Vanderbilt University Medical Center, Nashville, TN, USA
e-mail: hannah.r.burnette@vumc.org; douglas.b.johnson@vumc.org

Y. Wang (ed.), *Challenging Cases in Immunotherapy Related Organ Toxicities*, https://doi.org/10.1007/978-3-031-83533-9_56

completing his 1 year course of nivolumab) he noted several new erythematous skin lesions. An outside dermatologist noted a 1 cm keratotic plaque on his left anterior lower leg, a 5 mm keratotic papule on his right forearm, and a 1 cm brightly erythematous scaly patch on his right anterior lower leg. Biopsies were consistent with psoriasiform dermatitis with neutrophilic infiltrate (Fig. 56.1). ICI-induced psoriasiform dermatitis was suspected particularly given multiple concurrent irAEs (hypothyroidism, mucositis). Six months after completing nivolumab, his lesions flared further, and he presented to the emergency department with numerous tender, well-defined, red plaques with overlying silvery scale and excoriations throughout the scalp, trunk, extremities, hands, and feet (covering 15% body surface area (BSA)). He received 0.1% triamcinolone ointment wet wraps, clobetasol 0.05% solution for his scalp, and oral apremilast.

Two months later, his psoriasis and mucositis persisted with only modest improvement, and he was admitted to an outside hospital for nausea/vomiting and endoscopy/biopsy showed gastritis. He received a prednisone taper, apremilast was discontinued (due to gastrointestinal symptoms), and he was started on acitretin. However, his gastritis persisted, and it was felt that given the clinical and histological appearance, that this was related to nivolumab. Throughout the subsequent 5 months, his gastritis was recurrently treated with steroids, sucralfate, and pantoprazole. Given refractory irAEs in multiple organs despite front line treatment (Fig. 56.2), he received infliximab (300 mg intravenously, one dose) to treat for multi-organ toxicities 1 month later [1].

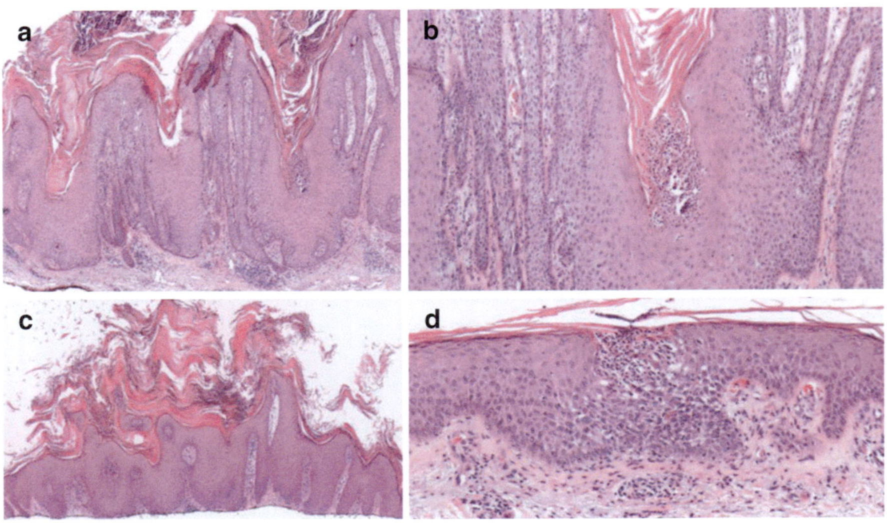

Fig. 56.1 Skin biopsy. (**a**, **b**). Psoriasiform dermatitis of right forearm and left anterior lower leg skin with regular acanthosis and parakeratosis (4×). (**c**) Higher power view of right forearm skin with neutrophilic collection. (**d**) Right anterior lower leg skin with spongiotic dermatitis and neutrophilic collection (4×)

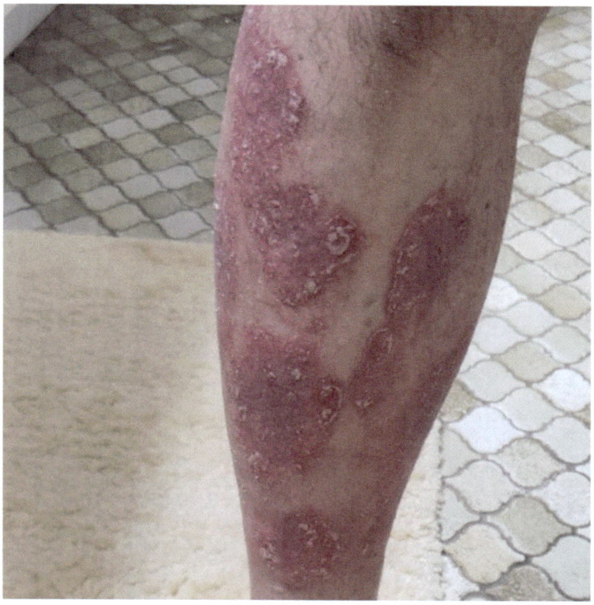

Fig. 56.2 Right anterior leg demonstrating numerous coalescing 3–10 cm well-defined, erythematous plaques with overlying white scale and excoriation

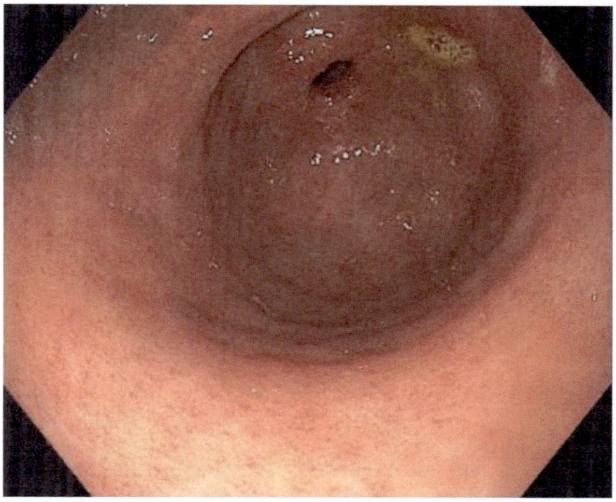

Fig. 56.3 Endoscopy showing erythematous gastric mucosa despite steroids and infliximab therapy

One month after infliximab, his psoriasis largely resolved (1% BSA), but his gastritis recurred upon tapering steroids with worsening nausea and abdominal pain. He underwent repeat endoscopy with erythematous gastric mucosa (Fig. 56.3); pathology demonstrated reactive gastropathy and chronic peptic-duodenitis-like changes. He transitioned to adalimumab for one dose which resulted in continuing control of his psoriasis and GI symptoms. However, he still required ongoing prednisone at 5–10 mg daily at last follow up approximately 6 months later.

Summary

In summary, this patient had stage III melanoma treated with adjuvant nivolumab. Acutely, his course was complicated by hypothyroidism, mucositis, and rash, with onset of treatment refractory gastritis and psoriasis which required biologic treatment.

This case is remarkable in that psoriasis and gastritis significantly worsened after ICI discontinuation and were steroid-refractory, flaring even after biologic administration. Ultimately this patient achieved remission from additional biologic treatment although still requires low-dose prednisone for gastrointestinal symptoms. Summary of the timeline events is shown in Fig. 56.4.

Discussion

Anti-PD-1 therapy has improved outcomes in high-risk and metastatic melanoma [2]. Despite its efficacy, anti-PD-1 treatments may cause immune-related adverse events (irAEs) across various organ systems. IrAEs generally begin within 3 months following immune checkpoint inhibitor (ICI) initiation, with a minority experiencing multi-organ involvement [3]. While delayed irAEs (onset >1 year post-ICI initiation) are occasionally reported, it is unclear how long the risk of irAEs persists following cessation of treatment [4]. While ICI is frequently associated with individual irAE, the multi-organ involvement, delayed onset, worsening off-treatment, and refractory nature are unusual.

Usually cutaneous irAEs arise early on treatment and occur in up to 72% of patients with median onset of 4 weeks after ICI initiation [5]. Anti-PD-1-induced psoriasis largely occurs in patients with pre-existing psoriasis and arise during treatment [6]. There are few reports of delayed (onset >12 months after treatment initiation) anti-PD-1-induced psoriasis, which, unlike our patient, did not require

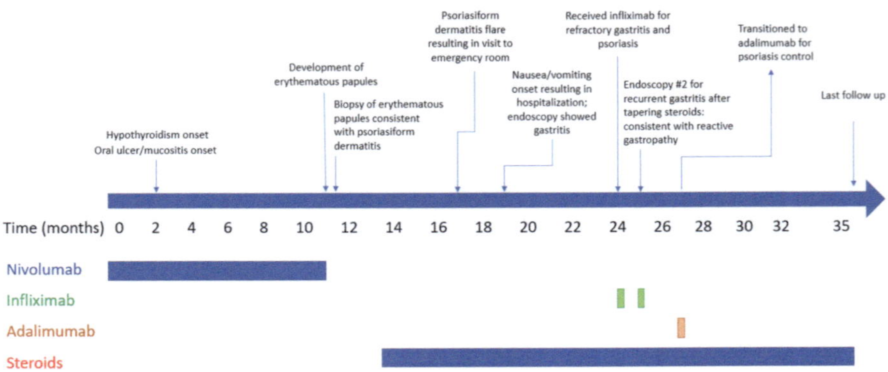

Fig. 56.4 Summary of timeline events (timepoint of 0 is the starting point of nivolumab)

additional immunosuppression [4] and improved after treatment cessation [7]. His psoriasis was treated with topical triamcinolone and clobetasol, as well as apremilast and acitretin with unclear response due to brief courses. It persisted despite systemic corticosteroid administration and ultimately improved with anti-TNF therapy, which reinforces other studies supporting the efficacy of infliximab for PD-1 inhibitor-induced psoriasis [8]. ICI-associated oral mucositis is less common, and symptoms usually subside with steroids and remain controlled when tapered [9]. Despite improvement with dexamethasone, this patient's oral ulcers were unusually persistent, recurring for almost 2 years when steroids were tapered. ICI-induced gastritis) increasingly reported [10] and was unusually refractory to steroids.

This case illustrates the potential for significant, delayed, worsening off-treatment, and persistent multi-organ system irAEs associated with nivolumab. It raises challenging questions surrounding the optimal management of patients with chronic irAEs. Should patients receive chronic steroids (e.g. 5–10 mg per day)? In our experience, some chronic, "smoldering" toxicities are well managed with such a strategy, that allows continuing of ICI therapy in appropriate cases. It is not clear whether ongoing use of steroids has any impact on long-term efficacy of ICI therapy. Studies have largely suggested that, if there is an effect, it is mostly for use of high-dose steroids or perhaps steroids at baseline [11]. Or perhaps biologics for steroid sparing should be used, though these raise questions surrounding immunosuppression and perhaps cancer recurrence. At least one study suggested that anti-tumor necrosis factor-α and/or α4β7 integrin agents can be used concurrently with ICI to allow for continued therapy along with suppression of gastrointestinal toxicity, although some patients still flared [12]. Some studies suggest that steroid-sparing immunosuppressives may be associated with inferior survival [13], although other studies do not show this effect [14, 15]. This case suggests the efficacy of TNF-alpha inhibitors in this setting, although it was effective at controlling his psoriasis, but only modestly effective at inducing gastritis control. Thus, selection of immunosuppression may be important for patients with ongoing multi-organ irAEs to heighten the chances of symptom control across organ systems (e.g. vedolizumab would not be a good choice in this patient, given the skin and GI involvement).

The case also raises the possibility of chronic irAEs arising after nivolumab discontinuation, a critically important issue to be monitored by clinical providers and patients following completion of therapy and also at the time of resumption. Of note, chronic irAEs may be associated with superior survival, although the possibility of bias is also high (given that patients with early progression and death do not have chronic irAEs by definition) [16, 17]. Individualized risk of cancer recurrence with indication of adjuvant ICI treatment should be carefully weighed against risk of morbid toxicities. Further research is thus needed to further characterize the incidence, timing, spectrum, and effective management strategies for delayed and persistent multi-organ system irAEs associated with ICI therapy.

References

1. Zou F, Faleck D, Thomas A, et al. Efficacy and safety of vedolizumab and infliximab treatment for immune-mediated diarrhea and colitis in patients with cancer: a two-center observational study. J Immunother Cancer. 2021;9:e003277.
2. Hemstock M, Amadi A, Kupas K, et al. Indirect treatment comparison of nivolumab versus placebo for the adjuvant treatment of melanoma. Eur J Cancer. 2020;132:176–86.
3. Haanen J, Carbonnel F, Robert C, et al. Management of toxicities from immunotherapy: ESMO clinical practice guidelines for diagnosis, treatment and follow-up. Ann Oncol. 2017;28:iv119–iv42.
4. Owen CN, Bai X, Quah T, et al. Delayed immune-related adverse events with anti-PD-1-based immunotherapy in melanoma. Ann Oncol. 2021;32:917–25.
5. Schneider BJ, Naidoo J, Santomasso BD, et al. Management of immune-related adverse events in patients treated with immune checkpoint inhibitor therapy: ASCO guideline update. J Clin Oncol. 2021;39:4073–126.
6. Sibaud V. Dermatologic reactions to immune checkpoint inhibitors. Am J Clin Dermatol. 2018;19:345–61.
7. Hofmann L, Forschner A, Loquai C, et al. Cutaneous, gastrointestinal, hepatic, endocrine, and renal side-effects of anti-PD-1 therapy. Eur J Cancer. 2016;60:190–209.
8. Hansen I, Heidrich I, Abeck F, et al. Successful treatment of PD-1 inhibitor-induced psoriasis with infliximab. J Eur Acad Dermatol Venereol. 2022;37:e621.
9. Sheth H, Pragya R, Kovale S, et al. Oral mucositis—case series of a rare adverse effect associated with immunotherapy. Support Care Cancer. 2021;29:4705–9.
10. Woodford R, Briscoe K, Tustin R, Jain A. Immunotherapy-related gastritis: two case reports and literature review. Clin Med Insights Oncol. 2021;15:11795549211028570.
11. Goodman RS, Johnson DB, Balko JM. Corticosteroids and cancer immunotherapy. Clin Cancer Res. 2023;29:2580–7.
12. Badran YR, Zou F, Durbin SM, et al. Concurrent immune checkpoint inhibition and selective immunosuppressive therapy in patients with immune-related enterocolitis. J Immunother Cancer. 2023;11:e007195.
13. Dearden H, Au L, Wang DY, et al. Hyperacute toxicity with combination ipilimumab and anti-PD1 immunotherapy. Eur J Cancer. 2021;153:168–78.
14. Tomsitz D, Ruf T, Zierold S, French LE, Heinzerling L. Steroid-refractory immune-related adverse events induced by checkpoint inhibitors. Cancers (Basel). 2023;15:2538.
15. Johnson DH, Zobniw CM, Trinh VA, et al. Infliximab associated with faster symptom resolution compared with corticosteroids alone for the management of immune-related enterocolitis. J Immunother Cancer. 2018;6:103.
16. Zou F, Abu-Sbeih H, Ma W, et al. Association of chronic immune-mediated diarrhea and colitis with favorable cancer response. J Natl Compr Cancer Netw. 2020;19:700–8.
17. Goodman RS, Lawless A, Woodford R, et al. Extended follow-up of chronic immune-related adverse events following adjuvant anti-PD-1 therapy for high-risk resected melanoma. JAMA Netw Open. 2023;6:e2327145.

Index

Y. Wang (ed.), *Challenging Cases in Immunotherapy Related Organ Toxicities*, https://doi.org/10.1007/978-3-031-83533-9

MIX
Papier aus verantwortungsvollen Quellen
Paper from responsible sources
FSC® C105338

If you have any concerns about our products,
you can contact us on
ProductSafety@springernature.com

In case Publisher is established outside the EU,
the EU authorized representative is:
Springer Nature Customer Service Center GmbH
Europaplatz 3, 69115 Heidelberg, Germany

Printed by Libri Plureos GmbH
in Hamburg, Germany